AGING AND THE ELDERLY:

PSYCHOLOGY, SOCIOLOGY AND HEALTH

AGING AND THE ELDERLY:

PSYCHOLOGY, SOCIOLOGY AND HEALTH

L. O. RANDAL
EDITOR

Nova Science Publishers, Inc.
New York

For permission to use material from this book please contact us:
Telephone 631-231-7269; Fax 631-231-8175
Web Site: http://www.novapublishers.com

LIBRARY OF CONGRESS CATALOGING-IN-PUBLICATION DATA
Available upon request

ISBN 13 978-1-60021-190-4
ISBN 10 1-60021-190-9

Published by Nova Science Publishers, Inc. ✦ New York

CONTENTS

PREFACE

The aging process involves many problems associated with decline whether it be in health, psychology or lifestyle or all three. This new book brings together new research on each these aspects.

Tip-of-the-tongue (TOT) states occur when a word is temporarily inaccessible for retrieval, despite a feeling of knowing the word. TOTs occur for people of all ages, but are particularly frustrating for older adults, most likely because TOTs increase across the lifespan and therefore become more noticeable to older adults, both in naturalistic and laboratory studies. One explanation for this increase is the Transmission Deficit model, where older adults have greater difficulty activating the necessary phonology, i.e., sounds, to facilitate word retrieval (e.g., Burke, MacKay, Worthley, and Wade, 1991). The authors of chapter review studies on the role of phonology in both inducing and resolving TOTs and present new data from 327 young adults and 132 older adults that categorizes TOTs on two dimensions: (1) the percent of "know" responses, "TOT" responses, and "don't know" responses that occur following a definition-like general knowledge question, and (2) the most common alternative words that come to mind instead of the to-be-retrieved word. Norms of this type do not exist for either young or older adults, and the chapter helps to identify stimuli that are most effective at inducing and resolving TOTs in both age groups.

The negative priming effect gained the attention of researchers interested in cognition and aging following the reports of several studies that older adults demonstrated smaller negative priming effects than in younger adults. Recently, however, this enthusiasm has dramatically waned because: 1) controversy surrounds the appropriate theoretical interpretation of the negative priming effect, and 2) there are accumulating studies showing no difference between younger and older adults in negative priming. Chapter 2 reviews the negative priming and aging literature highlighting the controversy. Then, the authors provide a novel theoretical approach to interpreting repetition effects that may renew interest in the negative priming phenomenon. Their analytical approach allows researchers to discriminate between two components of performance, and the chapter highlights the results from four studies that demonstrate this novel method. In particular, they highlight that the presence and absence of age differences in response repetition effects reflect the relative contributions of two processes. Together, the results argue against the practice of attributing age differences in repetition effects to deficits in any single cognitive process.

A major paradox in psychology and aging is the finding that older people maintain their psychological well being despite undeniable physical and cognitive declines. Theories and research developed largely in the West explain this paradox in terms of age-related improvement in emotional regulation. Given the well-documented cultural differences between the East and the West, there have been suggestions that these Western findings may not be generalizable to Eastern cultures. In chapter 3, the authors first review Western theories and empirical findings on age differences in emotional regulation. Then, they describe whether these findings are replicated in the East. Finally, they discuss the implications for studying emotional regulation in both Eastern and Western cultures, and suggest future directions for cross-cultural research in this area.

In chapter 4 the authors review the research examining the effects of the complexity of paid work and leisure time activities on older people's intellectual functioning. They find that much of the research does not take sufficient account of the possibility that correlations found between intellectual functioning and the complexity of paid work and leisure time activities may reflect the possibility that having a high level of intellectual functioning increases the likelihood that an individual may want to, or be in a position where they are expected to, engage in cognitively demanding tasks. Nevertheless, the research evidence is at least congruent with the possibility that carrying out intellectually demanding activities positively effects older individuals' intellectual functioning. The authors find stronger evidence for the positive effects of cognitively complex activities on older people's intellectual functioning in studies that employ statistics permitting the separation of the effects of complex activities on individuals' intellectual functioning from the effects of individuals' intellectual functioning on their likelihood carrying out complex intellectually demanding activities at work or at leisure. The tenor of findings from relevant animal and human experimental studies, as well as the outcomes of intervention studies with both normal individuals and those suffering from dementia, provide further support for the positive effects of cognitively complex activities on the intellectual functioning of the elderly. They conclude by discussing the theoretical and practical implications of the evidence that environmental complexity has a positive effect on the intellectual functioning of older people.

The numbers of older adults is increasing every year (U.S Census Bureau, 2004). As the population grows older and life expectancy increases, it becomes even more important to identify factors that reduce the incidence of chronic illnesses of middle and later adulthood and aid in coping (Smith, Kendall, & Keefe, 2002; Siegler, Bashan, Steffens, Bosworth, & Costa, 2002). One of the most critical factors is social support and social networks which have positive effects on the health and well-being of adults of all ages (Antonucci & Jackson, 1987; Bowling, 1994; Fratiglioni, Wang, Ericsson, Mayten, & Wimblad, 2000; Gotlib & Whiffen, 1992; Helgeson & Cohen, 1996; House, Umberson, & Landis, 1988; Kriegsman, Pennix, & Van Eijk, 1995; Reifman, 1995; Sarason, Sarason & Gurung, 2001; Schwarzer & Leppin, 1992).

In chapter 5 the authors first, following Bruner's (1990) call for understanding behavior within the context in which occurs, expand on ecological frameworks used to illuminate causes of behavior (e.g., Bronfenbrenner, 1986; Revenson, 1990, 1994), positing a contextually oriented framework as an analytic structure for describing and explicating social support processes. In a selective review of the literature, influences of intra- and interpersonal characteristics as well as cultural factors that mediate perceptions of social support and influence behavior are discussed. Next, they describe a longitudinal study of changes in social support that illustrates the utility of a contextual approach.

The results of Gurung et al., (2003) illustrate the dynamic nature of social support in a healthy aging cohort over time and across different sources. More broadly, it also highlights the utility of factoring in different contexts. The MacArthur Study data nicely capture people operating different independent and overlapping contexts: an intrapersonal context, an interpersonal context, and a temporal context. Clearly, each context overlaps with others and all influence behavior. Further studies of support and efforts to provide it might be especially attuned to the different contexts that social support is transacted in.

Independence and self–esteem are strongly related to physical and mental function which in turn are largely determined by nutritional status and physical activity, as reported in chapter 6. Food is an integral part of our well-being and quality of life. It extends beyond simply satisfying hunger and providing nourishment. Specific foods have a symbolic meaning and particular food habits are influenced by religious, cultural, social and emotional experience. Elderly people showing interest towards food, nourishment and keeping a good appetite, in most cases still are vital human beings full of interests and quite independent. Behavioural characteristics before mentioned describe the picture of the elderly aging with "a good health", known in medical literature as *Healthy Aging*. Aging is normally associated with body weight gain in individuals who fail to decrease food intake in proportion to the age-related decline in energy expenditure. However, decreases in body weight are common in elderly individuals (over 70 years of age) who do not eat enough to meet energy demands. Age related reduction in energy intake is largely a physiologic effect of healthy aging and reveals itself with a loss of eating need and pleasure. This reduction intake may predispose to the harmful anorexic effect of psychological, social and physical problems that become increasingly frequent with aging. The physiological anorexia of aging increases the propensity for developing pathological anorexia and weight loss when an older person falls ill with either a medical or a psychological illness. A 10% loss of body weight over 10 years is consistently associated with increased mortality and functional disability. Weight loss is one of the pathognomonic signs of malnutrition (whether energetic or protein-energy) which may negatively influence the clinical outcome of rehabilitation programmes, confirming that a convenient nutritional status helps the achievement of such a condition and it is absolutely essential when recovering from acute illnesses. A further demonstration of the importance of nutritional status has been pointed out by several studies showing that, after sixties of age, weight loss is associated to a decline in muscle mass and consequently in muscle strength. The picture just mentioned is well-known as *sarcopenia*, which plays a main role in the beginning of: frailty, functional and metabolic impairments, physical disabilities that expose the elderly to an increased risk of falls and protein-energy malnutrition. The obese elderly also affected by protein malnutrition configure the so called *fat frail* who obtains worse outcomes in rehabilitation programmes.

As reported in chapter 7, old age is the major risk factor for vascular disease, and as the population ages, is also becoming the most prevalent risk factor. There are few mechanistic explanations for the association of old age with vascular disease. Old age is associated with changes in the endothelium within the hepatic sinusoid, consisting of loss of fenestrations, thickening of the endothelium, deposition of basal lamina and increased expression of various antigens such as von Willebrands factor. These endothelial changes have been observed in humans, non-human primates and rats and may have a unique pathogenesis because of the role of the liver in detoxification and its exposure to gut-derived toxins and dietary substances. The age-related loss of hepatic sinusoidal endothelial fenestrations is particularly significant because fenestrations have an important role in the transfer of lipoproteins, especially chylomicron remnants, from sinusoidal blood to the hepatocytes (the 'liver sieve'). The loss of fenestrations with old age may explain the association of old age with impaired chylomicron remnant clearance and postprandial hyperlipidaemia. Given the ability to modulate fenestrations with various pharmacological and endogenous substrates, the hepatic sinusoidal endothelium may be a therapeutic target for the prevention and treatment of age-related dyslipidaemia and vascular disease.

Chapter 8 reviews that older Americans are an economically diverse group. In 2004, the median income of individuals age 65 and older was $15,199, but incomes varied widely around this average. Twenty-eight percent of Americans 65 or older had incomes of less than $10,000 in 2004, while 10% had incomes of $50,000 or more. As Congress considers reforms to Social Security and the laws governing pensions and retirement savings plans, it may be helpful to consider how changes to one income source would affect each of the others, and thus the total income of older Americans. Older persons receive income from a variety of sources, including earnings, pensions, personal savings, and public programs such as Social Security and Supplemental Security Income. Using data from the March 2005 *Current Population Survey,* the chapter describes the number of elderly receiving income from each of these sources and the extent to which income from each source is either concentrated at the high- or low-end of the income distribution or is evenly distributed. Retirement benefits from Social Security and pensions are the most common source of income among the aged. In 2004, Social Security paid benefits to 88% of Americans age 65 and older. Social Security is also the largest single source of income among the aged. Sixty-nine percent of Social Security beneficiaries age 65 or older receive more than half of their income from Social Security. For 39% of elderly recipients, Social Security contributes more than 90% of their income, and for nearly one-quarter of recipients, it is their *only* source of income. In 2004, 35% of people age 65 and older received income from a private or public pension. Among people age 65 and older who reported income from a government pension, the median annual amount was $15,600. Among recipients of private pensions, the median amount received in 2004 was just $6,720. Many Americans prepare for retirement by saving and investing some of their income while they are working. Of the 35.2 million Americans age 65 or older who were living in households in 2004, 19.7 million (56%) received income from assets, such as interest, dividends, rent, and royalties. Most received small amounts of income from the assets they owned. Of all individuals age 65 or older who received income from assets in 2004, half received less than $952. Earnings from work continue to be an important source of income for older Americans, especially those under age 70. Although there was a trend toward earlier retirement from about 1960 to 1985, over the past 20 years more Americans have continued to work at older ages. In 2004, median earnings for individuals age 55-6 1 who worked were $34,000, while median earned income for workers age 62-64 was $27,000. For workers 65 and older, the median earned income was $15,000. Poverty among those age 65 and older has fallen from one-in-three older persons in 1960 to one-in-ten today. While the overall rate of poverty is relatively low, it remains high for women, minorities, the less-educated, and those older than 80.

In: Aging and the Elderly: Psychology, Sociology and Health ISBN 1-60021-190-9
Editor: L. O. Randall, pp. 1-41

Chapter 1

RESOLVING TIP-OF-THE-TONGUE STATES IN YOUNG AND OLDER ADULTS: THE ROLE OF PHONOLOGY

Lise Abrams,* Dunja L. Trunk and Sara J. Margolin
University of Florida, FL, USA

ABSTRACT

Tip-of-the-tongue (TOT) states occur when a word is temporarily inaccessible for retrieval, despite a feeling of knowing the word. TOTs occur for people of all ages, but are particularly frustrating for older adults, most likely because TOTs increase across the lifespan and therefore become more noticeable to older adults, both in naturalistic and laboratory studies. One explanation for this increase is the Transmission Deficit model, where older adults have greater difficulty activating the necessary phonology, i.e., sounds, to facilitate word retrieval (e.g., Burke, MacKay, Worthley, and Wade, 1991). The present chapter reviews studies on the role of phonology in both inducing and resolving TOTs and presents new data from 327 young adults and 132 older adults that categorizes TOTs on two dimensions: (1) the percent of "know" responses, "TOT" responses, and "don't know" responses that occur following a definition-like general knowledge question, and (2) the most common alternative words that come to mind instead of the to-be-retrieved word. Norms of this type do not exist for either young or older adults, and this chapter helps to identify stimuli that are most effective at inducing and resolving TOTs in both age groups.

* Please address correspondence to: Dr. Lise Abrams, Department of Psychology, University of Florida, P.O. Box 112250, Gainesville, FL 32611-2250; Phone: (352) 392-2191; Fax: (352) 392-7985; Email: abrams@ufl.edu

INTRODUCTION

The tip-of-the-tongue (TOT) experience is a phenomenon that refers to a type of word retrieval failure, where a word is known but cannot be produced at a particular time (R. Brown and McNeill, 1966). Even when the word itself cannot be retrieved, people often have access to some phonological information about the word. Specifically, people can sometimes report the initial letter or sound, the first syllable, the final letter, number of syllables, and stress pattern (e.g., R. Brown and McNeill, 1966; Burke, MacKay, Worthley, and Wade, 1991; Harley and Bown, 1998; Koriat and Lieblich, 1975; Miozzo and Caramazza, 1997; Rubin, 1975). The importance of phonology in causing TOTs has been documented theoretically in the Transmission Deficit model (e.g., Burke et al., 1991; Burke and Shafto, 2004; James and Burke, 2000; MacKay and Burke, 1990; Rastle and Burke, 1996), which proposes that TOTs occur when connections to a word's phonological nodes are weakened and transmit insufficient priming to enable activation and retrieval of the word. These connections to phonology weaken as a function of two factors, frequency and recency of use; as a result, TOTs typically occur for low-frequency words and words not used recently (e.g., Burke et al., 1991; Vitevitch and Sommers, 2003). The Transmission Deficit model can also explain the availability of phonological information during TOTs, which occurs when some of the phonological nodes receive enough priming to become activated. However, *all* phonological nodes must become activated for the entire word to be retrieved.

A third factor that reduces connection strength and transmission of priming is the normal aging process, resulting in older adults having more TOTs both in the laboratory and in everyday life (e.g., Brown and Nix, 1996; Burke et al., 1991; Cohen and Faulkner, 1986; Cross and Burke, 2004; Evrard, 2002; Heine, Ober, and Shenaut, 1999; Maylor, 1990b). This increase in TOTs is accompanied by a decrease in availability of phonological information: Compared to young adults, older adults report less phonological information about the target word (e.g., Burke et al., 1991; Cohen and Faulkner, 1986; Heine et al., 1999). Older adults also are less likely to have an alternate word in mind when in a TOT state (e.g., Burke et al., 1991). These alternates, referred to as blockers (Reason and Lucas, 1984), interlopers (Jones, 1989), or persistent alternates (Burke et al., 1991), refer to an incorrect word that involuntarily comes to mind, instead of the intended word, and these alternates often overlap in phonology with the TOT word. Older adults' inability to retrieve partial phonological information and alternates to the same degree as young adults suggests that older adults have greater difficulty activating the necessary phonology to facilitate word retrieval (e.g., Burke et al., 1991; James and Burke, 2000).

Under the Transmission Deficit model's assumption that weakened connections to phonology cause TOTs, strengthening these connections should reduce TOTs and facilitate word retrieval as well as help resolve TOTs, both in young and older adults. This idea has been tested in two ways: (1) presenting a word's phonology prior to inducing a TOT and then assessing the incidence of a TOT for that word, or (2) presenting a word's phonology after a TOT has occurred and measuring whether the TOT word can now be retrieved.

PRESENTING PHONOLOGY BEFORE INDUCING TOTS

The general methodology in these studies involves presentation of a word(s) phonologically related to the target word (i.e., words that contain some of the target's phonology, such as the first phoneme, first syllable, stress pattern, or number of syllables), followed by a definition-like, general knowledge question intended to elicit retrieval of the target. If less TOTs are reported following phonologically related words relative to unrelated words, then this result would support the Transmission Deficit model's claim that recent presentation of a word phonologically related to the target strengthens phonological connections to the target, facilitating its retrieval. Only a few studies have been conducted solely with young adults, and these have led to mixed results. Bowles and Poon (1985) found that phonologically related words increased word retrieval and therefore reduced TOTs, relative to unrelated words, whereas Jones (1989) showed that phonologically related words decreased word retrieval and increased TOTs (but see Meyer and Bock, 1992, and Perfect and Hanley, 1992, for critiques of Jones' stimuli).

Research with both young and older adults has demonstrated support for the Transmission Deficit model. Rastle and Burke (1996) exposed participants to a target's phonology by having them complete a pronunciation task, where a list of words was shown one at a time, and participants read each word aloud. Following a ten-minute delay, participants heard a list of definitions corresponding to targets and were asked whether they knew the word, did not know the word, or were having a TOT. Half of the targets corresponding to the definitions had been presented during the pronunciation task, while the other half were words not seen recently. They found that more correct retrievals and fewer TOTs were experienced following words presented in the pronunciation task relative to nonpresented words, and this reduction in TOTs was equivalent for both young and older adults.

James and Burke (2000, Experiment 1) presented the target's phonology within the context of different words. They asked participants to read words aloud that cumulatively contained all of the syllables of the target word. For example, if participants had a TOT for the target word *abdicate*, they read aloud primes that included the following words: *ab*stract, in*di*gent, trun*cate*, tra*di*tion, and lo*cate*. They then saw the general knowledge question and attempted to retrieve the target. Prior production of the target's phonology via phonologically related words increased correct retrieval of targets and reduced TOTs. Similar to Rastle and Burke (1996), young and older adults benefited similarly from prior presentation of the to-be-retrieved phonology.

Burke, Locantore, Austin, and Chae (2004) investigated retrieval of proper names in young and older adults using homophones, words that sound the same but are spelled differently, to present a target's phonology in the prior production task. Using fill-in-the-blank statements, participants named either homophones (e.g., pit) or words phonologically unrelated to the target and then attempted to name a picture of a famous person whose name corresponded to the other spelling of the homophone (e.g., Brad Pitt). Prior production of the homophone increased retrieval of the proper names and reduced TOTs; however, this facilitation occurred only for older adults, not young adults. Their explanation for this age difference lies in the increased difficulty of retrieving proper names relative to object names. Within the Transmission Deficit model, proper names have virtually no connections to nodes in the semantic system, which makes them vulnerable to deficits in the transmission of priming to their lexical nodes and corresponding phonological nodes. For example, the proper name "Pitt" has no semantic connections except to the full name of people possessing that name, such as "Brad Pitt". In contrast, the object name "pit" connects to its many semantic properties, where "holds seed", "found in fruit", and "is hard" represent only a few of these properties. Although retrieving proper names is more difficult than retrieving object names for both young and older adults, this difficulty is exacerbated in older adults because of their weakened connections, resulting in more TOTs for proper names (e.g., Burke et al., 1991; Evrard, 2002). However, older adults are therefore able to benefit more than young adults from the strengthening of connections caused by production of the homophone, as found in Burke et al. (2004).

PRESENTING PHONOLOGY AFTER TOTS HAVE OCCURRED

Measuring the influence of phonology after a TOT has occurred has been tested using both cueing and priming paradigms. In both types of studies, the general knowledge question is presented first, and participants are asked to indicate whether they know, don't know, or are having a TOT for the target, which is the question's answer. Words phonologically related to the target are then presented, and participants are again presented with the question and asked to retrieve the target. The logic is that presenting the general knowledge question first can induce TOTs; therefore, presentation of a word's phonology in this methodology addresses whether phonology facilitates word retrieval by resolving TOTs.[1] The fundamental difference between cueing and priming paradigms is that in cueing paradigms, participants may be aware that the phonologically related words are related to the target word. This awareness of the relation between the cues and the target could cause participants to use a directed memory search for the target, using the cue's phonological properties. In contrast, priming studies present phonologically related words in a context where the words are seemingly "unrelated" to the general knowledge questions. Priming studies more closely reflect the spontaneous resolution processes that occur in everyday life, where the TOT word seems to "pop" into mind without conscious effort (see James and Burke, 2000, for further discussion of cueing vs. priming).

Studies on resolving TOTs in young adults have shown that both phonological cues and primes typically increase TOT resolution: Word retrieval is more likely to occur if words or letters that share phonology with the target word are presented during a TOT state (e.g., Abrams, White, and Eitel, 2003; Meyer and Bock, 1992). However, Abrams and Rodriguez (2005) found that a phonological prime's syntactic class determined the effect on TOT resolution. Participants read general knowledge questions and indicated whether they knew, did not know, or were having a TOT for the target. Following "TOT" and "don't know" responses, participants saw five words, four of which were phonologically unrelated filler words and one that was either a phonological prime or another phonologically unrelated filler.

[1] A few studies (Jones, 1989; Jones and Langford, 1987; Maylor, 1990a) do not explicitly ask participants whether or not they are experiencing a TOT before presenting the phonologically related words. Therefore, these studies cannot address TOT resolution and instead can only look at the occurrence of TOTs following phonologically related words.

Phonological primes contained the target's first syllable and either shared or did not share the target's part of speech. For example, the target "rosary" (a noun) was primed either with "robust" (an adjective) or "robot" (a noun). Retrieval of the target was attempted again after presentation of the five-word list. Different part-of-speech primes facilitated resolution of TOTs and increased target retrieval relative to phonologically unrelated words, whereas same part-of-speech primes had no effect on TOT resolution. The only evidence for an inhibitory effect, where phonologically related words increased TOTs, comes from Jones and his colleagues (e.g., Jones, 1989; Jones and Langford, 1987), but these studies have been criticized for improper counterbalancing that artificially inflated TOTs following phonologically related words (Meyer and Bock, 1992; Perfect and Hanley, 1992).

With respect to older adults, phonological cueing studies have also demonstrated mostly facilitation from phonologically related cues, although Maylor (1990a) demonstrated more TOTs following phonologically related cues relative to unrelated cues in 50 year-olds, similar to Jones (1989) and Jones and Langford (1987)'s studies with young adults. However, Maylor (1990a) found no effect of phonologically related words in 60 and 70 year-olds. Heine et al. (1999) found that cues consisting of the target's first letter (as well as dashes to indicate word length) increased retrieval of targets relative to semantic cues (words related to the target in meaning) for college students, young-old adults (ages 60-74), and old-old adults (ages 80-92), with young-old adults having more facilitation relative to the other two age groups. Differences in older adults' retrieval as a function of phonological cues in the above studies above may be a function of the cueing paradigm. Older adults generally are less able to use conscious recollection strategies as effectively as young adults (e.g., Light and LaVoie, 1993), which suggests that cueing studies may adversely affect older adults' ability to consistently demonstrate either inhibition or facilitation from phonology (see also Burke et al., 2004).

Using phonological primes, several studies have demonstrated that both young and older adults have increased word retrieval following phonological primes presented during TOT states. James and Burke (2000, Experiment 2) presented general knowledge questions, and following retrieval failures, they asked participants to read aloud and rate the pronunciation difficulty of primes cumulatively containing the phonology of the target (see the earlier description of Experiment 1 for sample primes). Both young and older adults resolved more TOTs after pronouncing the phonologically related list relative to an unrelated list, and the size of this priming effect was equivalent in both age groups.

White and Abrams (2002) tested young adults and two groups of older adults, a young-old group (aged 60-72) and an old-old group (aged 73-83), using a phonological priming paradigm. After presentation of general knowledge questions, participants read primes that shared a single syllable with the target, either the first, middle, or last syllable. The results showed that resolution of TOTs was greater following first-syllable primes relative to unrelated words, and this increased word retrieval occurred for young and young-old adults, but not old-old adults.

In sum, the data from studies with phonological cues and primes suggest that exposure to phonology, both before and after a TOT experience, influences word retrieval (most often by increasing it) in both young and older adults, although old-old adults are less likely to benefit to the same degree. These results support the Transmission Deficit model, where recent presentation of a word's phonology facilitates retrieval of the TOT word by transmitting bottom-up priming to other lexical nodes connected to it. Since the TOT word is connected phonologically to the related word, it accumulates enough priming to become activated and retrieved. Although older adults' connection strength is reduced, making them more susceptible to retrieval failures, the similarity between young and older adults in phonological priming of TOTs suggests that the benefits of activation through recent presentation are similar across age.

However, there are still a number of unanswered questions about characteristics inherent in the primes and targets that affect young and older adults' word retrieval and the degree to which young and older adults are differentially influenced by these characteristics. Several recent studies have begun to explore some of these factors. Vitevitch and Sommers (2003) found that both neighborhood density (the number of words that differ from a target by only one phoneme; see also Harley and Bown, 1998) and neighborhood frequency (the mean word frequency of all of a target's neighbors) influenced the occurrence of TOTs, with differential effects for young and older adults. Young adults had more TOTs for words with sparse neighborhoods than for words with dense neighborhoods, independent of neighborhood frequency. In contrast, older adults exhibited more TOTs for words with sparse neighborhoods only when the word had low neighborhood frequency.

With respect to phonological priming of TOT resolution, Abrams and Rodriguez (2005) showed that in young adults, a prime's word frequency was related to the likelihood of target retrieval following presentation of the prime. There were significant correlations between a prime's Francis and Kucera (1982) word frequency and the probability of resolving TOTs for its corresponding target. For different part-of-speech primes, the correlation was positive such that TOT resolution increased when the phonological prime was higher in frequency. For same part-of-speech primes, the correlation was negative, where TOT resolution decreased as the phonological prime increased in frequency. Whether the same pattern emerges for older adults is an empirical question that has yet to be tested.

These studies illustrate that there are many other factors to be explored in research on TOTs and TOT resolution. The present study provides a set of stimuli to facilitate future research in these areas.

The Present Study

Despite age equivalence in phonological priming of word retrieval, young and older adults do not necessarily qualitatively experience TOTs in the same way. Using data from five experiments conducted by Abrams and her colleagues, the purposes of the present study were: (1) to distinguish the definitions that are effective at consistently inducing TOTs from those that do not regularly elicit TOTs, (2) to examine which words induce TOTs in young and older adults, and (3) to identify the words that come to mind as alternate words when the target is not retrieved. By examining a large number of young and older adults' responses, the present study provides a set of extensive stimuli, which is especially significant given that there are relatively few published studies of normative data from both young and older adults (e.g., see White and Abrams, 2004). Our compilation of responses can be used to facilitate future studies with TOTs and phonologically related words by overcoming certain obstacles.

One issue in TOT research is that people experience TOTs on only a small number of trials, approximately 8-18% of the time (A. Brown, 1991). As a result, only a small percentage of the overall data can be analyzed, reducing the statistical power of the design (see Brown and McNeill, 1966, and Burke et al., 1991, for a discussion of the data loss problem). For example, if 80 targets are used in a study, then participants will experience TOTs for only 10 targets, on average. There are several reasons why TOTs occur infrequently. Some target words may have been less susceptible to TOTs, either because they were too easy and participants knew the words, or because they were too difficult and participants did not contain these words and definitions in their vocabulary. Comparing young and older adults complicates this picture because older adults generally have more "know" responses and less "don't know" responses than young adults (e.g., Burke et al., 1991; Vitevitch and Sommers, 2003; White and Abrams, 2002), which is most likely due to older adults' larger vocabularies (e.g., Kemper and Sumner, 2001; Verhaeghen, 2003). Thus, TOT research is most likely comparing young and older adults' responses on different stimuli. Another issue relevant to TOT research is that people sometimes experience TOTs for a word different from the target, usually a synonym, e.g., "kerchief" instead of "bandanna". These TOTs are then categorized as incorrect TOTs and are excluded from analyses, resulting in even less data that can be analyzed.

A second issue involves alternate words, which we are defining as words that participants were either incorrectly thinking of upon hearing the definition or that came to mind when participants were unable to retrieve the intended word. Just as targets may differ in susceptibility to TOTs for young and older adults, the types of alternate words that come to mind may also have age differences. Whereas previous research has established that older adults are less likely to think of alternates during TOTs, no one has categorized the words that are produced by young and older adults or assessed whether certain TOTs are more likely to produce predictable alternates than others.

In consideration of the above issues, the present study compiled a list of targets, their corresponding general knowledge questions, first-syllable primes, alternate words, and the percent of time young and older adults experienced TOTs on these targets. This list indicates targets on which words young and older adults had similar opportunities for TOTs as well as targets that were not effective for inducing TOTs in either or both age groups. These data can also be used to determine the general knowledge questions that should be modified to increase the likelihood of TOTs as well as the targets that should be excluded from use in future studies.

Method

Participants

Data from 327 young adults and 132 older adults were collected across five experiments. Table 1 presents each experiment and the age characteristics of its participants. Three experiments are with young adults only and come from Abrams et al. (2003) and Abrams and Rodriguez (2005), and two experiments tested both young and older adults; these come from White and Abrams (2002) and Abrams, Bahrick, and Robinson (2006).

Table 1. Age Demographics of Participants from Experiments Included in the Present Study

Experiment	Young Adults				Older Adults			
	N	Mean	SD	Range	N	Mean	SD	Range
White and Abrams (2002)	60	20.3 yrs	1.6	18-26	80	72.0 yrs	6.3	60-83
Abrams, Bahrick, and Robinson (2006)	60	18.8 yrs	0.9	18-21	52	74.0 yrs	7.0	61-91
Abrams, White, and Eitel (2003)[a]:								
Experiment 1	60	18.9 yrs	1.5	17-25				
Experiment 3	87	18.6 yrs	0.9	18-23				
Abrams and Rodriguez (2005)	60	18.8 yrs	1.0	17-21				

[a]Experiment 2 used the same young adult participants in White and Abrams (2002), so their age demographics are not repeated here.

Materials

All studies used definition-like questions to elicit TOTs for specified target words. Across studies, 163 different targets were tested, some of which were taken from previous studies (Burke et al., 1991; Francis and Kucera, 1982; Jones, 1989; Kohn et al., 1987; Meyer and Bock, 1992; Nelson and Narens, 1980) and others that were created by Abrams and her colleagues. All target words were 1-5 syllables in length, low frequency as measured by Francis and Kucera (1982), and none were proper names.

Primes consisted of either phonologically related words containing the target's first syllable (Abrams and Rodriguez, 2005; Abrams et al., 2003, Experiments 2 and 3; White and Abrams, 2002), middle or last syllable (White and Abrams, 2002), or first letter and/or phoneme (Abrams et al., 2003, Experiments 1 and 3). Abrams et al. (2006) was not designed as a priming study and therefore did not include primes.

The appendix presents the general knowledge questions, corresponding targets, and up to five first-syllable primes used in four of the five experiments detailed here. For targets that shared the same first syllable (e.g., "abacus" and "abdicate"), only one set of primes is listed because primes can be used for both targets. As can be seen in this appendix, primes consisted of both high- and low-frequency words whenever possible. For example, for the target "affidavit", "after" is a high-frequency prime (699 per million; Francis and Kucera, 1982), whereas "affable" is a low-frequency prime (1 per million; Francis and Kucera, 1982). Because researchers tend to use a variety of word frequency databases, we did not list frequency in the appendix; however, we refer the reader to available frequency databases (e.g., Baayen, Piepenbrock, and van Rijn, 1993; G. Brown, 1984; Francis and Kucera, 1982; Lund and Burgess, 1996; Thorndike and Lorge, 1944).

A few issues should be noted when selecting stimuli from this appendix. First, primes were designed to overlap in phonology with the target, but not necessarily orthography. For example, the target "acapella" had primes such as "octopus", which shares sound but not spelling with the target. Second, the phonological overlap between a prime and target's first syllable was assessed using Webster's New World College Dictionary (Neufeldt and

Guralnik, 1997). However, dictionaries can vary slightly in their phonetic descriptions, so future studies using these primes in conjunction with primes not listed here should verify all primes' phonology using the same reference. Third, Abrams et al. (2003) showed that retrieval of targets whose first syllable comprised of a single letter, e.g., aorta, was not facilitated by primes that overlapped solely in first phoneme/letter. Therefore, most of these targets were later paired with primes that also contained the second phoneme, e.g., "atrocity" was a prime for "atone". However, some of the targets were not used in later studies and therefore do not have these modified primes; these exceptions are indicated in the appendix.

Procedure

All experiments used the same initial procedure, which involved presenting a general knowledge question on the computer screen, and participants were instructed to say "know" if they knew the word, "don't know" if they did not know the word, or, "TOT" if they were having a TOT for the word. After responding "know," participants stated the retrieved word, which may or may not have been the intended target. In all but one experiment (Abrams et al., 2006), after a "don't know" or "TOT" response, phonological primes intermixed with unrelated words were displayed one word at a time[2], followed by the same general knowledge question. Participants again responded whether they knew, did not know, or were having a TOT. Participants who were still unable to retrieve the target were asked to state any other words that were in mind. After all questions had been presented, a recognition test was administered to determine whether or not the participant had experienced unresolved TOTs for the intended target. This test consisted of the questions for which the participant never retrieved an answer, along with four possible answers to choose from. Its purpose was to identify incorrect TOTs, corresponding to targets that were not identified correctly on the recognition test, so that they could be excluded from analyses relevant to each individual experiment.

Results

Responses to General Knowledge Questions

Table 2 displays the means and standard deviations for the overall percent of "TOT", "know", and "don't know" responses given by each age group following the first presentation of the general knowledge question. TOTs and "know" responses were further categorized as either correct or incorrect. Incorrect "know" responses occurred when participants retrieved a word other than the target after responding "know". TOTs were categorized as incorrect when a word other than the target was retrieved following the priming manipulation or when the target was not chosen on the recognition test.[3] T-tests were conducted on each type of response to assess age differences, and $p < .05$ was used as the criterion for significance in all analyses. Older adults overall exhibited more correct TOTs, more correct "know" responses, and fewer "don't know" responses than young adults. For incorrect responses, young adults

[2] As a control, some questions were followed by all phonologically unrelated words instead of primes.

[3] Abrams et al. (2006) did not use a method for identifying the correctness of TOTs, so we arbitrarily categorized all of them as correct TOTs, which slightly raises the ratio of correct TOTs to incorrect TOTs. This is justified by the finding that TOTs are more often correct than incorrect (e.g., White and Abrams, 2002).

had more incorrect TOTs than older adults, whereas older adults had more incorrect "know" responses.

Table 2. Overall Percent of Responses to General Knowledge Questions by Age Group

Response	Young Adults		Older Adults	
	Mean	SD	Mean	SD
Correct TOT	13.6	8.6	19.4	11.3
Correct Know	30.2	24.7	41.0	24.7
Don't Know	38.7	21.6	19.3	15.9
Incorrect TOT	3.4	3.8	2.0	3.1
Incorrect Know	14.1	12.8	18.2	17.6

Table 3 lists the percent of time young and older adults responded "TOT", "know", or "don't know" for each individual target. Note that there were 28 targets that were not used in the experiments with older adults, and these targets are indicated by a 0 in the number of participants column. There was considerable variability in targets' capability for inducing TOTs, both for young and older adults, such that stimuli induced TOTs anywhere from 0% (for "numismatist") to 47.9% (for "pawn") of the time in young adults and 0% (for "amorous") to 52.5% (for "planetarium") in older adults. The table also illustrates variability between the age groups in inducing TOTs because young and older adults exhibited greater amounts of TOTs on different words. For example, "philatelist" induced correct TOTs in older adults 30.4% of the time, but only 9.3% of the time in young adults. Conversely, there were virtually no age differences for "dowry", which produced correct TOTs 25% of the time in young adults and 24.4% of the time in older adults.

Table 3. Percent of "TOT", "Know", and "Don't Know" Responses to General Knowledge Questions for Each Target Word

Target	# of Participants	Age Group	Correct TOT (%)	Correct Know (%)	Don't Know (%)	Incorrect TOT (%)	Incorrect Know (%)
abacus	294	young	27.9	24.5	37.8	6.5	3.4
abacus	118	older	26.3	66.1	3.4	2.5	1.7
abdicate	294	young	12.6	16.0	53.1	8.8	9.5
abdicate	116	older	14.7	75.0	9.5	0.0	0.9
acapella	103	young	14.6	57.3	9.7	1.9	16.5
acapella	75	older	10.7	64.0	6.7	0.0	18.7
actuary	293	young	7.2	2.0	67.9	6.5	16.4
actuary	117	older	35.9	33.3	19.7	2.6	8.5
affirmation	158	young	3.8	0.6	82.3	2.5	10.8
affirmation	117	older	17.9	13.7	45.3	2.6	20.5
agnostic	294	young	9.5	21.8	32.3	8.8	27.6
agnostic	117	older	13.7	56.4	5.1	0.0	24.8
albatross	294	young	8.5	11.2	53.7	3.7	22.8
albatross	117	older	16.2	58.1	18.8	1.7	5.1
alchemy	243	young	10.7	34.2	52.7	0.4	2.1

Table 3. Continued

Target	# of Participants	Age Group	Correct TOT (%)	Correct Know (%)	Don't Know (%)	Incorrect TOT (%)	Incorrect Know (%)
alchemy	41	older	24.4	56.1	19.5	0.0	0.0
amber	59	young	5.1	33.9	49.2	1.7	10.2
amber	0	older					
ambergris	100	young	12.0	2.0	47.0	4.0	35.0
ambergris	42	older	31.0	11.9	45.2	0.0	11.9
ambrosia	48	young	12.5	16.7	64.6	0.0	6.3
ambrosia	42	older	21.4	11.9	50.0	0.0	16.7
amnesty	59	young	6.8	0.0	79.7	6.8	6.8
amnesty	0	older					
amorous	135	young	5.2	3.0	60.7	5.2	25.9
amorous	75	older	0.0	22.7	24.0	4.0	49.3
anachronistic	59	young	6.8	6.8	74.6	6.8	5.1
anachronistic	0	older					
anagram	294	young	13.9	11.9	64.3	1.7	8.2
anagram	117	older	23.9	22.2	42.7	0.9	10.3
anarchist	235	young	17.4	45.5	25.5	5.1	6.4
anarchist	117	older	23.9	37.6	22.2	0.0	16.2
anecdote	251	young	9.6	12.7	54.2	6.4	17.1
anecdote	117	older	20.5	6.0	35.9	3.4	34.2
aorta	103	young	13.6	30.1	24.3	5.8	26.2
aorta	75	older	5.3	60.0	5.3	5.3	24.0
astrology	59	young	6.8	40.7	39.0	1.7	11.9
astrology	0	older					
atone	84	young	8.3	1.2	40.5	0.0	50.0
atone	42	older	31.0	42.9	11.9	0.0	14.3
bandanna	162	young	3.7	22.8	11.7	2.5	59.3
bandanna	75	older	4.0	33.3	0.0	0.0	62.7
barnacle	246	young	8.1	53.3	20.3	1.6	16.7
barnacle	75	older	12.0	80.0	2.7	0.0	5.3
barter	48	young	10.4	83.3	6.3	0.0	0.0
barter	42	older	7.1	85.7	2.4	0.0	4.8
beaver	59	young	0.0	88.1	8.5	0.0	3.4
beaver	0	older					
biography	59	young	1.7	86.4	1.7	0.0	10.2
biography	0	older					
boomerang	151	young	15.2	76.2	5.3	0.7	2.6
boomerang	117	older	27.4	66.7	1.7	2.6	1.7
cadaver	59	young	22.0	40.7	22.0	3.4	11.9
cadaver	0	older					
caduceus	235	young	7.7	1.3	75.7	10.2	5.1
caduceus	117	older	18.8	37.6	33.3	1.7	8.5

Table 3. Continued

Target	# of Participants	Age Group	Correct TOT (%)	Correct Know (%)	Don't Know (%)	Incorrect TOT (%)	Incorrect Know (%)
calibration	235	young	12.8	14.9	48.9	4.3	19.1
calibration	117	older	14.5	30.8	30.8	2.6	21.4
calisthenics	242	young	9.5	6.2	29.3	7.0	47.9
calisthenics	117	older	17.1	7.7	19.7	7.7	47.9
calligraphy	293	young	11.6	57.3	15.7	0.7	14.7
calligraphy	117	older	20.5	52.1	11.1	2.6	13.7
canonize	59	young	6.8	10.2	67.8	3.4	11.9
canonize	0	older					
capillary	235	young	18.3	34.0	40.4	1.7	5.5
capillary	117	older	13.7	48.7	23.1	1.7	12.8
carcinogen	294	young	15.6	37.1	26.9	3.4	17.0
carcinogen	116	older	14.7	40.5	17.2	0.9	26.7
cartographer	183	young	18.6	26.8	39.9	4.4	10.4
cartographer	116	older	16.4	52.6	17.2	0.9	12.9
castanets	235	young	10.6	10.2	56.6	5.1	17.4
castanets	116	older	9.5	61.2	14.7	0.9	13.8
catharsis	111	young	3.6	6.3	67.6	8.1	14.4
catharsis	0	older					
chameleon	243	young	12.3	67.9	5.8	2.5	11.5
chameleon	41	older	14.6	82.9	2.4	0.0	0.0
cherub	59	young	5.1	49.2	39.0	0.0	6.8
cherub	0	older					
contingency	194	young	7.2	1.0	67.5	6.7	17.5
contingency	75	older	5.3	0.0	18.7	17.3	58.7
contraband	246	young	24.0	15.0	43.5	7.7	9.8
contraband	75	older	17.3	32.0	20.0	4.0	26.7
corona	294	young	7.1	8.5	71.1	6.1	7.1
corona	116	older	11.2	14.7	51.7	2.6	19.8
coroner	59	young	6.8	6.8	25.4	10.2	50.8
coroner	0	older					
cosmonaut	187	young	4.3	28.3	45.5	0.0	21.9
cosmonaut	75	older	9.3	52.0	9.3	1.3	28.0
covenant	235	young	9.8	15.7	46.0	5.5	23.0
covenant	116	older	21.6	15.5	40.5	0.0	22.4
decanter	294	young	8.8	3.4	49.3	8.2	30.3
decanter	116	older	19.8	38.8	4.3	3.4	33.6
desecrate	48	young	22.9	16.7	58.3	0.0	2.1
desecrate	41	older	34.1	31.7	29.3	0.0	4.9
determinist	241	young	12.4	5.8	62.2	5.8	13.7
determinist	116	older	15.5	6.9	37.9	5.2	34.5
detonate	235	young	11.1	27.7	30.2	3.4	27.7

Table 3. Continued

Target	# of Participants	Age Group	Correct TOT (%)	Correct Know (%)	Don't Know (%)	Incorrect TOT (%)	Incorrect Know (%)
detonate	116	older	14.7	44.0	6.9	3.4	31.0
dowry	48	young	25.0	37.5	35.4	0.0	2.1
dowry	41	older	24.4	75.6	0.0	0.0	0.0
egocentric	51	young	11.8	3.9	15.7	17.6	51.0
egocentric	75	older	13.3	6.7	12.0	2.7	65.3
ellipsis	210	young	9.5	22.9	54.8	5.2	7.6
ellipsis	116	older	14.7	2.6	64.7	4.3	13.8
embryo	294	young	18.4	37.1	21.8	2.4	20.4
embryo	116	older	19.0	37.9	33.6	0.0	9.5
emerald	59	young	1.7	66.1	11.9	0.0	20.3
emerald	0	older					
encrypt	59	young	6.8	6.8	67.8	0.0	18.6
encrypt	0	older					
endorse	107	young	18.7	47.7	29.9	0.0	3.7
endorse	41	older	12.2	87.8	0.0	0.0	0.0
ephemeral	51	young	5.9	5.9	23.5	21.6	43.1
ephemeral	75	older	2.7	0.0	13.3	17.3	66.7
epidermis	102	young	7.8	73.5	8.8	2.9	6.9
epidermis	75	older	5.3	68.0	12.0	0.0	14.7
epilogue	131	young	32.8	27.5	23.7	1.5	14.5
epilogue	41	older	26.8	24.4	12.2	0.0	36.6
equestrian	162	young	3.7	21.0	41.4	4.9	29.0
equestrian	75	older	8.0	38.7	5.3	0.0	48.0
esoteric	135	young	13.3	1.5	60.0	7.4	17.8
esoteric	75	older	5.3	6.7	29.3	6.7	52.0
estrogen	59	young	13.6	61.0	20.3	0.0	5.1
estrogen	0	older					
euphemism	211	young	9.5	8.5	70.6	2.4	9.0
euphemism	117	older	22.2	9.4	51.3	5.1	12.0
evangelist	109	young	5.5	11.9	35.8	3.7	43.1
evangelist	75	older	2.7	18.7	1.3	0.0	77.3
filament	296	young	7.8	29.4	56.4	1.7	4.7
filament	116	older	11.2	62.1	19.8	0.9	6.0
foal	48	young	31.3	18.8	18.8	0.0	31.3
foal	41	older	4.9	48.8	17.1	0.0	29.3
fovea	48	young	45.8	27.1	20.8	0.0	6.3
fovea	41	older	26.8	2.4	31.7	0.0	39.0
fratricide	48	young	27.1	6.3	62.5	0.0	4.2
fratricide	41	older	24.4	56.1	19.5	0.0	0.0
gazebo	58	young	10.3	41.4	31.0	1.7	15.5
gazebo	0	older					

Table 3. Continued

Target	# of Participants	Age Group	Correct TOT (%)	Correct Know (%)	Don't Know (%)	Incorrect TOT (%)	Incorrect Know (%)
gerrymander	151	young	18.5	9.9	62.3	4.0	5.3
gerrymander	118	older	20.3	50.0	22.9	0.8	5.9
haiku	191	young	12.0	66.0	19.9	1.0	1.0
haiku	43	older	23.3	23.3	53.5	0.0	0.0
hemophilia	191	young	35.6	27.7	24.6	1.6	10.5
hemophilia	43	older	46.5	37.2	11.6	0.0	4.7
hemorrhage	48	young	35.4	10.4	50.0	0.0	4.2
hemorrhage	43	older	18.6	60.5	14.0	0.0	7.0
heretic	135	young	15.6	7.4	40.7	11.1	25.2
heretic	75	older	10.7	18.7	12.0	10.7	48.0
hieroglyphics	246	young	11.8	76.8	9.3	0.8	1.2
hieroglyphics	75	older	16.0	70.7	6.7	1.3	5.3
hydrogen	110	young	2.7	40.0	23.6	8.2	25.5
hydrogen	75	older	4.0	42.7	8.0	1.3	44.0
hypochondriac	191	young	29.8	40.3	24.6	2.6	2.6
hypochondriac	43	older	27.9	69.8	2.3	0.0	0.0
imminent	59	young	5.1	11.9	67.8	3.4	11.9
imminent	0	older					
incisors	246	young	9.8	39.0	32.9	6.1	12.2
incisors	75	older	4.0	73.3	6.7	1.3	14.7
incubate	234	young	17.1	54.7	26.1	0.9	1.3
incubate	118	older	16.1	67.8	6.8	0.8	8.5
insomnia	294	young	23.8	63.6	5.8	1.4	5.4
insomnia	118	older	21.2	63.6	8.5	0.0	6.8
intransitive	194	young	5.7	2.1	69.1	5.2	18.0
intransitive	75	older	6.7	28.0	26.7	6.7	32.0
javelin	103	young	19.4	56.3	10.7	3.9	9.7
javelin	75	older	9.3	72.0	8.0	0.0	10.7
jettison	48	young	20.8	4.2	70.8	0.0	4.2
jettison	43	older	51.2	18.6	25.6	0.0	4.7
kaleidoscope	191	young	20.9	59.7	18.3	0.0	1.0
kaleidoscope	43	older	48.8	44.2	7.0	0.0	0.0
lampoon	48	young	22.9	0.0	70.8	0.0	6.3
lampoon	43	older	41.9	0.0	48.8	0.0	9.3
liaison	103	young	4.9	14.6	13.6	4.9	62.1
liaison	75	older	10.7	29.3	2.7	5.3	52.0
libretto	48	young	8.3	2.1	85.4	0.0	4.2
libretto	43	older	18.6	30.2	44.2	0.0	7.0
ligament	187	young	8.6	33.7	18.2	4.8	34.8
ligament	75	older	8.0	29.3	4.0	4.0	54.7

Table 3. Continued

Target	# of Participants	Age Group	Correct TOT (%)	Correct Know (%)	Don't Know (%)	Incorrect TOT (%)	Incorrect Know (%)
lynch	48	young	10.4	41.7	47.9	0.0	0.0
lynch	43	older	37.2	51.2	4.7	0.0	7.0
malevolence	246	young	9.3	4.1	45.1	6.5	35.0
malevolence	75	older	14.7	2.7	41.3	6.7	34.7
manna	107	young	6.5	19.6	66.4	0.9	6.5
manna	43	older	4.7	88.4	7.0	0.0	0.0
marinade	195	young	15.9	60.0	15.9	1.5	6.7
marinade	0	older					
marsupials	294	young	20.7	52.7	25.5	0.3	0.7
marsupials	118	older	32.2	43.2	21.2	1.7	1.7
mausoleum	103	young	10.7	18.4	29.1	14.6	27.2
mausoleum	75	older	8.0	64.0	0.0	1.3	26.7
mercenary	294	young	12.2	24.1	57.8	1.7	4.1
mercenary	118	older	25.4	56.8	8.5	2.5	6.8
meteorology	59	young	3.4	74.6	20.3	1.7	0.0
meteorology	0	older					
meticulous	135	young	12.6	10.4	21.5	10.4	45.2
meticulous	75	older	14.7	9.3	9.3	10.7	56.0
metronome	235	young	20.4	38.3	31.9	4.3	5.1
metronome	118	older	19.5	66.9	6.8	3.4	3.4
mince	48	young	25.0	10.4	27.1	0.0	37.5
mince	43	older	18.6	37.2	7.0	0.0	37.2
minstrel	59	young	6.8	5.1	52.5	6.8	28.8
minstrel	0	older					
misdemeanor	107	young	10.3	75.7	13.1	0.0	0.9
misdemeanor	43	older	30.2	65.1	4.7	0.0	0.0
misogynist	242	young	11.2	9.5	47.5	8.3	23.6
misogynist	118	older	11.9	28.0	36.4	6.8	16.9
molasses	242	young	6.6	30.6	44.6	2.1	16.1
molasses	118	older	7.6	50.8	26.3	0.0	15.3
molt	48	young	33.3	37.5	27.1	0.0	2.1
molt	41	older	36.6	56.1	7.3	0.0	0.0
mutiny	235	young	17.4	25.1	23.0	11.5	23.0
mutiny	116	older	15.5	44.0	8.6	5.2	26.7
narcissism	184	young	9.8	17.9	47.3	7.1	17.9
narcissism	41	older	26.8	34.1	12.2	0.0	26.8
negotiable	51	young	17.6	0.0	49.0	3.9	29.4
negotiable	75	older	12.0	0.0	41.3	8.0	38.7
nepotism	151	young	22.5	12.6	51.7	7.3	6.0
nepotism	116	older	37.1	58.6	3.4	0.0	0.9

Table 3. Continued

Target	# of Participants	Age Group	Correct TOT (%)	Correct Know (%)	Don't Know (%)	Incorrect TOT (%)	Incorrect Know (%)
numismatist	59	young	0.0	0.0	86.4	0.0	13.6
numismatist	0	older					
omniscient	246	young	13.8	19.5	31.3	4.5	30.9
omniscient	75	older	10.7	13.3	24.0	4.0	48.0
omnivore	184	young	15.2	48.4	21.2	2.2	13.0
omnivore	41	older	31.7	36.6	19.5	0.0	12.2
onomatopoeia	191	young	22.0	46.6	22.5	4.2	4.7
onomatopoeia	41	older	24.4	12.2	53.7	0.0	9.8
origami	209	young	19.6	67.9	11.5	0.5	0.5
origami	116	older	19.0	52.6	21.6	4.3	2.6
ornithology	58	young	17.2	5.2	69.0	0.0	8.6
ornithology	0	older					
orthodontist	107	young	5.6	91.6	2.8	0.0	0.0
orthodontist	40	older	10.0	80.0	7.5	0.0	2.5
oscillation	51	young	5.9	11.8	62.7	5.9	13.7
oscillation	75	older	9.3	4.0	45.3	8.0	33.3
palindrome	235	young	28.9	11.9	48.9	7.2	3.0
palindrome	116	older	41.4	8.6	40.5	3.4	6.0
pantomime	48	young	31.3	8.3	50.0	0.0	10.4
pantomime	41	older	29.3	56.1	9.8	0.0	4.9
papyrus	245	young	12.7	37.6	44.5	2.9	2.4
papyrus	75	older	6.7	77.3	5.3	1.3	9.3
paradox	242	young	18.6	8.7	56.6	3.7	12.4
paradox	41	older	34.1	4.9	56.1	0.0	4.9
parasite	293	young	16.0	56.7	17.1	3.4	6.8
parasite	117	older	20.5	64.1	8.5	0.0	6.8
parody	48	young	27.1	16.7	35.4	0.0	20.8
parody	40	older	37.5	7.5	32.5	0.0	22.5
parsimony	106	young	14.2	0.0	81.1	0.9	3.8
parsimony	40	older	32.5	0.0	65.0	0.0	2.5
pasteurize	235	young	17.0	29.8	38.7	4.7	9.8
pasteurize	115	older	11.3	68.7	9.6	0.9	9.6
pawn	48	young	47.9	0.0	31.3	0.0	20.8
pawn	40	older	47.5	5.0	15.0	0.0	32.5
pendulum	294	young	7.5	46.6	39.8	0.3	5.8
pendulum	116	older	10.3	59.5	25.9	0.9	3.4
perjury	294	young	23.1	41.8	24.5	1.7	8.8
perjury	117	older	20.5	68.4	4.3	0.0	6.8
perpendicular	59	young	5.1	40.7	23.7	3.4	27.1
perpendicular	0	older					
petrify	48	young	16.7	8.3	72.9	0.0	2.1

Table 3. Continued

Target	# of Participants	Age Group	Correct TOT (%)	Correct Know (%)	Don't Know (%)	Incorrect TOT (%)	Incorrect Know (%)
petrify	41	older	34.1	14.6	39.0	0.0	12.2
philatelist	183	young	9.3	0.5	78.1	1.6	10.4
philatelist	115	older	30.4	38.3	15.7	3.5	12.2
placebo	235	young	15.7	63.0	17.0	1.7	2.6
placebo	41	older	29.3	65.9	4.9	0.0	0.0
plagiarize	235	young	16.6	80.4	1.7	0.0	1.3
plagiarize	40	older	20.0	80.0	0.0	0.0	0.0
planetarium	132	young	33.3	15.9	34.8	4.5	11.4
planetarium	40	older	52.5	25.0	15.0	0.0	7.5
potpourri	294	young	7.8	83.7	6.1	0.0	2.4
potpourri	115	older	40.0	40.0	9.6	2.6	7.8
pride	48	young	27.1	33.3	25.0	0.0	14.6
pride	40	older	17.5	75.0	0.0	0.0	7.5
procrastinate	294	young	8.2	80.6	8.8	0.0	2.4
procrastinate	115	older	14.8	66.1	9.6	5.2	4.3
proselytize	59	young	10.2	3.4	64.4	16.9	5.1
proselytize	0	older					
reincarnate	246	young	11.8	66.3	8.1	1.2	12.6
reincarnate	75	older	6.7	37.3	6.7	0.0	49.3
reiterate	294	young	21.1	14.3	46.9	3.4	14.3
reiterate	114	older	23.7	13.2	39.5	2.6	21.1
rhetorical	194	young	13.9	51.0	23.7	1.0	10.3
rhetorical	75	older	9.3	32.0	33.3	4.0	21.3
rosary	59	young	6.8	69.5	20.3	3.4	0.0
rosary	0	older					
samurai	48	young	6.3	64.6	27.1	0.0	2.1
samurai	39	older	7.7	84.6	7.7	0.0	0.0
seismology	48	young	27.1	16.7	50.0	0.0	6.3
seismology	41	older	31.7	39.0	22.0	0.0	7.3
serenade	48	young	4.2	25.0	68.8	0.0	2.1
serenade	40	older	15.0	65.0	20.0	0.0	0.0
serrated	187	young	10.2	26.2	49.2	3.2	11.2
serrated	75	older	10.7	37.3	25.3	2.7	24.0
silhouettes	235	young	16.6	23.4	42.1	1.7	16.2
silhouettes	115	older	14.8	36.5	28.7	4.3	15.7
silo	59	young	8.5	35.6	45.8	1.7	8.5
silo	0	older					
simile	293	young	9.9	70.3	7.2	4.1	8.5
simile	115	older	24.3	21.7	21.7	6.1	26.1
sloop	47	young	6.4	0.0	89.4	0.0	4.3
sloop	40	older	17.5	10.0	65.0	0.0	7.5

Table 3. Continued

Target	# of Participants	Age Group	Correct TOT (%)	Correct Know (%)	Don't Know (%)	Incorrect TOT (%)	Incorrect Know (%)
soliloquy	191	young	23.6	19.4	17.8	6.3	33.0
soliloquy	40	older	25.0	37.5	30.0	0.0	7.5
spatula	52	young	5.8	88.5	3.8	0.0	1.9
spatula	0	older					
spelunker	100	young	16.0	20.0	51.0	1.0	12.0
spelunker	42	older	35.7	42.9	19.0	0.0	2.4
stamina	51	young	7.8	19.6	58.8	2.0	11.8
stamina	75	older	9.3	33.3	22.7	5.3	29.3
subscription	59	young	5.1	33.9	42.4	1.7	16.9
subscription	0	older					
synagogue	59	young	5.1	45.8	13.6	3.4	32.2
synagogue	0	older					
toga	106	young	8.5	64.2	21.7	0.0	5.7
toga	38	older	5.3	81.6	10.5	0.0	2.6
torpedo	210	young	6.2	40.0	46.7	1.9	5.2
torpedo	116	older	17.2	41.4	20.7	1.7	19.0
tranquilize	294	young	19.4	7.1	32.3	4.8	36.4
tranquilize	115	older	28.7	19.1	11.3	4.3	36.5
translucent	187	young	11.8	13.4	32.6	17.6	24.6
translucent	75	older	12.0	28.0	8.0	6.7	45.3
tsunami	294	young	10.2	43.9	36.4	1.4	8.2
tsunami	115	older	14.8	47.0	19.1	4.3	14.8
utopia	210	young	15.7	39.5	28.1	1.4	15.2
utopia	114	older	26.3	32.5	12.3	1.8	27.2
venison	246	young	8.1	50.4	32.1	2.4	6.9
venison	75	older	9.3	90.7	0.0	0.0	0.0

We calculated the percent of targets on which young and older adults experienced correct TOTs at least 8% of the time (the lower end of the range of TOT rates reported by A. Brown, 1991). Young adults experienced TOTs on 71% of the targets, whereas older adults experienced TOTs on 86% of the targets. Similarly, 73% of the targets produced correct TOTs at least 8% of the time in *both* young and older adults, suggesting that the majority of general knowledge questions were useful in inducing TOTs in both age groups.

To identify general knowledge questions that were not specific enough in inducing retrieval of the intended target, we compared the percent of targets that yielded more incorrect responses than correct TOTs. Young and older adults had more incorrect "know" responses than correct TOTs for 43% and 42% of targets, respectively. Young adults experienced more incorrect TOTs than correct TOTs for 6% of targets, whereas older adults exhibited more incorrect TOTs on only 3% of targets. This relatively large number of incorrect responses given by both age groups suggests that many of the definitions often elicited retrieval of a word different from the target.

ALTERNATE WORDS AVAILABLE DURING TOTS OR INCORRECTLY RETRIEVED AS TARGETS

Table 4 lists alternate words that were in mind during TOTs as well as alternates incorrectly retrieved as targets after a "know" response. It is important to clarify that unlike previous studies, the goal of the present study was not to determine the percent of time that alternates occurred in young and older adults during TOT states. Instead, we were interested in using alternates to see whether any consistencies existed between young and older adults in retrieving a specific alternate. The top three alternates[4] are listed along with the number of people who gave that response.[5] A response was required to be given at least twice for inclusion in this table. Targets for which young and older adults gave the same most frequent alternate are marked with an asterisk. As can be seen in this table, there is remarkable similarity in the alternate words produced by young and older adults: young and older adults retrieved at least one of the same alternates 86% of time. However, both age groups retrieved the same most frequent alternate only 46% of the time, suggesting that there are age differences in the most available alternate. Alternates also shared phonological overlap with the target on some occasions, e.g., the alternate "scramble" shares /am/ with the target "anagram", although the amount of overlap is not as high as reported in previous studies. This result most likely occurred because our alternates included words incorrectly retrieved following a "know" responses, which were most often synonyms that were not necessarily phonologically related to the target.

Table 4. Alternate Words Available During TOTs or Incorrectly Retrieved as Targets Following "Know" Responses

Target	Age Group	Most Frequent Alternate (N)	Alternate (N)	Alternate (N)	Alternate (N)
abacus	young	sliderule/r (12)	calculator (11)	meniscus (3)	
abacus	older	calculator (2)			
abdicate	young	resign (31)	dethrone (20)	step down (13)	
abdicate	older	abduct (2)	renounce (2)		
acappella*	young	solo (34)	acoustic (4)	vocal (3)	
acappella	older	solo (21)			
actuary	young	accountant (25)	insurance agent (23)	adjuster (13)	
actuary	older	adjuster (8)	statistician (5)	analyst (3)	
affirmation	young	taking the 5th (8)	promise (7)	testimony (3)	
affirmation	older	conscientious	objection (9)	taking the 5th (7)	objector (19)
agnostic*	young	atheist (166)	scientist (5)	skeptic/al (5)	
agnostic	older	atheist (54)			
albatross	young	seagull (81)	pelican (71)	dove (11)	
albatross	older	swan (3)	seagull (2)		
alchemy	young	chemistry (7)	melting (3)	blacksmith (2)	ore (2)
alchemy[a]	older	N/A			

[4] If there was a tie for 3rd place, a 4th alternate word was listed.

[5] More young adults were tested than older adults, which yielded more opportunities for young adults to produce alternates.

Table 4. Continued

Target	Age Group	Most Frequent Alternate (N)	Alternate (N)	Alternate (N)	Alternate (N)
ambergris	young	blubber (53)	oil (9)	fat (7)	
ambergris	older	sperm oil (2)			
amber	young	gold (8)			
amber[b]	older	------			
ambrosia[a]	young	N/A			
ambrosia	older	nectar (4)			
amnesty	young	pardon (11)	Clinton (2)		
amnesty[b]	older	N/A			
amorous*	young	affection (12)	romantic (10)	lust (9)	
amorous	older	affectionate (20)	lovable (12)	lover (8)	
anachronistic[a]	young	N/A			
anachronistic[b]	older	------			
anagram*	young	jumble (27)	scramble (22)	puzzle (9)	acronym (9)
anagram	older	jumble (5)	puzzle (5)	scramble (4)	
anarchist	young	communist (22)	radical (7)	monarchy (4)	
anarchist	older	liberalist (9)	radical (2)	revolutionary (2)	
anecdote	young	story (24)	summary (14)	biography (7)	
anecdote	older	essay (31)	story (14)	synopsis (9)	
aorta	young	heart (36)	coratid (12)	jugular (8)	
aorta	older	coratid (25)	heart (8)	coronary (5)	vein (5)
astrology	young	astronomy (7)	Gallileo (2)	horoscope (2)	
astrology[b]	older	------			
atone	young	apology (23)	repent (8)	reconciliation (4)	
atone	older	penance (4)	repent (2)		
bandanna	young	scarf (184)	kerchief (7)	tie (6)	
bandanna	older	kerchief (44)	scarf (38)		
barnacle	young	snail(s) (28)	clams (12)	crustacean (10)	
barnacle	older	mussels (5)	snail (2)		
barter[a]	young	N/A			
barter	older	swap (2)			
beaver[a]	young	N/A			
beaver[b]	older	------			
biography	young	autobiography (6)			
biography[b]	older	------			
boomerang	young	Frisbee (3)	Australian (2)		
boomerang[a]	older	N/A			
cadaver	young	corpse (6)	specimen (3)	carcass (2)	
cadaver[b]	older	------			
caduceus	young	blue cross blue shield (12)	red cross (8)	Hippocratic symbol (4)	physician(4)
caduceus	older	medusa/s (7)	doctor (6)		
calibration	young	in tune (34)	converting (14)	standardizing (13)	
calibration	older	synchronize (8)	standardizing (7)	alignment (2)	
calisthenics*	young	aerobics (64)	cardio (54)	yoga (41)	
calisthenics	older	aerobics (75)	dancing (7)	gymnastics (5)	

Table 4. Continued

Target	Age Group	Most Frequent Alternate (N)	Alternate (N)	Alternate (N)	Alternate (N)
calisthenics	older	aerobics (75)	dancing (7)	gymnastics (5)	
calligraphy	young	cursive (16)	penmanship (4)	manuscripts (3)	
calligraphy	older	penmanship (19)	spencercian (6)	palmer method (4)	
canonize	young	sanctify (3)	martyr (3)		
canonize[b]	older	------			
capillary*	young	blood vessels (16)	ventricle (9)	vesicle (5)	
capillary	older	blood vessels (5)	areolas (4)	corpuscle (4)	
carcinogen	young	tumor (23)	cancerous (19)	malignant (19)	
carcinogen	older	malignant (6)	cigarette(s) (5)	cell (4)	
cartographer	young	mapmaker (19)	topographer (15)	cipher (3)	geologist (3)
cartographer	older	cartologist (15)	cardiologist (4)		
castanets*	young	tambourine (26)	drums (24)	finger cymbals (15)	maracas (15)
castanets	older	tambourine (10)	maracas (8)	bongo (6)	
catharsis	young	therapy (8)	hypnosis (6)	confession (4)	
catharsis[b]	older	------			
chameleon	young	gecko (27)	iguana (20)	salamander (3)	
chameleon[a]	older	N/A			
cherub[a]	young	N/A			
cherub[b]	older	------			
contingency	young	coincidence (21)	fate (15)	luck (14)	
contingency	older	happenstance (21)	accident (16)	random (14)	
contraband	young	black-market (44)	smuggled (35)	bootlegged (10)	
contraband	older	smuggled (29)	black-market (6)	bootlegged (3)	illicit trade (3)
corona*	young	stratosphere (16)	ozone layer (11)	halo (5)	
corona	older	stratosphere (18)	ionosphere (13)	cornea (4)	ozone layer (4)
coroner	young	detective (20)	investigator (3)	forensics (2)	
coroner[b]	older	------			
cosmonaut*	young	astronaut (100)	captain (4)	aeronaut (4)	
cosmonaut	older	astronaut (37)			
covenant	young	contract (59)	commandment (12)	oath (10)	
covenant	older	commandment (15)	bible (4)	promises (3)	
decanter	young	bottle (99)	carafe (42)	flask (23)	
decanter	older	carafe (51)	bottle (9)	flask (3)	
desecrate[a]	young	N/A			
desecrate[a]	older	N/A			
determinist*	young	fate/fatalist (21)	predestination (9)		
determinist	older	fatalist (33)	predestination (6)	pessimist (5)	
detonate*	young	ignite (94)	trigger (15)	activate (8)	
detonate	older	ignite (48)	activate (4)	trigger (4)	
dowry[a]	young	N/A			
dowry[a]	older	N/A			
egocentric	young	selfish (27)	narcissistic (16)	egotistical (13)	
egocentric	older	egotist (39)	self-centered (20)	selfish (16)	
ellipsis*	young	ellipse (18)	etceteras (15)	asterisk(s) (7)	
ellipsis	older	ellipse/s (5)	dash (4)	pause (4)	

Table 4. Continued

Target	Age Group	Most Frequent Alternate (N)	Alternate (N)	Alternate (N)	Alternate (N)
embryo*	young	fetus (51)	zygote (41)	baby (5)	
embryo	older	fetus (11)	baby (7)	unborn child (3)	
emerald	young	jade (7)			
emerald[b]	older	------			
encrypt	young	encode (13)	codify (2)		
encrypt[b]	older	------			
endorse	young	verify (2)	sign (2)	authenticate (2)	
endorse[a]	older	N/A			
ephemeral	young	short (21)	fleeting (5)	quick (4)	shortly (4)
ephemeral	older	momentary (16)	instant (14)	fleeting (13)	
epidermis	young	endoderm (4)	ectoderm (4)		
epidermis	older	derma (15)			
epilogue	young	conclusion (11)	afterward (11)	prologue (6)	
epilogue	older	addendum (8)	afterward (2)	appendix (2)	postscript (2)
equestrian*	young	jockey (58)	horseback rider (26)	cowboy (14)	
equestrian	older	jockey (35)	horseback rider (12)	horseman (11)	
esoteric*	young	incomprehensible (14)	secret (11)	inside joke (10)	
esoteric	older	incomprehensible (21)	unfathomable (12)	mystery (8)	
estrogen	young	progesterone (2)	testosterone (2)		
estrogen[b]	older	------			
euphemism	young	censorship (12)	politically correct (12)	replacement (4)	
euphemism	older	politically correct (6)	tact (4)	polite (3)	
evangelist*	young	minister (21)	priest (20)	reverend (16)	
evangelist	older	minister (80)	pastor (14)	priest (10)	reverend (10)
filament	young	fuse (12)	wires (9)	flint (7)	
filament	older	tungsten (6)	element (5)	light (4)	
foal*	young	colt (5)	pony (4)	fawn (3)	
foal	older	colt (12)			
fovea	young	pupil (6)	cornea (3)		
fovea	older	macular (5)	cornea (3)	lens (2)	pupil (2)
fratricide	young	murder (2)			
fratricide[a]	older	N/A			
gazebo	young	pavilion (4)	canopy (2)		
gazebo[b]	older	------			
gerrymander	young	favoritism (4)	districts (3)	separate (3)	
gerrymander	older	redistricting (4)	districts (3)		
haiku	young	sonnet (3)			
haiku[a]	older	N/A			
hemophilia	young	anemia (15)	hemorrhage (5)	hemoglobin (3)	
hemophilia[a]	older	N/A			
hemorrhage[a]	young	N/A			
hemorrhage	older	hemophilia (2)			
heretic	young	nonconformist (28)	rebel (17)	atheist (14)	
heretic	older	agnostic (23)	atheist (14)	nonconformist (7)	
hieroglyphics	young	calligraphy (4)			

Table 4. Continued

Target	Age Group	Most Frequent Alternate (N)	Alternate (N)	Alternate (N)	Alternate (N)
hieroglyphics	older	cuneiform (3)	pictograph (3)		
hydrogen*	young	helium (24)	oxygen (14)	nitrogen (7)	
hydrogen	older	helium (35)	oxygen (20)	gas (4)	
hypochondriac	young	paranoia (6)	obsessive-compulsive(4)	delusion (2)	hallucination (2)
hypochondriac[a]	older	N/A			
imminent	young	omen (4)	impending (4)	perilous (2)	
imminent[b]	older	------			
incisors	young	canines (29)	bi/cuspids (26)		
incisors	older	cuspids (6)	canines (4)		
incubate	young	insulate (5)	hibernation (3)	fermentation (3)	
incubate	older	brooder (8)	nesting (4)		
insomnia	young	narcolepsy (19)	sleep apnea (11)	amnesia (4)	
insomnia	older	amnesia (7)	sleep apnea (7)		
intransitive*	young	adverb (41)	indirect object (8)	action (6)	passive (6)
intransitive	older	adverb (26)	indirect verb (7)	passive (5)	
javelin*	young	discus (5)	shot put (4)	disk (4)	
javelin	older	discus (8)	lance (4)	spear (3)	
jettison[a]	young	N/A			
jettison[a]	older	N/A			
kaleidoscope	young	telescope (3)	spectroscope (2)		
kaleidoscope[a]	older	N/A			
lampoon[a]	young	N/A			
lampoon[a]	older	N/A			
liaison*	young	mediator (117)	middleman (10)	ally (3)	ambassador (3)
liaison	older	mediator (28)	facilitator (13)	go between (10)	
libretto[a]	young	N/A			
libretto[a]	older	N/A			
ligaments	young	tendon/s (58)	muscles (33)	cartilage (27)	
ligaments	older	muscle/s (51)	cartilage (15)	tendon(s) (13)	
lynch[a]	young	N/A			
lynch[a]	older	N/A			
malevolence	young	malicious (53)	hatred (49)	evil (7)	mean (7)
malevolence	older	vindictive (6)	hatred (5)	malicious (4)	misfortune (4)
manna	young	ambrosia (4)	bread (3)		
manna[a]	older	N/A			
marinade	young	broth (6)	sauté (6)	oil (3)	seasoning (3)
marinade[b]	older	------			
marsupial	young	kangaroo (5)	pouch (4)	mammals (3)	kingdoms (3)
marsupial[a]	older	N/A			
mausoleum	young	tomb(stone)/s (60)	crypt/s (8)		
mausoleum	older	crypt/s (16)	tomb(stone) (14)		
mercenary*	young	spy (16)	guerilla (7)	soldier (5)	
mercenary	older	spy (6)	legionnaire (6)	soldier of fortune (3)	
meteorology[a]	young	N/A			

Table 4. Continued

Target	Age Group	Most Frequent Alternate (N)	Alternate (N)	Alternate (N)	Alternate (N)
meteorology[b]	older	------			
meticulous*	young	perfectionist (44)	anal (38)	obsessive compulsive disorder (7)	
meticulous	older	perfectionist (37)	picky (12)	precise (9)	
metronome	young	meter (13)	clock (9)	pendulum (7)	
metronome	older	pendulum (2)			
mince*	young	dice (17)			
mince	older	dice (15)			
minstrel	young	jester (14)	Shakespeare (2)	bard (2)	joker (2)
minstrel[b]	older	------			
misdemeanor[a]	young	N/A			
misdemeanor[a]	older	N/A			
misogynist*	young	chauvinist (47)	sexist (37)	anti-feminist (9)	
misogynist	older	chauvinist (15)	woman hater (12)	anti-feminist (6)	
molasses*	young	(maple) syrup (30)	sap (12)		
molasses	older	(cane) syrup (20)			
molt[a]	young	N/A			
molt[a]	older	N/A			
mutiny	young	coup (22)	revolution (18)	revolt (15)	
mutiny	older	insurrection (22)	coup (17)	revolution (12)	
narcissism	young	self-esteem (16)	conceited (15)	egotism (15)	
narcissism	older	egotism (8)	egocentric (2)		
negotiable*	young	debate (28)	topic (6)	controversial (4)	
negotiable	older	debate (22)	on the table (6)	moot (6)	
nepotism	young	bias (15)	discrimination (12)	favoritism (11)	
nepotism[a]	older	N/A			
numismatist	young	(coin) collector (19)			
numismatist[b]	older	------			
omniscient*	young	omnipotent (81)	genius (38)	wise (8)	
omniscient	older	omnipotent (34)	genius (12)	God (6)	wise (6)
omnivore*	young	carnivore (56)	herbivore (13)	mammal (4)	
omnivore	older	carnivore (5)			
onomatopoeia*	young	synonym (3)	oxymoron (3)	alliteration (2)	
onomatopoeia	older	synonym (3)			
origami	young	papier-mâché (3)			
origami[a]	older	N/A			
ornithology	young	aviary (2)			
ornithology[b]	older	------			
orthodontist[a]	young	N/A			
orthodontist[a]	older	N/A			
oscillation	young	wave/s (7)	rhythm (4)	sway (3)	vibrate (3)
oscillation	older	rhythm (7)	vibrate (6)	harmonic/s (4)	motion (4)
palindrome*	young	anagram (17)	acronym (6)	homonym (5)	idiom (5)
palindrome	older	anagram (10)			
pantomime	young	charade/s (2)			

Table 4. Continued

Target	Age Group	Most Frequent Alternate (N)	Alternate (N)	Alternate (N)	Alternate (N)
pantomime[a]	older	N/A			
papyrus	young	eucalyptus (8)	reed (7)	aloe (5)	paper (5)
papyrus	older	papaya (2)			
paradox	young	oxymoron (34)	ironic (12)	contradictory (9)	
paradox[a]	older	N/A			
parasite	young	symbiotic (11)	leech (7)	bacteria (7)	
parasite	older	leech (7)			
parody*	young	satire (10)			
parody	older	satire (6)	mimic (2)		
parsimony	young	simplicity (4)	concise (2)		
parsimony[a]	older	N/A			
pasteurize*	young	homogenization (13)	mold (8)	boiling (8)	
pasteurize	older	homogenization (10)	sterilizing (6)		
pawn*	young	collateral (8)			
pawn	older	collateral (19)			
pendulum	young	seesaw (13)	pulley (10)	lever (5)	
pendulum	older	fulcrum (5)			
perjury*	young	lie (80)	Clinton (5)	treason (2)	
perjury	older	lie (18)			
perpendicular	young	right angle (20)			
perpendicular[b]	older	------			
petrify[a]	young	N/A			
petrify	older	fossilize (2)			
philatelist	young	stamp collector (64)	hobby (3)	stampographer (3)	
philatelist	older	numismatist (13)	stamp collector (10)		
placebo	young	glucose (3)	diabetes (2)	pseudo (2)	
placebo	older	placenta (3)			
plagiarize[a]	young	N/A			
plagiarize[a]	older	N/A			
planetarium*	young	observatory (12)	projector (5)	IMAX theater (3)	Sistine Chapel (3)
planetarium	older	observatory (3)			
potpourri	young	incense (8)	fragrant (3)		
potpourri	older	sachet (10)	incense (6)	deodorant (3)	scents (3)
pride	young	pack (5)			
pride	older	den (3)			
procrastinate	young	tardiness (4)	delay (3)	lateness (3)	lazy (3)
procrastinate	older	stalling (4)	delay (3)		
proselytize	young	missionary (7)	convert (3)	Mormon (3)	evangelist (2)
proselytize[b]	older	------			
reincarnate*	young	resurrection (42)	rebirth (11)	evolution (2)	life after death (2)
reincarnate	older	resurrection (53)	reborn/rebirth (19)		
reiterate*	young	emphasize (52)	repetition (31)	stress (10)	
reiterate	older	emphasize (16)	stress (9)	restate (6)	

Table 4. Continued

Target	Age Group	Most Frequent Alternate (N)	Alternate (N)	Alternate (N)	Alternate (N)
rhetorical*	young	hypothetical (33)			
rhetorical	older	hypothetical (15)	redundant (4)	shocker (4)	
rosary	young	beads (3)			
rosary[b]	older	------			
samurai[a]	young	N/A			
samurai[a]	older	N/A			
seismology	young	geology (2)			
seismology	older	seismography (2)			
serenade[a]	young	N/A			
serenade[a]	older	N/A			
serrated*	young	jagged (30)	sharp (7)	rigid (6)	
serrated	older	jagged (12)	saw tooth (9)	segregated (3)	
silhouettes*	young	sketch (32)	shadow (22)	profile (14)	
silhouettes	older	sketch (17)	cartoon (5)	profile (2)	etching (2)
silo	young	barrel (2)			
silo[b]	older	------			
simile*	young	metaphor (34)	analogy (14)	synonym (2)	
simile	older	metaphor (15)	comparison (13)	analogy (11)	
sloop	young	catamaran (2)			
sloop[a]	older	N/A			
soliloquy	young	monologue (51)	aside (23)	narration (2)	dramatic irony (2)
soliloquy	older	aside (2)			
spatula[a]	young	N/A			
spatula[b]	older	------			
spelunker	young	archeologist (11)	excavist (8)	cave diver (7)	
spelunker[a]	older	N/A			
stamina	young	strength (14)	will (2)		
stamina	older	fortitude (11)	perseverance (9)	endurance (4)	faith (4)
subscription	young	contract (9)	ticket (2)		
subscription[b]	older	------			
synagogue	young	temple (20)	mosque (2)		
synagogue[b]	older	------			
toga	young	robe (4)			
toga[a]	older	N/A			
torpedo	young	missiles (15)	bomb (8)	projectile (3)	
torpedo	older	rocket (13)	missiles (9)	Polaris (8)	
tranquilize*	young	sedation (129)	anesthesia (18)	relaxed (12)	
tranquilize	older	sedation (52)	pacify (8)	medicate (6)	
translucent*	young	opaque (51)	prism (22)	transparent (13)	
translucent	older	opaque (43)	prism (12)	filter (4)	lens (4)
tsunami	young	monsoon (29)	typhoon (10)	transverse wave (4)	
tsunami	older	typhoon (8)	surge (5)		
utopia*	young	nirvana (23)	paradise (10)	bliss (6)	euphoria (6)
utopia	older	nirvana (27)	heaven (14)	paradise (12)	
venison	young	(deer) meat (15)	veal (9)		
venison[a]	older	N/A			

Note: The number of people who gave each alternate are shown in parentheses.

[a] These targets had no alternates given.

[b] These targets were never presented to older adults.

* These were targets where young and older adults had the same most frequent alternate.

Discussion

The results of the present study support the idea that there are both similarities and differences in the types of words on which young and older adults experience TOTs. In terms of similarities, both age groups demonstrated that some targets elicit TOTs more than others. Furthermore, young and older adults had the same alternate word in mind 86% of the time among their top three alternates, suggesting that when alternate words were retrieved, young and older adults were retrieving similar types of words. This finding can be especially useful for phonological priming studies given the overlap of alternates and targets in phonology; some of these alternates could also serve as primes, and they have the advantage of being equivalently represented in young and older adults' lexicons.

With respect to age differences, approximately 25% targets did not result in a sufficient number of correct TOTs for both age groups. In looking at targets where only one age group had TOTs at least 8% of the time, this result typically occurred because older adults knew the answer or young adults did not know the answer, resulting in fewer TOTs for that age group. This finding suggests that some of the targets are differentially susceptible to TOTs as a function of age group; therefore, future research should consider using our tables to select targets that overall are more equivalent in inducing TOTs in young and older adults. Dahlgren (1998) has suggested that older adults have more TOTs because they have a greater base of knowledge (i.e., vocabulary). If TOT studies equate young and older adults by giving them relatively equivalent opportunities to experience TOTs, then finding that older adults still experience increased TOTs would contradict Dahlgren's (1998) conclusion (see Cross and Burke, 1994, and Heine et al., 1999, for other arguments against this conclusion). Nonetheless, the fact that older adults consistently display larger vocabularies than young adults (e.g., Kemper and Sumner, 2001; Verhaeghen, 2003) may explain why they have fewer incorrect TOTs relative to young adults. By virtue of their reduced vocabularies, young adults do not know as many of the targets as older adults. Therefore, young adults may be more likely to say "TOT" when not experiencing one to reduce the number of times they say "don't know", for fear of appearing less intelligent to the experimenter.

The tables presented here also demonstrate that independent of age, some of the general knowledge questions used in TOT studies need revision. Questions that rarely result in correct TOTs because the targets are easily retrieved (a high percent of correct "know" responses) or not in participants' vocabulary (a high percent of "don't know" responses) may not be worth using, at least in their present form. Questions that elicit many incorrect responses (either "know" or TOT) should be modified to increase the likelihood that the target will be the to-be-retrieved word. Alternates can also provide significant information: Targets that have frequent alternates coming to mind indicate that the general knowledge questions are not precise enough to encourage retrieval of the intended target. Consideration of these factors will lead to a more useful set of general knowledge questions and targets.

Other factors besides the wording of the general knowledge question contribute to targets' susceptibility to TOTs and TOT resolution. A word's frequency influences TOTs, with more TOTs occurring for low-frequency words (e.g., Burke et al., 1991). A word's neighborhood density and neighborhood frequency interact with age to determine the rate of TOTs (Vitevitch and Sommers, 2003). A prime's part of speech in conjunction with a prime's word frequency influences TOT resolution following phonological priming (Abrams and Rodriguez, 2005). There are also individual differences in rates of TOTs; participants vary greatly in how many TOTs they experience and in the amount of phonological priming of TOT resolution. Using the data tabulated here to investigate new factors will extend our understanding of the role of phonology in lexical retrieval while overcoming some of the difficulties in conducting TOT research. Having more TOTs occur will decrease the variability that accompanies a small number of TOTs (e.g., Brown and McNeill, 1966; Burke et al., 1991). Most importantly, future studies will be able to assess potential age differences in TOTs and phonological priming of TOT incidence and resolution using an optimal set of stimuli.

APPENDIX: GENERAL KNOWLEDGE QUESTIONS, TARGETS AND FIRST-SYLLABLE PRIMES

Question	Target	Prime	Prime	Prime	Prime	Prime
What do you call an instrument for performing calculations by sliding beads along rods or grooves?	abacus	abstinence	abnormal	abdomen	absence	abhor
What word means to formally renounce a throne?	abdicate	*See abacus*				
What is the musical term that means 'without instrumental accompaniment'?	acappella	occupancy	octopus	octagon		
What do you call a person who computes insurance risk and premiums?	actuary	acrobat	accurate	activated	acronym	acknowledge ment
What is a sworn statement in writing, made under oath?	affidavit	affirmation	affluent	after	affable	
What do you call a solemn declaration made by a person who conscientiously declines taking an oath?	affirmation	*See affidavit*				
What do you call someone who believes that we cannot know whether or not God exists?	agnostic	agony	aggravate	agriculture		
What is a large seabird, sometimes used as a metaphor for spiritual burden?	albatross	alibi	allocate	alfalfa	albino	altruistic
What is a medieval chemical science concerned primarily with the conversion of the base metals into gold?	alchemy	*See albatross*				
What is the term for a brownish-yellow fossil resin used for making jewelry and ornaments?	amber	ammunitio n	amphibian	amateur	amplify	amputate
What is the name of the substance derived from a whale that is used to make perfume?	ambergris	*See amber*				
What is the food of the Greek and Roman gods?	ambrosia	*See amber*				
What do you call a pardon for political offenses against a government?	amnesty	*See amber*				

APPENDIX - CONTINUED

Question	Target	Prime	Prime	Prime	Prime	Prime
What do you call being full of love or fond of loving?	amorous	*See amber*				
What word is used to describe something that exists or seems to exist outside of its proper time?	Anachronistic	anonymous	anesthetize			
What is a word or phrase made from another word by rearranging its letters?	Anagram	ancestor	annual	analyze	antenna	animate
What do you call someone who believes there should be no organized government?	Anarchist	*See anagram*				
What do you call a short account of an incident (especially a biographical one)?	Anecdote	*See anagram*				
What is the largest artery in the human body?	Aorta[a]	able	agency	alien		
What do you call the study of the positions of celestial bodies with the belief that they have an influence on the course of natural earthly occurrences and human affairs?	Astrology	assumption	assemble			
What is the term for making amends for a sin?	Atone	attenuate	atrocity			
What is the name for a large, bright colored handkerchief or square of material usually worn around the neck?	Bandanna	bandit	banish	banner	banjo	
What do you call small, shelled animals which accumulate on the underside of a ship?	Barnacles	bartender	barbaric	barbecue	bargain	
What word means to trade by exchanging goods for others' goods rather than money?	Barter	*See barnacles*				
What is the name of the animal that builds canals or dams?	Beaver	beacon	beyond			
What do you call an account of a person's life written, produced, or composed by another?	Biography	biceps	bisect			
What is a flat, curved, wooden weapon which returns to the thrower?	Boomerang	bootlegger	booty	booster		
What do you call a dead body used for dissection?	Cadaver	colonial	canary	communicate	cathedral	*See also corona*
What is the medical symbol consisting of two snakes entwined on a winged rod?	Caduceus	*See cadaver or corona*				
What is the process of adjusting a measuring instrument to a standard?	Calibration	calcium	calendar	calorie	calculus	calculate

Appendix – Continued

Question	Target	Prime	Prime	Prime	Prime	Prime
What do you call exercises that are designed to develop muscular tone and to promote physical well-being, and are performed without an apparatus (e.g., running)?	Calisthenics	*See calibration*				
What do you call the art of elegant, highly decorative handwriting?	Calligraphy	*See cadaver or corona*				
What term means to declare a deceased person a saint?	Canonize	cancel	candid			
What do you call a tiny vessel that connects an artery and a vein?	Capillary	capture	captain	capsule	captivate	
What do you call a substance that tends to cause a cancer?	Carcinogen	cartilage	cardiac	carnation	carbohydrate	cartridge
What do you call a person who makes maps?	Cartographer	*See carcinogen*				
What do you call a percussion instrument used especially by dancers that consists of two small shells of hard wood, ivory, or plastic?	Castanets	cascade	casserole	castle		
In psychology, what is the term for a technique used to relieve tension and anxiety by bringing repressed feelings and fears to consciousness, i.e., a purging of emotions?	Catharsis	*See cadaver or corona*				
What is a small lizard noted for its ability to change color to resemble its environment?	Chameleon	*See cadaver or corona*				
What do you call a representation of a small angel, portrayed as a child with a chubby rosy face?	Cherub	cherry	cherish			
What is the term for a usually prepared for possibility whose occurrence depends on chance or uncertain conditions?	Contingency	conspiracy	conspicuous	consumer	conversion	conductive
What do you call illegal trade, or smuggling goods into or out of a country contrary to law?	Contraband	consequenc e	contemplate	contact	connotation	conscious
What is the outermost part of the sun's atmosphere called?	Corona	comedian	cocoon	collection	commander	*See also cadaver*
What do you call a public officer whose primary function is to investigate by inquest any death thought to be of other than natural causes?	Coroner	corsage	cordial			

APPENDIX - CONTINUED

Question	Target	Prime	Prime	Prime	Prime	Prime
What is the name for a person trained to pilot, navigate, or otherwise participate in the Soviet space program?	cosmonaut	costume	cosmetic			
What do you call a formal, binding agreement, or the word meaning the promises from God to humans?	covenant	cover	covet			
What is a stoppered glass vessel in which wine or liquor is brought to the table?	decanter	decision	defiant	deceptive	design	deteriorate
What is the term for violating the sanctity of a shrine or holy place?	desecrate	detriment	debtor			
What do you call someone who believes that there is no such thing as free will and that our fates are directed by forces that we cannot control?	determinist	*See decanter*				
What is the word that means to cause to explode or to set off, e.g., a bomb?	detonate	*See desecrate*				
What is the term for the money or property that a bride brings to her husband at marriage?	dowry	*No primes used*				
What do you call someone who is concerned only with him or herself, rather than the society?	egocentric[a]	edict	emu			
What do you call the three periods (...) used to indicate an omission or a pause?	ellipsis	electron	elongate	elastic		
What do you call the developing fetus before birth?	embryo	emperor	emphasize	empire	embassy	employ
What is the name of a green precious stone used in jewelry, such as necklaces or rings?	emerald	*See embryo*				
What word means to put into code or cipher?	encrypt	enhance	enzyme	entice	entire	
What is the term for writing one's signature on the reverse side of a check?	endorse	*See encrypt*				
What word means lasting only a very brief time?	ephemeral	*No primes used*				
What is the outermost layer of skin called?	epidermis	epic	epoch			
What do you call a closing section added to a novel providing further comment or information?	epilogue	*See epidermis*				
What is the word for someone who rides on horseback?	equestrian	equivalence	equivocal	equipment		
What do you call something that is intended for, or understood by, only a small group of people?	esoteric	escalator	espionage	estimate	escapade	

APPENDIX – CONTINUED

Question	Target	Prime	Prime	Prime	Prime	Prime
What do you call any of several hormones produced chiefly by the ovaries that act to regulate certain female reproductive functions?	Estrogen	*See esoteric*				
What is a substitution of an inoffensive term for one considered offensive?	Euphemism[a]	eulogy	euthanize	eucalyptus	euphoria	
What do you call a preacher of the gospel who holds large, often televised, public services?	Evangelist	event	evict	evaporate		
What is the glowing wire inside a light bulb?	Filament	filler	filthy	filtering		
What do you call a newborn horse?	Foal	*No primes used*				
What is the name of the central area of the retina where vision is most acute?	Fovea	*No primes used*				
What do you call the act of killing one's own brother?	Fratricide	*No primes used*				
What do you call a small, usually open-sided roofed structure in a garden or park?	Gazebo	garage	galore			
What word means to divide an area into electoral districts in order to give special advantage to one political party?	Gerrymander	gerund	geriatric	gerontology		
What is the name of the unrhymed Japanese poem having 3 lines containing 5, 7, and 5 syllables?	Haiku	hyena	hydraulic	hibernate	hypothesis	highway
What is the name of the disease in which blood does not clot normally, resulting in excessive bleeding?	Hemophilia	helium	helix			
What word means to bleed heavily or uncontrollably?	Hemorrhage	*No primes used*				
What do you call someone who holds beliefs contrary to the beliefs of the church, or anyone who does not conform with an established doctrine, principle or attitude?	Heretic	heritage	heroine			
What is an ancient Egyptian picture-writing system?	Hieroglyphics	*See haiku*				
What is the colorless, highly flammable gaseous element that is the most abundant and lightest element in the universe?	Hydrogen	*See haiku*				

APPENDIX - CONTINUED

Question	Target	Prime	Prime	Prime	Prime	Prime
What do you call a person who is unnecessarily anxious about his or her health and often suffers from imaginary illnesses?	hypochondria c	*See haiku*				
What word describes something that is threatening to occur immediately, said especially of misfortune or peril?	imminent	immature	imagine			
What are the front cutting teeth called?	incisors	industry	indicate	intensity	infinity	innocence
What does it mean to keep eggs warm (as by body heat, e.g., chickens) until they hatch?	incubate	*See incisors*				
What do you call a chronic difficulty in falling asleep?	insomnia	*See incisors*				
What do you call a verb that does not require a direct object to complete its meaning?	intransitive	*See incisors*				
What is a light spear commonly used in athletic contests for distance throwing?	javelin	*No primes used*				
What word means to voluntarily sacrifice (e.g., cargo) in order to lighten a ship or aircraft's load in time of distress?	jettison	jetliner	jet-propelled			
What do you call the tubular viewing toy that produces symmetrical designs through an arrangement of colored chips and mirrors?	kaleidoscope	catastrophe	commemor ate	capacity	*See cadaver and corona*	
What is the term for a light, mocking satire directed against an individual?	lampoon	*No primes used*				
What do you call someone who functions as a connection or link between two groups or persons, so that they can work together effectively?	liaison	leakage	legalese	lesion		
What is the term for the words or text of an opera?	libretto	*No primes used*				
What do you call the band of tissues that connects bones and keeps organs in place?	ligament	*No primes used*				
What is the term to hang or kill by mob action?	lynch	*No primes used*				
What do you call having or showing ill will towards someone, or the desire to do evil to others?	malevolence	marina	majestic	machine	magenta	majority

APPENDIX. CONTINUED

Question	Target	Prime	Prime	Prime	Prime	Prime
What is the term for the food miraculously supplied from heaven?	manna	manor	manage			
What do you call a savory sauce in which meat, fish, or a vegetable is soaked before cooking to enhance the flavor?	marinade	marrow	marry	marathon	marigold	
What is the name of the mammals (including kangaroos and opossums) that carry their young in an abdominal pouch?	marsupials	margarine	marvelous	marmalade	marketing	
What do you call a stone building (often found in a cemetery) with places for entombment of the dead above ground?	mausoleum	*No primes used*				
What do you call a professional soldier hired by a foreign country?	mercenary	mermaid	murky	mercy		
What is the science of investigating the weather?	meteorology	measles	meager			
How would you describe someone who is extremely careful and precise about minute details?	meticulous	medallion	metabolize	memorial	menagerie	meridian
What is the ticking device that musicians use for keeping time?	metronome	medical				
What word means to cut or chop food into very small pieces?	mince	*No primes used*				
What do you call a medieval entertainer who traveled from place to place, especially to sing and recite poetry?	minstrel	minivan	minimize			
What is the name of the criminal offense that has a lesser punishment than a felony?	misdemeanor	misfortune	miscarry			
What do you call someone who hates women?	misogynist	millenium	miraculous	militia	mirage	
What do you call any thick, brown syrup produced during the refining of sugar?	molasses	medallion	malignant	monopoly	morality	
What word means to shed hair, feathers, or an outer layer periodically, as with the changing seasons?	molt	*No primes used*				
What is the term for a revolt against authority, or a rebellion of soldiers against their officers?	mutiny	muted	mutilate	mutation	musical	

APPENDIX - CONTINUED

Question	Target	Prime	Prime	Prime	Prime	Prime
What is the psychiatric term for excessive admiration of oneself?	narcissism	narcotic				
What is the term that describes an issue that is open to discussion?	negotiable	neglect	negate	necessity		
What is favoritism in hiring based on family relationships?	nepotism	*No primes used*				
What is the term for a person who collects coins?	numismatist	nudity	nuclear			
What is the term for having complete or infinite knowledge, awareness or understanding, or for being all-knowing?	omniscient	ominous	ombudsman	omelette		
What do you call an animal that eats every type of food, including meat and vegetables?	omnivore	*See omniscient*				
What do you call a word which describes a sound, where the sound made pronouncing the word is the same as the sound it describes, for example, 'bang', 'thud', and 'screech'?	onomatopoeia	onlooker	ongoing	oncology	onset	
What is the name of the art of Japanese paper folding?	origami	orchard	ordain	ordinary	organizer	orchestra
What is the term for the scientific study of birds?	ornithology	*See origami*				
What is the name of a dentist who specializes in fitting braces on teeth?	orthodontist	*See origami*				
What is the word that describes back and forth vibration in a steady uninterrupted fashion?	oscillation	osmosis	ostracism	ostentatious		
What do you call a word or sentence that reads the same backward or forward, such as 'Madam, I'm Adam'?	palindrome	palisade	pallet	palimony	palpable	
What is the term for telling a story without words using only symbolic, exaggerated bodily movements?	pantomime	*No primes used*				
What is the name of the Egyptian plant that is cut into strips and pressed into a material to write on?	papyrus	pajamas	paternal	pacific	parade	parabola
What do you call a statement that appears contradictory, but may be true?	paradox	paragraph	paralyze	parenting	parish	paranoia

APPENDIX – CONTINUED

Question	Target	Prime	Prime	Prime	Prime	Prime
What is the term for the organism that lives on or in another, obtaining nourishment from it?	Parasite	*See paradox*				
What is a literary work that imitates the characteristic style of an author or a work for comic effect or ridicule?	Parody	*See paradox*				
What is the term for the principle that the simplest explanation is best?	Parsimony	parfait	partial			
What do you call the end product of exposing milk, cheese, or fermented liquids to a high temperature, killing bacteria and arresting fermentation?	Pasteurize	pastoral	passage	passport	passive	
What word means to deposit something valuable as a security for money borrowed?	Pawn	*No primes used*				
What is a long suspended body, lever, etc, whose lower end moves to and fro in an arc under the influence of gravity (e.g., the swinging metal piece on a grandfather clock)?	Pendulum	penalty	penetrate	pension	pentagon	
What do you call false testimony while under oath?	Perjury	percentage	perceptive	perform	permanent	perhaps
What word describes something that is at 90 degree angles to a given plane or line?	Perpendicular	*See perjury*				
What is the term for converting into stone?	Petrify	*No primes used*				
What do you call a person who collects and studies stamps?	Philatelist	philanthropy	philosopher	phenomenon	facilitate	
What do you call the sugar pill given as medicine to a patient either to humor him/her, or used as a control in testing the efficacy of another, medicated substance?	Placebo	placenta	platoon	plunder		
What word means to steal the writings or ideas of another and pass them off as one's own?	Plagiarize	plaintiff	player	playwright	playful	
What is the name of the building where one can view projected images of celestial bodies on the inner surface of a dome?	Planetarium	planning	plantation			
What is the name for a mixture of dried spices and flowers used for perfuming a room?	Potpourri	poet	polar	ponytail		
What do you call a group or family of lions?	Pride	*No primes used*				

APPENDIX - CONTINUED

Question	Target	Prime	Prime	Prime	Prime	Prime
What is the word that means to put off doing something, especially habitually, until a future time?	procrastinate	profess	profound	procedural	proficiently	proportional
What word means to seek to convert others, especially to one's religion?	proselytize	prosecute	prosthetic			
What is the term for being born again, after one has already died?	reincarnate	recycle	reaction	reimburseme nt	reunion	
What is it called when you repeat something for emphasis?	reiterate	*See reincarnate*				
What do you call a question that is asked for effect with no answer expected?	rhetorical	resilient	recession	ricotta	risotto	ridiculous
What is a string of beads used in counting prayers?	rosary	robot	robust			
What is the term for the class of ancient Japanese warriors that wore two swords?	samurai	*No primes used*				
What is the science of investigating earthquakes?	seismology	*No primes used*				
What is the term for a performance usually given outdoors at night for a woman being courted?	serenade	serendipity	ceremony	seraphim		
What word means toothed or notched like a saw?	serrated	*See serenade*				
What is a drawing consisting of the outline of something (e.g., a face profile), usually filled with a black color?	silhouette	silicon	silly	silver		
What do you call a tall cylindrical structure, usually beside a barn, in which grain is stored?	silo	psychiatrist	psychedelic			
What is the figure of speech in which one thing is likened to another, by the use of 'like' or 'as' (e.g., a heart as big as a whale)?	simile	symposium	symmetrical	simple	symbolic	simulate
What do you call a sailboat with one mast and two sails?	sloop	*No primes used*				
What do you call the lines in a drama in which a character reveals his or her thoughts, only to himself (e.g., Hamlet's 'To be or not to be' speech)?	soliloquy	solicitor	solidify	societal	sophisticated	
What is an instrument that is used for turning pancakes, eggs, etc.?	spatula	*No primes used*				
What do you call a person who explores caves?	spelunker	*No primes used*				

Appendix - Continued

Question	Target	Prime	Prime	Prime	Prime	Prime
What do you call the physical or moral power of endurance?	stamina	stampede	stammer			
What do you call a formal agreement to receive and pay for a periodical, books, theater tickets, etc. for a specified period of time?	subscription	submarine	subdivide			
What is the name of a building or place of meeting for worship and religious instruction in the Jewish faith?	synagogue	synthesis	synthetic			
What is the term for a loose outer garment worn by citizens of ancient Rome?	toga	toenail	tonal			
What do you call a missile, launched from a submarine?	torpedo	tortoise	torrid	torso	torture	tortilla
What is to make calm or serene or to reduce agitation, especially by use of a drug?	tranquilize	transcript	transcend	transfer	transmitter	transference
What do you call something that permits light to pass through it, but diffuses it enough so the object on the other side is not completely visible?	translucent	*See tranquilize*				
What is the proper name for a 'tidal wave'?	tsunami	suicide	suitable	supersede	supreme	superscript
What is the term for an idealized state, place, or situation of perfection?	utopia	utensil	utilize	utility		
What do you call the meat from a deer used for food?	venison	venue	vengeful	venomous	ventilate	

[a] These targets have a single phoneme as their first syllable, and their primes shared only that phoneme with the target.

Authors' Notes

We thank Katherine White for her helpful comments on a draft of this chapter, and we thank Stacy Eitel and Vanessa Robinson for their assistance in organizing the data presented here. Correspondence concerning this article should be sent to Lise Abrams, Department of Psychology, University of Florida, Gainesville, FL 32611-2250. Email: abrams@ufl.edu.

References

Abrams, L., Bahrick, H. P., & Robinson. V. B. (2006, April). *Restoring young and older adults' access to words following retrieval failures.* Poster presented at the 11th biennial Cognitive Aging Conference, Atlanta, GA.

Abrams, L., and Rodriguez, E. L. (2005). Syntactic class influences phonological priming of tip-of-the-tongue resolution. *Psychonomic Bulletin and Review, 12,* 1018-1023.

Abrams, L., White, K. K., and Eitel, S. L. (2003). Isolating phonological components that increase tip-of-the-tongue resolution. *Memory and Cognition, 31,* 1153-1162.

Baayen, R. H., Piepenbrock, R., and van Rijn, H. (1993). *The CELEX lexical database.* Philadelphia, PA: Linguistic Data Consortium, University of Pennsylvania.

Bowles, N. L., and Poon, L. W. (1985). Effects of priming in word retrieval. *Journal of Experimental Psychology: Learning, Memory, and Cognition, 11,* 272-283.

Brown, A. S. (1991). A review of the tip-of-the-tongue experience. *Psychological Bulletin, 109,* 204-223.

Brown, A. S., and Nix, L. A. (1996). Age-related changes in the tip-of-the-tongue experience. *American Journal of Psychology, 109,* 79-91.

Brown, G. D. A. (1984). A frequency count of 190,000 words in the London-Lund corpus of English conversation. *Behavior Research Methods, Instruments, and Computers, 16,* 502-532.

Brown, R. and McNeill, D. (1966). The "tip of tongue" phenomenon. *Journal of Verbal Learning and Verbal Behavior, 5,* 325-337.

Burke, D. M., Locantore, J. K., Austin, A. A., and Chae, B. (2004). Cherry pit primes Brad Pitt: Homophone priming effects on young and older adults' production of proper names. *Psychological Science, 15,* 164-170.

Burke, D. M., MacKay, D.G., Worthley, J.S., and Wade, E. (1991). On the tip of the tongue: What causes word finding failures in young and older adults? *Journal of Memory and Language, 30,* 542-579.

Burke, D. M., and Shafto, M. A. (2004). Aging and language production. *Current Directions in Psychological Science, 13,* 21-24.

Cohen, G., and Faulkner, D. (1986). Memory for proper names: Age differences in retrieval. *British Journal of Developmental Psychology, 4,* 187-197.

Cross, E. S., and Burke, D. M. (2004). Do alternative names block young and older adults' retrieval of proper names? *Brain and Language, 89,* 174-181.

Dahlgren, D. J. (1998). Impact of knowledge and age on tip-of-the-tongue rates. *Experimental Aging Research, 24,* 139-153.

Evrard, M. (2002). Ageing and lexical access to common and proper names in picture naming. *Brain and Language, 81,* 174-179.

Francis, W. N., and Kucera, H. (1982). *Frequency analysis of English usage: Lexicon and Grammar.* Boston: Houghton and Mifflin.

Harley, T. A., and Bown, H. E. (1998). What causes a tip-of-the-tongue state? Evidence for lexical neighbourhood effects in speech production. *British Journal of Psychology, 89,* 151-174.

Heine, M. K., Ober, B. A., and Shenaut, G. K. (1999). Naturally occurring and experimentally induced tip-of-the-tongue experiences in three adult age groups. *Psychology and Aging, 14,* 445-457.

James, L. E., and Burke, D. M. (2000). Phonological priming effects on word retrieval and tip-of-the-tongue experiences in young and older adults. *Journal of Experimental Psychology: Learning, Memory, and Cognition, 26,* 1378-1391.

Jones, G. V. (1989). Back to Woodworth: Role of interlopers in the tip-of-the-tongue phenomenon. *Memory and Cognition, 17,* 69-76.

Jones, G. V., and Langford, S. L. (1987). Phonological blocking in the tip of the tongue state. *Cognition, 26,* 115-122.

Kemper, S., and Sumner, A. (2001). The structure of verbal abilities in young and older adults. *Psychology and Aging, 16,* 312-322.

Kohn, S. E., Wingfield, A., Menn, L., Goodglass, H., Gleason, J. B., and Hyde, M. (1987). Lexical retrieval: The tip-of-the-tongue phenomenon. *Applied Psycholinguistics, 8,* 245-266.

Koriat, A. and Lieblich, I. (1975). Examination of the letter serial position effect in the "TOT" and the "don't know" states. *Bulletin of the Psychonomic Society*, 6, 539-541.

Light, L. L., and LaVoie, D. (1993). Direct and indirect measures of memory in old age. In P. Graf and M. E. J. Masson (Eds.), *Implicit memory: New directions in cognition, development, and neuropsychology* (pp.207-230). Hillsdale, NJ: Lawrence Erlbaum.

Lund, K., and Burgess, C. (1996). Producing high-dimensional semantic spaces from lexical co-occurrence. *Behavior Research Methods, Instruments, and Computers, 28,* 203–208.

MacKay, D. G., and Burke, D. M. (1990). Cognition and aging: A theory of new learning and the use of old connections. In T. Hess (Ed.), *Aging and cognition: Knowledge organization and utilization* (pp. 213-263). Amsterdam: North Holland.

Maylor, E. A. (1990a). Age, blocking and the tip of the tongue state. *British Journal of Psychology, 81,* 123-134.

Maylor, E. A. (1990b). Recognizing and naming faces: Aging, memory retrieval, and the tip of the tongue state. *Journals of Gerontology, 45,* P215-P226.

Meyer, A. S., and Bock, K. (1992). The tip-of-the-tongue phenomenon: Blocking or partial activation? *Memory and Cognition, 20,* 715-726.

Miozzo, M., and Caramazza, A. (1997). Retrieval of lexical-syntactic features in tip-of-the-tongue states. *Journal of Experimental Psychology: Learning, Memory, and Cognition, 23,* 1410-1423.

Nelson, T. O., and Narens, L. (1980). Norms of 300 general-information questions: Accuracy of recall, latency of recall, and feeling-of-knowing ratings. *Journal of Verbal Learning and Verbal Behavior, 19,* 338-368.

Neufeldt, V., and Guralnik, D. B. (Eds.). (1997). *Webster's New World College Dictionary* (3rd ed.). New York: Simon and Schuster.

Perfect, T. J., and Hanley, J. R. (1992). The tip-of-the-tongue phenomenon: Do experimenter-presented interlopers have any effect? *Cognition, 45,* 55-75.

Rastle, K. G., and Burke, D. M. (1996). Priming the tip of the tongue: Effects of prior processing on word retrieval in young and older adults. *Journal of Memory and Language, 35,* 585-605.

Reason, J. T., and Lucas, D. (1984). Using cognitive diaries to investigate naturally occurring memory blocks. In J. E. Harris and P. E. Morris (Eds.), *Everyday memory actions and absent-mindedness* (pp. 53-70). London: Academic Press.

Rubin, D. C. (1975). Within word structure in the tip-of-the-tongue phenomenon. *Journal of Verbal Learning and Verbal Behavior*, 14, 392-397.

Thorndike, E. L., and Lorge, I. (1944). *The teacher's word book of 30,000 words*. New York: Teacher's College, Columbia University.

Verhaeghen, P. (2003). Aging and vocabulary scores: A meta-analysis. *Psychology and Aging, 18,* 332-339.

Vitevitch, M. S., and Sommers, M. S. (2003). The facilitative influence of phonological similarity and neighborhood frequency in speech production in younger and older adults. *Memory and Cognition, 31,* 491-504.

White, K. K., and Abrams, L. (2002). Does priming specific syllables during tip-of-the-tongue states facilitate word retrieval in older adults? *Psychology and Aging, 17,* 226-235.

White, K. K., and Abrams, L. (2004). Free associations and dominance ratings of homophones for young and older adults. *Behavior Research Methods, Instruments, and Computers, 36,* 408-420.

In: Aging and the Elderly: Psychology, Sociology and Health ISBN 1-60021-190-9
Editor: L. O. Randall, pp. 43-62

Chapter 2

AGING AND REPETITION EFFECTS

Cecile A. Marczinski *
University of Kentucky, Lexington, KY, USA

ABSTRACT

The negative priming effect gained the attention of researchers interested in cognition and aging following the reports of several studies that older adults demonstrated smaller negative priming effects than in younger adults. Recently, however, this enthusiasm has dramatically waned because: 1) controversy surrounds the appropriate theoretical interpretation of the negative priming effect, and 2) there are accumulating studies showing no difference between younger and older adults in negative priming. Thus, this chapter reviews the negative priming and aging literature highlighting the controversy. Then, we provide a novel theoretical approach to interpreting repetition effects that may renew interest in the negative priming phenomenon. Our analytical approach allows researchers to discriminate between two components of performance, and this chapter highlights the results from four studies that demonstrate this novel method. In particular, we highlight that the presence and absence of age differences in response repetition effects reflect the relative contributions of two processes. Together, the results argue against the practice of attributing age differences in repetition effects to deficits in any single cognitive process.

OVERVIEW

This chapter focuses on repetition effects in performance tasks and on how these effects can be used to study age differences in cognition. This research was motivated in particular by prior research that used the negative priming method. In a typical computerized negative

* Address correspondence to: Cecile A. Marczinski, Ph.D., Department of Psychology, Rm. 012I Kastle Hall, University of Kentucky, Lexington, KY, 40506-0044; Phone: (859) 257-4977; Fax: (859) 323-1979; E-mail: cecile.marczinski@uky.edu

priming task, participants are presented with a prime display and then a probe display. For both displays, a response is required to a target stimulus (e.g., a red word), while a distractor stimulus (e.g., a green word) is ignored. On ignored repetition trials, the target in the probe display is identical (or related) to the distractor in the preceding prime display. Responses of younger adults on these trials are often slower than on control trials in which the probe target is unrelated to both the prime target and the prime distractor (Dalrymple-Alford and Budayr, 1966; Lowe, 1979; Neill, 1977; Tipper, 1985). This difference in performance between ignored repetition trials and control trials is known as *negative priming* (Tipper and Cranston, 1985).

The negative priming effect gained the interest of researchers of cognition and aging following several studies that reported smaller negative priming effects in older adults than in younger adults (Hasher, Stoltzfus, Zacks, and Rypman, 1991; McDowd and Oseas-Kreger, 1991; Tipper, 1991). A conclusion that might reasonably be drawn from this finding is that older adults are deficient in the mechanisms responsible for the negative priming effect. However, this conclusion assumes that negative priming is a pure measure of a single process. In fact, recent studies suggest that negative priming cannot be explained adequately by any single process account (Kane, May, Hasher, Rahhal, and Stoltzfus, 1997; Milliken, Joordens, Merikle, and Seiffert, 1998; Neill and Mathis, 1998). Together with some contradictory empirical findings, the insufficiency of single process accounts has made it increasingly difficult to use negative priming as a tool to study cognition and aging. Thus, the primary purpose of this chapter is to highlight a conceptual framework for interpreting repetition effects that addresses this problem.

Negative Priming and Aging

The negative priming task has been used as a tool to investigate cognitive deficits associated with various special populations. Children (Tipper, Bourque, Anderson, and Brehaut, 1989), patients with schizophrenia (Beech, Powell, McWilliam, and Claridge, 1989; LaPlante, Everett, and Thomas, 1992), and patients with frontal lobe lesions (Metzler and Parkin, 2000) have all been documented as producing smaller negative priming effects than appropriate control participants. The focus of this chapter is the corresponding finding in older adults; several studies have reported smaller negative priming effects for older adults than for younger adults (Hasher et al., 1991; Kane et al., 1997; McDowd and Oseas-Kreger, 1991; Tipper, 1991). A difference in negative priming between older and younger adults is a potentially important observation, as it may help to identify processing mechanisms that decline in efficiency with age. However, the perceived importance of this finding has been tempered recently by debate over the processing mechanisms that cause negative priming.

The inhibitory model attributes negative priming to the inhibition of internal representation of distractors. According to this view, when a distractor reappears as a target in a following probe display, the prior inhibition of this item's memory representation results in slowed responding relative to a control condition. Thus, an absence of negative priming in older adults has been used as evidence that inhibitory mechanisms decrease in efficiency with increasing age (Tipper, 1991).

By contrast, the episodic-retrieval model attributes negative priming to memory retrieval processes. By this view, attention to a probe triggers the retrieval of information about past episodes involving similar stimuli. If response information is encoded as part of these episodes, and if that response information is incompatible with current task demands, then its retrieval may interfere with performance (Neill and Mathis, 1998; Neill, Valdes, Terry, and Gorfein, 1992; Wood and Milliken, 1998; for related episodic-memory-based views see Milliken et al., 1998; Park and Kanwisher, 1994). However this episodic-retrieval approach was not specifically designed to address age differences in negative priming (but see Pesta and Sanders, 2000). However, it could be argued that the specificity of encoding (or retrieval) is lower for older adults than for younger adults. Consequently, any effect that depends on specific episodic encoding would be larger for younger adults than for older adults.

Kane et al. (1997) proposed that both inhibition and episodic retrieval can cause negative priming. This dual mechanism hypothesis was offered to explain the emerging variable findings that negative priming sometimes did and sometimes did not differ between younger and older adults. Kane et al. assumed that older adults have an inhibitory processing deficit. Consequently, in tasks for which inhibition is responsible for negative priming, one ought to find larger negative priming effects for younger than for older adults. By contrast, younger and older adults are assumed to not differ in terms of the contribution of episodic retrieval to performance. Thus, in tasks for which episodic retrieval is responsible for negative priming, one ought to observe equivalent negative priming effects for younger and older adults. In support of this view, Kane et al. demonstrated that age differences in negative priming depended on the proportion of trials that contained identical targets for prime and probe displays. Kane et al. assumed that a high proportion of these repeated target trials would encourage participants to rely on retrieval of the immediately prior episode to generate a response. Under such conditions, negative priming ought to reflect the contribution of episodic retrieval processes. Consistent with this view, Kane et al. found age differences in negative priming when the proportion of repeated target trials was low but not when it was high.

Although consistent with the view that older adults suffer from inhibitory processing deficits, a concern with the dual mechanism hypothesis is that researchers are saddled with the problem of determining which of two mechanisms is responsible for negative priming in any particular case. This issue has become increasingly critical to resolve, as the results of numerous studies accumulate showing no difference between younger and older adults in negative priming. For example, negative priming has been observed for both younger and older adults in a location-based negative priming task (Connelly and Hasher, 1993). Likewise, there have been recent reports of negative priming for both younger and older adults in a Stroop Color-Word interference task (Little and Hartley, 2000), a letter identification task (Gamboz, Russo, and Fox, 2000; Grant and Dagenbach, 2000), and a conceptual (semantic) negative priming task (Schooler, Neumann, Caplan, and Roberts, 1997). A meta-analysis on adult age differences in 29 negative priming studies (21 identity negative priming and 8 location negative priming) revealed that both younger and older adults produce reliable negative priming effects, yet the effect is often reduced in older adults (Verhaeghen and De Meersman, 1998). Further disconcerting was the results of an updated meta-analysis of 36 identity negative priming studies (the analysis included the studies found in Verhaeghen and De Meersman's meta-analysis). This further quantitative review on the effect of aging on the magnitude of the negative priming effect resulted in the authors concluding that the negative priming effect was not significantly different between younger and older adults (Gamboz, Russo and Fox, 2002). These findings appeared to have dramatic implications not only empirically, but also theoretically, as the authors further analyzed the results from studies where the experimental conditions should allegedly foster inhibitory processes separately from those that should allegedly foster episodic retrieval. There were no age differences in the size of the negative priming effect between younger and older adults when this effect was measured with experimental conditions that should have, allegedly, differentially promoted inhibition or episodic retrieval. As such, the Kane et al. approach of suggesting that inhibition or episodic retrieval could cause negative priming, accounting for the variability in age differences in negative priming effects, appeared to be unsatisfactory.

In summary, then, although age differences in the negative priming effect are observed at least in some cases, there are a host of situations in which age differences in the negative priming effect are not evident. This is particularly problematic, as the existing theoretical explanation of inhibitory versus episodic contributions to the negative priming effect do not delineate the conditions where age differences in negative priming, should or should not, be present. As such, we are at a crossroads. We can decide that the negative priming effect in unreliable and uninteresting as a model to study age differences in cognitive processing and look at other paradigms. That choice has been made by many aging researchers, as the number of citations of studies on age differences in negative priming have dropped dramatically in the last few years, perhaps reflecting the existing frustration with the state of the literature and the current theoretical explanations trying to account for the variable results. However, the alternative approach is to take heed of Thomas Murner's 16th century German proverb, "Don't throw the baby out with bathwater". Following his advice, we decided to look at the variable results that currently existed and then look at this question with new eyes and a fresh approach.

RESEARCH STRATEGY

The research strategy we used to address this issue assumes that performance measures, such as negative priming, are unlikely to provide pure measures of a single cognitive process. Consequently, some alternative to categorizing negative priming effects as caused by inhibition or caused by episodic retrieval is necessary to understand how negative priming and cognitive aging are related. Further, we assume that processes that contribute to negative priming effects also contribute to repetition effects using other methods. We were encouraged to adopt this approach by mounting evidence that negative priming in selective attention tasks is not a direct by-product of dedicated selective attention processes. In particular, a variety of recent studies have shown that negative priming is not as directly related to a selective ignoring process as was once thought (MacDonald and Joordens, 2000; MacDonald, Joordens, and Seergobin, 1999; Milliken and Joordens, 1996; Milliken et al., 1998; Neill and Kahan, 1999; Wood and Milliken, 1998). Thus, we assumed that performance in tasks that do not have a selective attention requirement might well have some of the same properties as performance in a conventional negative priming task. By examining the underlying cognitive processes of similar performance tasks, we thought we might gain new information that could be applied to the negative priming literature.

To that end, we used a two-alternative forced-choice (2-AFC) task in all of the experiments described in this chapter. This task produces an interference effect that we propose is a conceptual analog to the negative priming effect. In support of this proposal, we demonstrate that this interference effect can be smaller in older adults than in younger adults and that this age difference can be eliminated by a variable that also eliminates age differences in negative priming. To the extent that the results from the 2-AFC task are analogous to those reported in studies of negative priming, the explanatory focus can be sharpened to those processes that contribute to performance in both types of tasks.

THE REPETITION EFFECT IN TWO-ALTERNATIVE FORCED-CHOICE TASKS

In the experiments presented in this chapter, participants were presented with a prime display and a probe display on each trial. Both prime and probe displays contained a single colored rectangle. A rule was given to the participant, such as *Red and yellow rectangles belong to one category, and blue and green rectangles belong to the other category.* The participant's task was to give the correct categorical response to the colored rectangle in each display. This procedure produces three types of trials, which are depicted in Figure 1. On same stimulus trials (SSTs), the same color is presented in prime and probe displays. For example, the participant might respond to a red rectangle and then make the same response to a second red rectangle. On same response trials (SRTs), different colors are presented in prime and probe displays, but they require the same categorical response. In this case, if the participant learned the rule that red and yellow belonged to the same category, then he or she might respond to a red rectangle and make the same response to a yellow rectangle. On different trials (DTs), different colors are presented in prime and probe displays, and they require different categorical responses. Here, the participant might respond to a red rectangle and then make a different response to a blue rectangle. Prior studies of younger adults have revealed that response times (RTs) are consistently faster on SSTs than on DTs in this type of task. We called this difference a *stimulus repetition effect (DT – SST)*. More important in the present context as it relates the negative priming effect, responses are often slower for SRTs than for DTs (Pashler and Baylis, 1991; Smith, 1968; Terry, Valdes, and Neill, 1994). We paid particular attention to this latter difference, which we called a *response repetition effect (DT – SRT)*.

Further, we propose that there are two separate influences that contribute to stimulus repetition and response repetition effects in a 2-AFC task. We assume one of these influences to be episodic in nature, in the sense that retrieval of a prior stimulus and its associated response contribute to performance. For example, assume that the colors red and yellow belong to one response category, and the colors blue and green belong to the other response category. Now consider an experimental trial in which the colors red and yellow are responded to consecutively as the prime and probe. The responses required to these two colors are the same, but the stimuli to which these responses are made are different. This partial overlap in the processing requirements for consecutive stimuli holds the potential for interference. In particular, it may be difficult to link an action to a percept when it has just recently been linked with a different percept. We view this source of interference as analogous to that in a negative priming study in which a stimulus is ignored on one trial and then attended on a subsequent trial. In effect, both negative priming and negative response repetition effects can be thought of as caused, at least in part, by the retrieval of a prior processing episode that is inappropriate for transfer to the current task (Neill and Mathis, 1998; Wood and Milliken, 1998). We use the short label *specific* to describe this component in the remainder of this chapter, which captures the idea that this influence depends not just on the prior response but on the specific stimulus to which a prior response was made.

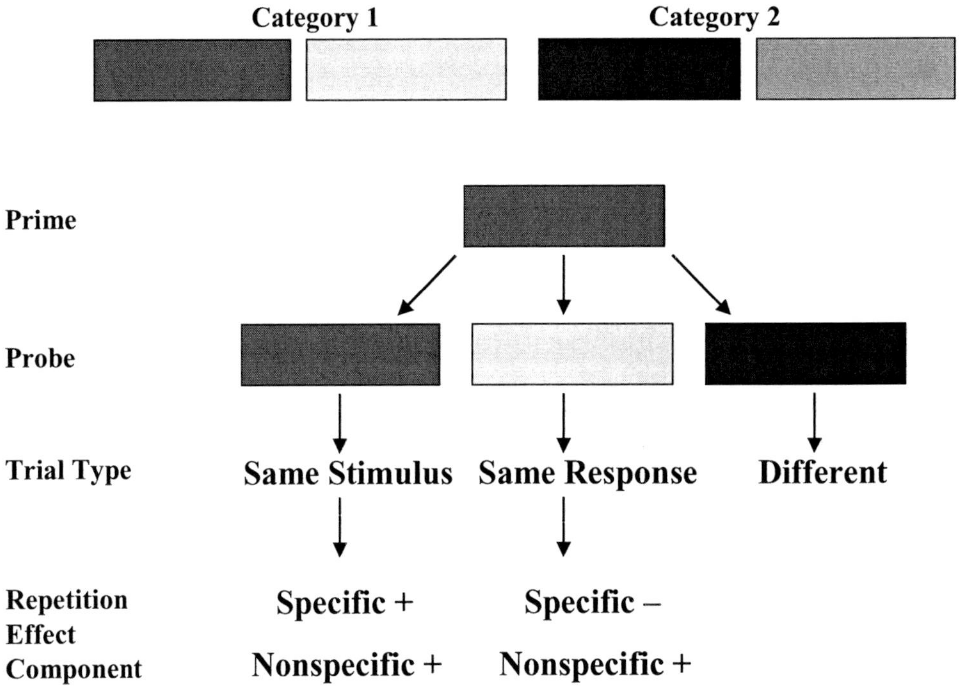

Figure 1. The design used in all experiments described in this chapter. In the same stimulus condition, the same color is presented in prime and probe displays. Consequently, both the specific (perception and action) and the nonspecific (action) components speed performance (indicated with a + sign) in this condition relative to the different condition. In the same response condition, different colors are presented in the prime and probe, but they require the same response. In this case, the specific repetition component interferes with performance (indicated by a – sign), whereas the nonspecific component speeds performance (indicated with a + sign) relative to the different condition.

In addition to this specific influence on performance, we assumed that performance on a 2-AFC task is affected by response repetition independent of the perceptual match between the prior and the current stimuli. We use the short label *nonspecific* to describe this second influence, which captures the idea that this influence does not depend on the specific stimulus to which a prior response was made. It seems possible that this nonspecific influence is related to response perseveration effects that have been reported in other literatures. Response perseveration involves an immediate and sometimes inappropriate repetition of a prior response (Sandson and Albert, 1984, 1987; Shindler, Caplan, and Hier, 1984). Interesting to note, there is substantial overlap in the clinical and developmental populations that have demonstrated reduced negative priming on the one hand and a tendency to perseverate a prior response on the other hand. Older adults have greater difficulty than younger adults in stopping an overt response and adopting a new response on the Wisconsin Card Sorting Test (WCST; Kramer, Humphrey, Larish, Logan and Strayer, 1994). Various patient populations, such as patients with schizophrenia and patients with frontal lobe lesions, also tend to perseverate prior responses on the WCST (Annoni, Pegna, Michel, Estade, and Landis, 1998; Elliott, McKenna, Robbins, and Sahakian, 1995). Finally, patients with dementia have been observed to perseverate prior responses compared with age-match controls, with greater severity of dementia associated with greater perseveration (Bayles, Tomoeda, Kaszniak, Stern, and Eagans, 1985).

Results from studies using the stop-signal method also suggest that older and younger adults differ in ability to prevent execution of an activated response. The stop-signal paradigm was developed to determine a participant's ability to suppress well-practiced, but momentarily inappropriate, responses. On most trials on the stop-signal task, the participant makes categorization responses as quickly as possible. The ability to suppress responses can be assessed when a tone sounds to indicate that a response should be withheld, and indeed older adults are less successful than younger adults at stopping responses (May and Hasher, 1998). Experimental manipulations that constrain information processing capacity similarly demonstrate that slowed information processing is associated with increased impulsive responding (Marczinski and Fillmore, 2003a, 2003b). Therefore, increased response perseveration in the elderly is consistent with models that advanced age is associated with rate reductions in information processing (Salthouse, 1991). Together, the results from these studies of response perseveration and response stopping suggest that the tendency to repeat the prior response in our 2-AFC task may be larger for older than for younger adults.

Two Influences in Concert or Opposition

To illustrate how two components jointly contribute to performance in the present 2-AFC task, we consider first a SST. When two identical stimuli repeat within a trial, both the component that is stimulus specific (because of a link between perception and action) and the component that is not stimulus specific (because of response perseveration) produce a tendency to repeat the prior response. In other words, the two components act *in concert.* By contrast, when two different stimuli from the same category appear consecutively, the specific influence interferes with the correct response, whereas the nonspecific influence again favors the correct response. Here, the two components act *in opposition* to one another, and the relative strength of the two components determines whether RTs are slowed or speeded relative to the different condition.

An analogous argument can be made concerning performance in a negative priming task. In this case, the effect of stimulus repetition can be thought of as having two components: a specific component that depends on how a prime was encoded (i.e., attended versus ignored) and a nonspecific component that affects performance independent of how a prime was encoded. When the same target appears consecutively, specific processes associated with how an item was encoded match. Assuming that the nonspecific component speeds performance on repeated trials independent of how a prime was encoded, the specific and nonspecific components work in concert on these repeated target trials. By contrast, when the prime distractor becomes the probe target, specific processes associated with how an item was encoded may interfere with performance on repeated trials (Neill et al., 1992). Again, assuming that the nonspecific component speeds performance on repeated trials independent of how a prime was encoded, the specific and nonspecific components work in opposition on these ignored repetition trials. Consequently, as described earlier for the 2-AFC task, whether negative priming occurs would depend on the relative strength of the two processes that work in opposition.

In the experiments described in this chapter, we applied this logic to performance in the 2-AFC task. This application involved estimating the specific component of the repetition effect by calculating the difference in performance between SRT (specific and nonspecific processes in opposition) and SST (specific and nonspecific processes in concert) conditions (SRT – SST). Because participants make the same response to prime and probe stimuli in these conditions, the nonspecific influence for these two conditions ought to be the same. Therefore, the difference in performance between these two conditions removes this nonspecific component, leaving a measure of the component that is specific to the stimulus to which a response is made (see Lindsay and Jacoby, 1994, for a similar analysis of Stroop Color – Word performance).

Note that the relative contributions of the specific and nonspecific influences dictate whether negative response repetition effects are observed. A large nonspecific component could potentially override the contribution of the specific influence, resulting in a positive response repetition effect. As described earlier, older adults perseverate responses and have difficulty stopping prepotent responses on various tasks. If there is a larger contribution of the perseveration of prior responses, a nonspecific influence, in older adults compared with younger adults, and then this could potentially outweigh the specific contribution to performance, if it were the same between older and younger adults. By the same logic, an experimental manipulation that increases the contribution of the specific influence could outweigh an opposing nonspecific influence, resulting in a negative response repetition effect.

Research Findings Comparing Older and Younger Adults

To demonstrate an age difference in the response repetition effect, analogous to an age difference in the negative priming effect, we recruited 16 older adults (mean age = 76.0 years) and 32 younger adults (mean age of 18.8 years), who all had normal or corrected-to-normal visual acuity and normal color vision. Participants completed the 2-AFC task at their optimal arousal time (May and Hasher, 1998), as circadian cycles of arousal differ across the lifespan, with the optimal performance of older adults observed in the morning and the optimal performance of younger adults observed in the later afternoon to evening. As testing during nonoptimal times exacerbates age differences in cognitive performance, we attempted to test all participants at their optimal times (Hasher, Zacks, and Rahhal, 1999).

A research assistant unaware of the research hypotheses tested each participant individually. Testing occurred in a laboratory room that contained a desk with a computer and normal room illumination. Stimuli were presented by a microcomputer using Micro Experimental Laboratory (MEL) software (Schneider, 1988) and responses were spoken aloud into a microphone that was clipped onto the participant's shirt. The stimuli were four colored rectangles (red, yellow, blue, and green). The participants were required to categorize the color of the rectangle that appeared in the prime display and then do so again for the color that appeared in the probe display. The two categories were arbitrarily called *cat* and *dog*, with the intention that the category labels were not systematically or semantically related to the colors. Colors assignments were counterbalanced across participants. The 2-AFC task consisted of 32 practice trials followed by 320 experimental trials. Each of the four prime colors was paired with each of the four probe colors. Thus, the proportion of SSTs was .250, the proportion of SRTs was .250, and the proportion of DTs was .500. Each trial contained the following sequence of events: (a) a fixation cross for 500 ms, (2) a 500 ms blank interval, (c) the prime display presented until the participant responded, (d) a 500 ms blank interval, and (e) a probe display until the participant responded (see Figure 2). Participants were instructed to respond to each prime and probe display by saying aloud either 'cat' or 'dog' and the instructions emphasized that responses should be fast as well as accurate.

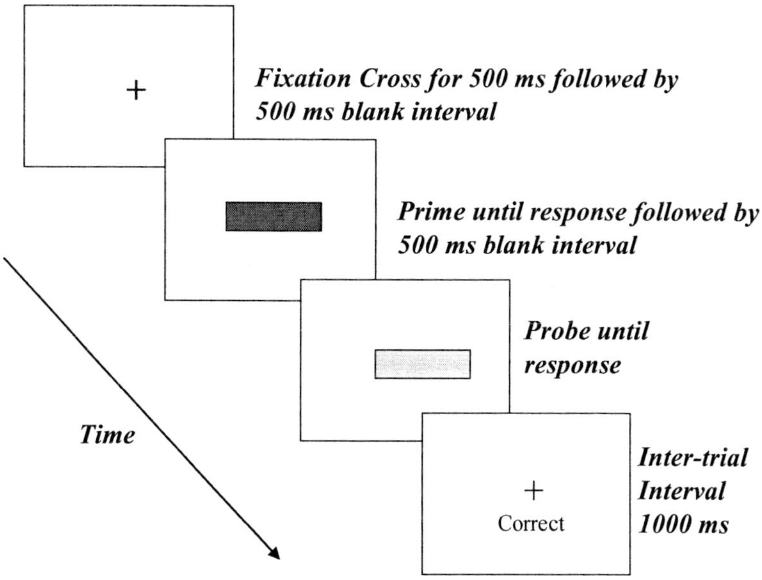

Figure 2. The sequence of displays in the 2-AFC task used in all experiments of this chapter.

The results of this study are shown in Tables 1 and 2 (see also Marczinski, Milliken, and Nelson, 2003, Experiment 1). To address issues related to slower overall performance in older adults, we conducted data analyses on both raw mean RTs and on a proportion transformation of the mean RTs (to account for slowing associated with advanced age) with equivalent results. As such, all tables show the raw mean RTs.

In Table 1, the younger adults showed a reliable negative response repetition effect, while the older adults actually showed a slightly positive response repetition effect. As such, an age difference in response repetition effects was observed similar to age differences in negative priming effects previously reported in the literature. Note that this age difference was obtained in a task that did not incorporate a selective attention component (an important finding as recent negative priming studies have noted that selective attention may not be the critical task detail that determines the negative priming effect).

Table 1. Mean Response Times (RT) and Standard Deviations in Milliseconds and Error Percentages (ERR) for the Older and Younger Groups in Experiment 1

	Older			Younger		
	RT		*ERR*	RT		*ERR*
	M	*SD*		*M*	*SD*	
Priming Condition						
SST	515.0	82.0	0.4	484.0	59.5	0.3
SRT	638.0	117.9	1.8	588.0	94.3	4.8
DT	649.0	115.6	1.0	558.0	75.2	0.8
Stimulus Repetition Effect (DT – SST)	**+134**	67.0		**+74**	43.7	
Response Repetition Effect (DT – SRT)	**+11**	45.4		**-30**	37.2	

SST = same stimulus trial; SRT = same response trial; DT = different trial.

Recall that we proposed that a nonspecific influence reflecting response perseveration might contribute to repetition effects to a greater degree in older adults compared to younger adults. As shown in Figure 1, this nonspecific influence would facilitate response times in both Same Stimulus and Same Response trials. If this were the case, then more positive Response Repetition effects in older adults should coincide with more positive Stimulus Repetition effects in older adults compared to the younger adults. As shown in Table 1, this was observed.

In our two-component model, we proposed that the measure of the specific component of performance could be calculated by looking at the difference in performance between Same Response and Same Stimulus trials (as this calculation removed the nonspecific influence that contributed equally to both conditions). As shown in Table 2, there was no significant difference between the older and younger adults for the specific component of performance.

Table 2. A measure of the specific component of performance (Same Response Trial – Same Stimulus Trial) in milliseconds for Experiments 1 and 2

	Specific Component (SRT – SST)	
	Older	Younger
Experiment 1		
M	**+123**	**+104**
SD	67.5	65.0
Experiment 2		
M	**+247**	**+143**
SD	173.1	78.8

In summary, age differences in response repetition effects (DT – SRT) observed in this experiment appeared to parallel age differences that have been observed in the negative priming effect (Kane et al., 1997). We proposed that response repetition effects have two components: a specific component that depends on the stimulus to which a response was made, and a nonspecific component that does not depend on the stimulus to which a response was made. Our measure of the specific component (SRT – SST) that removed the nonspecific component of performance, was not significantly different for the younger and older adults. As such, we can infer that the age difference in response repetition effects owes to differences between younger and older adults in the nonspecific influence. This finding is consistent with other reports that the tendency to repeat a prior response appears to be greater for the older adults than for the younger adults.

Now that we had demonstrated an age difference in response repetition effects, we were now interested in demonstrating no age difference in response repetition effects so that we could fully address the variability in the negative priming literature. Kane et al. (1997) demonstrated that negative priming in older adults is sensitive to the proportion of target repeated trials. In particular, whereas only younger adults produced a reliable negative priming effect when the proportion of target repetitions was low, both younger and older adults produced reliable negative priming effects when the proportion of target repetitions was high.

As we have proposed that response repetition effects (DT – SRT) in the 2-AFC task are conceptually similar to negative priming effects, then a manipulation that removes age differences in the negative priming effect should similarly remove age difference in response repetition effects. Thus increasing target repetition trials in a negative priming task should be akin to increasing same stimulus trials (SST) in the 2-AFC task. By our model, there are two components that influence performance; specific and nonspecific. Increasing the number of SST should potentially increase the specific component, as this is the component that is perceptually specific and depends on the prior stimulus to which a response was made. Recent evidence from other performance tasks have reported the older adults show greater facilitation of target repetitions compared to younger adults (Castel, Chasteen, Scialfa and Pratt, 2003). However, there are no indications in the literature that older adults will not still show evidence of greater nonspecific influences, as there are no studies indicating that response perseveration effects can be absent in some experimental contexts in older adults.

Therefore, we considered two scenarios to account for equivalent response repetition effects in younger and older adults. Equivalent response repetition effects might reflect similar specific and nonspecific components to performance in younger and older adults. However, the alternative scenario is that the two components that make up the response repetition effect would be larger for older than for younger adults. Given that the two components of the response repetition effect produce opposite effects on behavior, the sum of two large influences could be equivalent to the sum of two small influences.

In Experiment 2, we examined how increasing the proportion of SST would influence the performance of younger and older adults in our 2-AFC task. The proportion of SSTs was .375, the proportion of SRTs was .125, and the proportion of DTs was again .500. Note that this proportion manipulation introduced a predictive relation between the colors of the prime and the colors of the probe but not between the responses required for the prime and the responses required for the probe. In other words, the prime response 'cat' was followed half of the time by the probe response 'cat' and half of the time by the probe response 'dog'. All other aspects of the procedure for this experiment were identical to the first experiment.

For this experiment, we recruited 16 older adults (mean age = 76.4 years) and 32 younger adults (mean age = 19.1 years), who had not participated in the first experiment. All aspects of this experiment were identical to the first experiment, except that the proportion manipulation in this experiment introduced a predictive relation between the prime color and the probe color. The results of this study are shown in Tables 2 and 3 (see also Marczinski et al., 2003, Experiment 2).

As predicted, increasing a predictive relation between the colors of the prime and the probe resulted in large and negative response repetition effects for both the older and the younger participants, as shown in Table 3. Thus, we had now demonstrated no age difference in response repetition effects analogous to the many findings in the negative priming literature of no age differences (Kane et al., 1997). As described earlier, we hypothesized that older adults would demonstrate greater nonspecific influences reflecting greater perseveration of prior responses, facilitating response times in both SST and SRT conditions. The older adults demonstrated dramatically larger stimulus repetition effects than the younger adults in this experiment.

Table 3. Mean Response Times (RT) and Standard Deviations in Milliseconds and Error Percentages (ERR) for the Older and Younger Groups in Experiment 2

	Older			Younger		
	RT		*ERR*	RT		*ERR*
	M	*SD*		*M*	*SD*	
Priming Condition						
SST	520.0	85.5	1.4	497.0	89.0	0.5
SRT	767.0	220.3	4.2	640.0	108.4	9.9
DT	709.0	169.2	1.2	591.0	112.9	1.2
Stimulus Repetition Effect						
(DT – SST)	**+189**	105.8		**+94**	65.2	
Response Repetition Effect						
(DT – SRT)	**-58**	105.2		**-49**	47.6	

SST = same stimulus trial; SRT = same response trial; DT = different trial.

In our model, response repetition effects may reflect the relative contributions of the specific and nonspecific influences. Equivalent and negative response repetition effects in both age groups, combined with greater stimulus repetition effects in the older adults suggest that there is a greater nonspecific component of performance in the older adults than in the younger adults. Thus, the equivalent response repetition effects in both age groups indicate that the specific component must be larger in the older adults compared to the younger adults. As shown in Table 2, the older adults did show a larger specific component.

In summary, there were two critical results in this second experiment. First, the response repetition effect (DT – SRT) for younger adults did not differ from that for older adults, and both were significantly less than zero. Note that this contrasts with the first experiment, in which the response repetition effects were significantly different for younger and older adults and significantly different from zero only for the younger adults. The second important result is that the specific component of the repetition effect (SRT – SST) was larger for older adults than for younger adults. Given the equivalent response repetition effects in both age groups and the larger stimulus repetition effects in the older adults, it appears that both the specific and nonspecific components of the repetition effect were larger for older than for younger adults and that these two influences offset each other.

RESEARCH FINDINGS COMPARING OPTIMAL AND NONOPTIMAL TESTING TIMES

In the final two experiments, we were interested in testing our two component model of repetition effects with May and Hasher's (1998) suggestion that comparing younger adults tested at their optimal time of circadian arousal (generally the late afternoon) with younger adults tested at their nonoptimal time of arousal (generally the early morning) may be an important tool for understanding processing changes that occur with increasing age (Hasher, Zacks, and Rahhal, 1999; Intons-Peterson, Rocchi, West, McLellan and Mackney, 1999; May, 1999; May, Hasher, and Stoltzfus, 1993). Circadian arousal does not remain consistent across the day, as there are peaks in arousal. For younger adults, the peaks are generally in the afternoon to evening. By contrast, the elderly show a reverse pattern with the peak occurring in the morning. For younger adults, EEG studies have identified reduced temporal and frontal activity during nonoptimal time of arousal compared with optimal time of arousal (Briere, Forest, Chouinard, and Godbout, 2003). Furthermore, fatigued individuals show increased perseverative errors compared to non-fatigued individuals (van der Linden, Frese, Meijman, 2003).

If comparisons of younger participants at optimal and non-optimal testing times reflect information processing changes analogous to the aging process, predictions can be made regarding response repetition effects and our two component model. We predicted that in an experiment design identical to Experiment 1 (where an age difference in response repetition effects was obtained), younger adults tested at optimal and nonoptimal times should not differ in the specific component of performance. By contrast, nonspecific influences should be greater at nonoptimal testing times compared to optimal testing times, analogous to the age differences obtained in Experiment 1.

Therefore, in Experiment 3, we tested 40 younger adults (mean age = 21.9 years), confirming that they conformed to the typical arousal pattern of this age group (e.g., preferred to take classes, write exams, and write essays in the afternoon or evening). Half of the participants performed the 2-AFC task in the morning between 8:30 and 10:00 a.m. (non-optimal testing) and the other half were testing between 3:30 and 5:00 pm. (optimal testing time). All aspects of the procedure were identical to Experiment 1.

As shown in Table 4, response repetition effects (DT – SRT) were smaller and closer to zero in the group tested at their non-optimal time of arousal compared to the group tested at their optimal time of arousal. Stimulus repetition effects were also larger and more positive in the non-optimal testing time group indicating that this group had larger nonspecific influences contributing to performance. Our analytic technique was utilized to calculate the specific component of performance (SRT – SST) for both groups. As shown in Table 5, equivalent specific influences were observed in both groups. Thus, it appeared that reduced response repetition effects in the group tested at their non-optimal arousal time reflected the greater relative contribution of nonspecific components of performance. By contrast, the specific component of performance was uninfluenced by the time of day manipulation. Note that the identical pattern of results was obtained in Experiment 1 whereby the older and younger adults differed in the nonspecific influence, but not the specific influence.

Table 4. Mean Response Times (RT) and Standard Deviations in Milliseconds and Error Percentages (ERR) for the Younger Participants Tested at Their Optimal and Nonoptimal Testing Times in Experiment 3

	Nonoptimal (a.m.)			Optimal (p.m.)		
	RT		*ERR*	RT		*ERR*
	M	SD		*M*	*SD*	
Priming Condition						
SST	463.9	65.2	0.4	451.8	51.8	0.4
SRT	567.8	105.1	5.1	552.8	84.2	4.6
DT	555.7	101.3	1.2	523.5	70.1	1.6
Stimulus Repetition Effect (DT – SST)	**+92**	44.7		**+72**	33.4	
Response Repetition Effect (DT – SRT)	**-12**	32.1		**-29**	41.2	

SST = same stimulus trial; SRT = same response trial; DT = different trial.

Table 5. A measure of the specific component of performance (Same Response Trial – Same Stimulus Trial) in milliseconds for Experiments 3 and 4 where younger participants were tested at their nonoptimal and optimal time of day

	Specific Component (SRT – SST)	
	Nonoptimal (a.m.)	Optimal (p.m.)
Experiment 3		
M	**+104**	**+101**
SD	51.6	56.6
Experiment 4		
M	**+151**	**+121**
SD	49.0	38.5

In the final experiment, younger adults tested at their optimal time of day were compared with younger adults tested at their non-optimal time of arousal using the same proportion manipulation described in Experiment 2 (that increased the predictive relation between the color of the prime and the color of the probe). There were three predictions based on the findings observed in Experiment 2. First, the younger adults tested at their non-optimal time of arousal and the younger adults tested at their optimal time should both demonstrate negative response repetition effects. Second, the non-optimal testing time group of participants should show greater facilitation in the stimulus repetition effect due to the greater relative contribution of the nonspecific component of performance. Finally, the non-optimal group of participants also should demonstrate greater contributions of the specific component of performance than the optimal group of participants.

The results were as predicted. Participants tested at non-optimal and optimal times of arousal both demonstrated large and negative response repetition effects (see Table 6). Greater facilitation of stimulus repetition effects was observed in the participants tested at their non-optimal time of arousal compared to the group tested at the optimal time of arousal, indicating that there were greater nonspecific influences on performance at the non-optimal time of testing. Finally, a larger specific component on performance was observed in the non-optimal time of arousal group compared to the optimal arousal group of participants (see Table 5). Replicating the observations of Experiment 2, equivalent response repetition effects did not indicate equivalence in the two components of performance. Greater contributions of both the specific and nonspecific components was observed in the group tested at the non-optimal testing time compared to the optimal testing time. This finding is analogous to the findings of Experiment 2, whereby the older adults demonstrated greater specific and nonspecific components compared to the younger adults.

Table 6. Mean Response Times (RT) and Standard Deviations in Milliseconds and Error Percentages (ERR) for the Younger Participants Tested at Their Optimal and Nonoptimal Testing Times in Experiment 4

	Nonoptimal (a.m.)			**Optimal (p.m.)**		
	RT		**ERR**	**RT**		**ERR**
	M	**SD**		**M**	**SD**	
Priming Condition						
SST	483.5	56.3	0.1	455.0	55.4	0.0
SRT	634.7	85.1	9.1	576.1	80.8	9.1
DT	569.4	84.5	1.1	516.4	58.3	0.4
Stimulus Repetition Effect						
(DT – SST)	**+86**	49.9		**+61**	30.9	
Response Repetition Effect						
(DT – SRT)	**-65**	58.8		**-60**	54.4	

Note. SST = same stimulus trial; SRT = same response trial; DT = different trial.

Summary of Findings

The results of the four experiments presented in this chapter suggest the following two conclusions. First, the effect of aging of response repetition effects observed in a 2-AFC task appear to parallel the effects of aging on negative priming effects. Older adults did not produce negative response repetition effects in one experimental context (Experiment 1), yet did produce large and negative response repetition effects in another context (Experiment 2). By contrast, younger adults demonstrated response repetition effects in both contexts. These findings bear importance, as the 2-AFC task does not incorporate a selective attention component. Therefore, our findings are consistent with recent suggestions that selective attention is not required to achieve negative priming type effects.

Second, the present chapter argues against the view that response repetition effects and negative priming effects reflect a process pure measure of some cognitive process (such as inhibition or episodic retrieval). Instead, we illustrate a new approach of separating two memory influences that jointly contribute to behavior in simple performance tasks. We view performance as incorporating two components: (a) a specific component that depends on the mapping between a particular prior stimulus and the response made to that stimulus and (b) a nonspecific component that depends on the prior response independent of the stimulus to which it was made. To measure the specific component, we assumed that the nonspecific component would be identical in both conditions in which a repeated response is required. As such, the difference in performance in these two conditions subtracts out the nonspecific component, leaving a measure that reflects just the specific component of the repetition effect. Our two-component model appears to be able to account for the variability in age differences in response repetition effects and may be a new alternative to the existing and unsatisfactory episodic/inhibitory dichotomy (Gamboz et al., 2002).

Why Two Influences?

Throughout this chapter, we proposed that there are specific and nonspecific memorial influences on performance in a 2-AFC task. An obvious question that arises is why these two influences contribute separately to performance? One answer to this question begins with the well-documented distinction between two parallel processing pathways for vision (Livingstone and Hubel, 1988; Milner and Goodale, 1996; Ungerleider and Mishkin, 1982). The dorsal and ventral processing streams are two pathways in the brain that have been argued to conduct visual information independently. Most recently, it has been recognized that these two pathways may be best understood by considering the purpose of vision (Milner and Goodale, 1996). In some situations, vision is needed for perception (the ventral stream), while in other cases, vision is needed for action (the dorsal stream). An example might be helpful to clarify the distinction between these two streams. Imagine that you are looking at a wooden block sitting on a table. If your task is predominantly perceptual in nature (e.g., you are looking at the block to determine whether the block is yellow or brown), you would be relying more on the ventral stream of processing. By contrast, if your task requires action (e.g., you are reaching out to pick up this wooden block), you would be relying more on the dorsal stream of processing. For this task of picking up the block, vision need only be accurate enough to complete the appropriate action.

Milner and Goodale (1996) provided compelling evidence to distinguish between the perception and action functions of these two processing streams. One source of this evidence comes from patients with brain lesions isolated in one processing stream or the other. For example, one case described by these researchers is patient D.F. With a large battery of diagnostic tests, the researchers determined that D.F. demonstrated intact visuomotor behavior despite profound perceptual deficits. For example, when 120 line drawings of everyday objects (such as an apple or a book) were presented to D.F., she was able to correctly name only 11% of these drawings. However, her preserved visuomotor function was indicated by her ability to reach out and grasp those objects with remarkable accuracy. For example, she could easily pick up different sized wooden blocks off a table. Furthermore, she was even able to catch a ball thrown at her by the experimenter. In essence, her deficits were perceptual, but she was able to use vision to guide her actions. The empirical support for the perception-action hypothesis has been widespread including results from neuroimaging experiments, human neuropsychology, monkey neurophysiology, and human psychophysical experiments (Goodale and Westwood, 2004).

In this chapter, evidence was provided that the effects of repetition can be specific to the link between perception and action or nonspecific and related solely to the prior action. The two memorial influences described may reflect the influences of memory involving the ventral and dorsal visual pathways, as described by Milner and Goodale (1996). The effects of repetition that are nonspecific may be due to processing in the dorsal visual pathway. The effects that are perceptually specific may be due to processing in the ventral visual pathway. Current innovations in brain imaging could be used to determine if this tentative hypothesis is plausible.

SUMMARY

The research reported in this chapter focused on the cognitive processes that contribute to the repetition effects in 2-AFC tasks and how these processes changes with age. We were motivated to address this issue with the controversial findings of variable age differences in the negative priming literature that were not being adequately addressed with the current theoretical models of negative priming. In this chapter, we argued that response repetition effects in a 2-AFC task are analogous to negative priming effects and that response repetition effects are determined by two separate memorial components. One component is *specific* to the prior perception and action, while the other component is *nonspecific* reflecting the prior action independent of the perceptual stimulus to which that action was made. Our two-component model may be the approach that might renew interest in studies of age differences in negative repetition effects and repetition effects in general.

AUTHOR'S NOTES

The author wishes to sincerely thank Dr. Bruce Milliken and Sarah Nelson at McMaster University, Canada, for significant contributions to the theoretical and empirical aspects of this research.

This research was supported by the Natural Sciences and Engineering Research Council of Canada.

REFERENCES

Annoni, G., Pegna, A., Michel, C., Estade, M., and Landis, T. (1998). Motor perseverations: A function of the side and the site of a cerebral lesion. *European Neurology, 40*, 84-90.

Bayles, K.A., Tomoeda, C.K., Kaszniak, A.W., Stern, L.Z., and Eagans, K.K. (1985). Verbal perseveration of dementia patients. Brain and Language, 25, 102-116.

Beech, A., Powell, T., McWilliam, J., and Claridge, G. (1989). Evidence of reduced "cognitive inhibition" in schizophrenia. *British Journal of Clinical Psychology*, 28, 110-116.

Briere, M.-E., Forest, G., Chouinard, S., and Godbout, R. (2003). Evening and morning EEG differences between young men and women adults. *Brain and Cognition, 53*, 145-148.

Castel, A.D., Chasteen, A.L., Scialfa, C.T., and Pratt, J. (2003). Adult age differences in the time course of inhibition of return. *Journal of Gerontology: Psychological Sciences, 58B*, P256-P259.

Connelly, S.L., and Hasher, L. (1993). Aging and the inhibition of spatial location. Journal of Experimental Psychology: *Human Perception and Performance, 19*, 1238-1250.

Dalrymple-Alford, E.C., and Budayr, B. (1966). Examination of some aspects of the Stroop Color-Word test. *Perceptual and Motor Skills, 23*, 1211-1214.

Elliott, R., McKenna, P.J., Robbins, T.W., and Sahakian, B.J. (1995). Neuropsychological evidence for frontostriatal dysfunction in schizophrenia. *Psychology and Medicine, 25*, 619-630.

Gamboz, N., Russo, R., and Fox, E. (2000). Target selection difficulty, negative priming and age. *Psychology and Aging, 15*, 542-550.

Gamboz, N., Russo, R., and Fox, E. (2002). Age differences in the identity negative priming effect: An updated meta-analysis. *Psychology and Aging, 17*, 525-531.

Goodale, M.A., and Westwood, D.A. (2004). An evolving view of duplex vision: separate but interacting cortical pathways for perception and action. *Current Opinions in Neurobiology, 14*, 203-211.

Grant, J.D., and Dagenbach, D. (2000). Further considerations regarding inhibitory processes, working memory, and cognitive aging. *American Journal of Psychology, 113*, 69-94.

Hasher, L., Stoltzfus, E.R., Zacks, R.T., and Rypma, B. (1991). Age and inhibition. *Journal of Experimental Psychology: Learning, Memory, and Cognition, 17*, 163-169.

Hasher, L., Zacks, R.T., and Rahhal, T.A., (1999). Timing, instructions, and inhibitory control: Some missing factors in the age and memory debate. *Gerontology, 45*, 355-357.

Intons-Peterson, M.J., Rocchi, P., West, T., McLellan, K., and Hackney, A. (1999). Age, testing at preferred or nonpreferred times (testing optimality), and false memory. *Journal of Experimental Psychology: Learning, Memory and Cognition, 25*, 23-40.

Kane, M.J., May, C.P., Hasher, L., Rahhal, T., and Stoltzfus, E.R. (1997). Dual mechanisms of negative priming. *Journal of Experimental Psychology: Human Perception and Performance, 23*, 632-650.

Kramer, A.F., Humphrey, D.G., Larish, J.F., Logan, G.D., and Strayer, D.L. (1994). Aging and inhibition: Beyond a unitary view of inhibitory processing in attention. *Psychology and Aging, 9*, 491-512.

LaPlante, L., Everett, J., and Thomas, J. (1992). Inhibition through negative priming with Stroop stimuli in schizophrenia. British Journal of Clinical Psychology, 31, 307-326.

Lindsay, D.S., and Jacoby, L.L. (1994). Stroop process dissociations: The relationship between facilitation and interference. *Journal of Experimental Psychology: Human Perception and Performance, 20*, 219-234.

Little, D.M., and Hartley, A.A. (2000). Further evidence that negative priming in the Stroop Color- Word task is equivalent in older and younger adults. *Psychology and Aging, 15*, 9-17.

Livingstone, M., and Hubel, D. (1988). Segregation of form, color, movement, and depth: Anatomy, physiology, and perception. *Science, 240*, 740-749.

Lowe, D.G. (1979). Strategies, context, and the mechanisms of response inhibition. *Memory and Cognition, 7*, 382-389.

MacDonald, P.A., and Joordens, S. (2000). Investigating a memory-based account of negative priming: Support for selection-feature mismatch. *Journal of Experimental Psychology: Human Perception and Performance, 26*, 1478-1496.

MacDonald, P.A., Joordens, S., and Seergobin, K.N. (1999). Negative priming effects that are bigger than a breadbox: attention to distractors does not eliminate negative priming, it enhances it. *Memory and Cognition, 27*, 197-207.

Marczinski, C.A., and Fillmore, M.T. (2003a). Pre-response cues reduce the impairing effects of alcohol on the execution and suppression of responses. *Experimental and Clinical Psychopharmacology, 11*, 110-117.

Marczinski, C.A., and Fillmore, M.T. (2003b). Dissociative antagonistic effects of caffeine on alcohol-induced impairment on behavioral control. *Experimental and Clinical Psychopharmacology, 11*, 228-236.

Marczinski, C.A., Milliken, B., and Nelson, S. (2003). Aging and repetition effects: Separate specific and nonspecific influences. *Psychology and Aging, 18*, 780-790.

May, C.P. (1999). Synchrony effects in cognition: the costs and a benefit. *Psychonomic Bulletin and Review, 6*, 142-147.

May, C.P., and Hasher, L. (1998). Synchrony effects in inhibitory control over thought and action. Journal of Experimental Psychology: Human Perception and Performance, 24, 363-379.

May, C.P., Hasher, L., and Stoltzfus, E.R. (1993). Optimal time of day and the magnitude of age differences in memory. *Psychological Science, 4*, 326-330.

McDowd, J.M., and Oseas-Kreger, D.M. (1991). Aging, inhibitory processes, and negative priming. *Journal of Gerontology: Psychological Sciences, 46*, 340-345.

Metzler, C., and Parkin, A.J. (2000). Reversed negative priming following frontal lobe lesions. *Neuropsychologia, 38*, 363-379.

Milliken, B., and Joordens, S. (1996). Negative priming without overt prime selection. *Canadian Journal of Experimental Psychology, 50*, 333-346.

Milliken, B., Joordens, S., Merikle, P.M., and Seiffert, A.E. (1998). Selective attention: A reevaluation of the implications of negative priming. Psychological Review, 105, 203-229.

Milner, A.D., and Goodale, M.A. (1996). *The Visual Brain in Action.* Oxford, Great Britain: Oxford University Press.

Neill, W.T. (1997). Inhibitory and facilitatory processes in attention. *Journal of Experimental Psychology: Human Perception and Performance, 3*, 444-450.

Neill, W.T., and Kahan, T.A. (1999). Response conflict reverses priming: A replication. *Psychonomic Bulletin and Review, 6*, 304-308.

Neill, W.T., and Mathis, K.M. (1998). Transfer-inappropriate processing: Negative priming and related phenomena. In D. L. Medin (Ed.), The psychology of learning and motivation: Advances in research and theory (Vol. 38, pp. 1-44). San Diego, CA: Academic Press.

Neill, W.T., Valdes, L.A., Terry, K.M., and Gorfein, D.S. (1992). The persistence of negative priming: II. Evidence for episodic trace retrieval. *Journal of Experimental Psychology: Learning, Memory, and Cognition, 18*, 993-1000.

Park, J., and Kanwisher, N. (1994). Negative priming for spatial location: Identity mismatching, not distractor inhibition. *Journal of Experimental Psychology: Human Perception and Performance, 20*, 613-623.

Pashler, H., and Baylis, G. (1991). Procedural learning: II. Intertrial repetition effects in speeded-choice tasks. *Journal of Experimental Psychology: Learning, Memory, and Cognition, 17*, 33-48.

Pesta, B.J., and Sanders, R.E. (2000). Aging and negative priming: Is ignored information inhibited or remembered? *Experimental Aging Research, 26*, 37-56.

Salthouse, T.A. (1991). *Theoretical perspectives on cognitive aging.* Hillsdale, NJ: Erlbaum.

Sandson, J., and Albert, M.L. (1984). Varieties of perseveration. *Neuropsychologia, 22*, 715-732.

Sandson, J., and Albert, M.L. (1987). Perseveration in behavioral neurology. *Neurology, 37*, 1736-1741.

Schneider, W. (1988). Micro Experimental Laboratory: An integrated system for IBM PC compatibles. *Behavior Research Methods, Instruments, and Computers, 20*, 206-217.

Schooler, C., Neumann, E., Caplan, L.J., and Roberts, B.R. (1997). Continued inhibitory capacity throughout adulthood: Conceptual negative priming in younger and older adults. *Psychology and Aging, 12*, 227-674.

Shindler, A.G., Caplan, L.R., and Hier, D.B. (1984). Intrusions and perseverations. *Brain and Language, 23*, 148-158.

Smith, M.C. (1968). Repetition effect and short-term memory. *Journal of Experimental Psychology, 77*, 435-439.

Terry, K.M., Valdes, L.A., and Neill, W.T. (1994). Does "inhibition of return" occur in discrimination tasks? *Perception and Psychophysics, 55*, 323-363.

Tipper, S.P. (1985). The negative priming effect: Inhibitory priming by ignored objects. *Quarterly Journal of Experimental Psychology: Human Experimental Psychology, 37(A)*, 571-590.

Tipper, S.P. (1991). Less attentional selectivity as a result of declining inhibition in older adults. *Bulletin of the Psychonomic Society, 29*, 45-47.

Tipper, S.P., Bourque, T.A., Anderson, S.H., and Brehaut, J.C. (1989). Mechanisms of attention: A developmental study. *Journal of Experimental Child Psychology, 48*, 353-378.

Tipper, S.P., and Cranston, M. (1985). Selective attention and priming: Inhibitory and facilitatory effects of ignored primes. *Quarterly Journal of Experimental Psychology: Human Experimental Psychology, 37(A)*, 591-611.

Ungerleider, L.G., and Mishkin, M. (1982). Two cortical visual systems. In D.J. Ingle,

M.A. Goodale, and R.J.W. Mansfield (Eds.), *Analysis of Visual Behavior*, (pp. 549-586). Cambridge, MA: MIT Press.

van der Linden, D., Frese, M., Meijman, T.F. (2003). Mental fatigue and the control of cognitive processes: effects on perseveration and planning. *Acta Psychologica, 113*, 45-65.

Verhaeghen, P., and De Meersman, L. (1998). Aging and the negative priming effect: A meta-analysis. *Psychology and Aging, 13*, 435-444.

Wood, T., and Milliken, B. (1998). Negative priming without ignoring. *Psychonomic Bulletin and Review, 5*, 470-475.

In: Aging and the Elderly: Psychology, Sociology and Health ISBN 1-60021-190-9
Editor: L. O. Randall, pp. 63-88

Chapter 3

AGE DIFFERENCES IN EMOTIONAL REGULATION: FINDINGS FROM WESTERN AND EASTERN CULTURES

Helene H. Fung,* Bob H. Ching and Dannii Y. Yeung
The Chinese University of Hong Kong, China

ABSTRACT

A major paradox in psychology and aging is the finding that older people maintain their psychological well being despite undeniable physical and cognitive declines. Theories and research developed largely in the West explain this paradox in terms of age-related improvement in emotional regulation. Given the well-documented cultural differences between the East and the West, there have been suggestions that these Western findings may not be generalizable to Eastern cultures. In this chapter, we first review Western theories and empirical findings on age differences in emotional regulation. Then, we describe whether these findings are replicated in the East. Finally, we discuss the implications for studying emotional regulation in both Eastern and Western cultures, and suggest future directions for cross-cultural research in this area.

INTRODUCTION

Growing old is associated with many undeniable declines and losses, such as poorer health, worse working memory, slower reaction time, and ageism in society. For many years, researchers and laypeople alike have believed that because of all these declines and losses, old age is characterized by depression and unhappiness. Indeed, aging in the emotional area has been presumed to follow the same downward trajectory that is evident in physical and cognitive areas. However, recent empirical findings do not support these beliefs. These

* Correspondence concerning the chapter should be directed to Helene Fung, Department of Psychology, The Chinese University of Hong Kong, Room 328 Sino Building, Chung Chi College, Shatin, New Territories, Hong Kong. Electronic mail may be sent to hhlfung@psy.cuhk.edu.hk.

findings reveal that older people enjoy the same, if not higher, levels of life satisfaction than are younger people (Diener and Suh, 1997). They also experience a more positive emotional profile (Carstensen, Pasupathi, Mayr, and Nesselroade, 2000; Gross, Carstensen, Pasupathi, Tsai, Gotestam-Skorpen, and Hsu, 1997; Mroczek, 2001). Socioemotional selectivity theory (Carstensen, 1992, 1995, 1998; Carstensen, Fung, and Charles, 2003; Carstensen, Isaacowitz, and Charles, 1999) explains this paradox in terms of people's increased motivation to regulate their emotions as they grow older. This theory has received considerable support in North American and European literatures, but has rarely been tested in the East. In this chapter, we will first describe the theory and its implications for emotional regulation. We will then use the theory as a framework to review Western empirical findings on age differences in emotional regulation. We will also be our own critics and discuss ways in which these findings may not be generalizable to Eastern cultures. Finally, we will describe the handful of studies that have attempted to replicate these findings in the East, and suggest future directions for cross-cultural research in this area. We acknowledge that the terms "Western" and "Eastern" cultures can each be used to describe a great variety of countries and regions. However, in view of the fact that most relevant studies were conducted in North America, Europe and the Greater China (Mainland China, Taiwan, Hong Kong), this chapter refers to empirical findings obtained from North America and Europe as "Western" findings, and those obtained from the Greater China as "Eastern" findings.

Before we review theories and empirical findings regarding age-related emotional regulation, a definition of emotional regulation is necessary. We adopt Diamond and Aspinwall (2003)'s definition that emotional regulation is "the internal and transactional processes through which individuals consciously or unconsciously modulate one or more components of emotion, by modifying either their own experience/behavior/expression or the emotion-eliciting situation" (p. 127). In other words, we argue that emotional regulation involves two primary processes. Before an emotion has occurred, emotional regulation entails proactively selecting social situations to maximize the likelihood of positive emotional experiences and minimize the likelihood of negative ones. Once an emotion has occurred, emotional regulation involves modifying the subjective experience, behavior or expression of the emotion to reduce its negative impact, if any, to the psychological well being of oneself and/or others. Consistent with Gross (1998), we call the first type of emotional regulation "antecedent-focused emotional regulation" and the second type "response-focused emotional regulation."

Socioemotional Selectivity Theory and its Implications for Emotional Regulation

Socioemotional selectivity theory (Carstensen et al., 1999, 2003; Carstensen, Gross, and Fung, 1997) argues that as people grow older, they prioritize and become better at emotional regulation. Specifically, the theory proposes that the same essential set of goals operates throughout life, but the relative importance of specific types of goals changes as a function of one's place in the life cycle. The theory focuses on two broad classes of goals: knowledge-related goals and emotionally meaningful goals. Knowledge-related goals are those that increase future preparedness by banking information about oneself and the world. Subsumed under this goal trajectory are information-seeking, social comparison, identity striving and achievement motivation in educational and occupational endeavors. In contrast, emotionally meaningful goals are present-oriented and are aimed at maximizing emotional satisfaction in the here and now. They include motives to feel good, derive emotional meaning from life, deepen intimacy and maintain the self. Knowledge-related goals are the most salient in young adulthood when time left in life is perceived as open-ended and people are allocating considerable resources to prepare for the long and undetermined future. Emotionally meaningful goals, in contrast, assume primacy in later life when future time is perceived as increasingly limited.

The focus on emotionally meaningful goals motivates older people to pursue social situations that are more likely to fulfill this type of goals. It also leads them to pay more attention to emotional information, and to show biases in cognitive processing that result in better emotional regulation. In addition, because emotions are of central importance to older people, they are more likely to engage in coping strategies that aim at regulating emotional states. They also display greater emotional control. Younger adults on average do not prioritize emotionally meaningful goals and thus do not show these preferences, leading to age differences in emotional regulation. Below we first describe empirical findings on age differences in situation selection, and cognitive processing. These differences enable aging individuals to put themselves in environments that aid their emotional regulation, and thus fit our definition of antecedent-focused emotional regulation. Then, we review findings on age differences in coping strategies and emotional control, describing how these age differences contribute to older adults' superior response-focused emotional regulation, relative to their younger counterparts. We first examine findings obtained from North America and Europe.

WESTERN EMPIRICAL FINDINGS ON AGE DIFFERENCES IN ANTECEDENT-FOCUSED EMOTIONAL REGULATION

Age Differences in Situation Selection

Regulating social interactions is one of the most effective emotional regulatory strategies (Carstensen et al., 1997). Social goals direct social behaviors. When knowledge-related goals are accentuated, novel and peripheral social partners are most appealing, because their unfamiliarity increases the likelihood that an individual will learn something new from them. When emotionally meaningful goals assume primacy, however, emotionally close social partners are preferred because they are more likely to provide predictable emotional experiences that facilitate feelings of social connectedness (Carstensen, et al, 1997). Hence, socioemotional selectivity theory predicts that older adults who place greater importance on emotionally meaningful goals prefer to interact with emotionally close social partners, whereas younger adults who attach greater importance to knowledge-related goals invest in novel and peripheral social partners.

Indeed, a number of studies using participants from a wide age range and various ethnic groups have consistently found that compared to younger people, old people have smaller social networks, yet these smaller networks are composed of a higher proportion of emotionally close social partners (Ajrouch, Antonucci, and Janevic, 2001; Antonucci,

Lansford, Schaberg, Smith, Baltes, Akiyama, Takahashi, and Fuhrer, 2001; Fung, Carstensen, and Lang, 2001; Lang and Carstensen, 1994; Lang, Staudinger, and Carstensen, 1998). A cross-cultural study examining social network characteristics of French, Germans, and Americans showed that younger people have larger social networks than their older counterparts (Antonucci et al., 2001). Older German adults also reported a greater number of emotionally close social partners in their networks than did their younger counterparts. These findings suggest that older adults' small networks are largely consisted of emotionally close social partners. Our own study comparing European Americans' and African Americans' social networks also revealed that older people, regardless of their ethnicity, reported as many emotionally close social partners as, but fewer peripheral partners, in their networks than did their younger counterparts (Fung, Lai, and Ng, 2001). Another study also found that among both the Blacks and the Whites, older adults had a greater proportion of family members in their networks than did younger adults (Ajrouch et al., 2001). Studies of Germans aged between 70-104 years further show that the decline in social contact with age is due to a reduction in the number of "less close" and "not close" social partners (i.e., peripheral partners) whereas the number of "very close" social partners does not differ between age groups (Lang and Carstensen, 1994, Lang et al., 1998). In fact, although older adults have less contact with their network members, they report a greater number of relatives or close friends as close social partners, and report higher levels of relationship satisfaction, than do younger people (Ajrouch, et al., 2001; Fingerman and Birditt, 2003; Lansford, Sherman, and Antonucci, 1998; Morgan, 1988). These age-related patterns remain unchanged even after controlling for structural factors such as whether the individual has nuclear family members, and personality factors like extraversion and openness to experience (Lang et al., 1998).

Results of longitudinal studies also reveal a similar pattern of age-related differences in social network composition. Carstensen (1992) examined interaction frequency, emotional closeness, and relationship satisfaction in six types of social relationships (i.e., acquaintance, sibling, parent, close friends, spouse, and child) at ages 18, 20, 40 and 50 years. Interactions with emotionally close social partners such as spouses, parents, and siblings remained relatively stable over time and satisfaction derived from these relationships increased with age. Yet, interaction and satisfaction with acquaintances declined. Field and Minkler (1988) compared the social support networks of old people aged between 74 and 93 over 14 years. They found that contact with children and siblings remained almost unchanged over time, and the feeling of closeness with children increased with age. In addition, Lang (2000) explored the change of personal networks of older adults longitudinally and revealed that the well-documented decline in network size with age was mainly due to the reduction of peripheral social relationships. In particular, when older adults perceived that their life was coming to an end, they intentionally discontinued relationship with peripheral social partners. At the same time, emotional closeness with family members and social companions increased. A four-year longitudinal study of older Dutch adults also showed that total network size of older adults was relatively stable over time, with an increasing number of close relatives and a decreasing number of friends in their social networks (van Tilburg, 1998). These research findings once again show that as one ages, relationships that are emotionally rewarding are maintained and fostered whereas relationships with peripheral partners are discontinued deliberately. These age-related changes serve emotion regulatory purposes. They enhance emotionally meaningful and gratifying experiences, and minimizes potentially negative social exchanges (Carstensen et al., 2003), thereby improving affective well being among older adults.

To further examine the voluntary nature of these age-related changes, studies were conducted to directly test the social preferences of older and younger adults (Fredrickson and Carstensen, 1990; Fung, Carstensen, and Lutz, 1999, Study 1). In these studies, participants from a wide range of age were asked to imagine that they had 30 minutes of free time and would like to spend that time with someone. They were given three potential social partners to choose from: (1) a member of your immediate family, (2) the author of a book, and (3) an acquaintance with whom you seem to have much in common. The immediate family member represents emotionally close social partner whereas both the author and acquaintance represent novel and peripheral social partners. Results of these studies repeatedly found that older adults showed a strong preference for spending time with emotionally close social partners whereas younger adults did not have such preferences. The smaller network size and the decline in social contact among older adults may simply reflect a proactive choice on the part of older adults to spend their precious time with the types of social partners they prefer.

In summary, reduction in the number of social partners in old age is mainly due to decreased contact with peripheral and novel social partners. Contacts with family member, relatives and close friends remain stable over time. These age-related changes are proactive. Older adults are actively involved in the selection of their social partners in order to maximize emotional satisfaction from the interactions. This form of antecedent-focused emotional regulation enables older adults to focus their resources on the handful of social relationships that truly matter, and to minimize negative and superficial social experiences, contributing to their higher levels of relationship satisfaction relative to their younger counterparts.

Age Differences in Cognitive Processing

Antecedent-focused emotional regulation is not only evident in how aging individuals structure their objective social world, but also in how they mentally represent, evaluate and process social information. As we review below, older adults, compared with their younger counterparts, put greater weights on emotional information when they evaluate, encode and process information. These age differences allow older adults to construe their social world as more emotionally meaningful and positive, and to avoid negative experience. In other words, while the strategies we reviewed in the previous section enable older adults to regulate their emotions by actively shaping their world, the strategies we describe in this section allow older adults to interpret their subjective experience as positive.

Fredrickson and Carstensen (1990) studied mental representations of social partners in older and younger adults. They asked Americans ranged from adolescents to octogenarians to categorize a set of 18 prospective social partners according to how similarly they would feel when they interacted with these social partners. Three general dimensions were revealed by the sorts: an emotional or "like/dislike" dimension, an informational dimension, and a dimension characterized by future possibilities. Older people weighted the emotional dimension most heavily, followed by middle-aged and younger people. This focus on the emotional quality of prospective social partners, even at the expense of other qualities, enables older adults to proactively avoid negative social experience.

In fact, once older adults have formed an evaluation of a person, it is very hard to change that first impression. Older American adults weigh negative information more heavily in evaluating hypothetical others than do their younger counterparts (Hess and Pullen, 1994).

Moreover, when this information is later counterbalanced by positive information about the same person, younger people modify their views in light of the positive information but older people do not. The pattern is the most evident when the information provided is about morality, as opposed to ability (Hess, Bolstad, Woodburn, and Auman, 1999). Older adults' greater tendencies to assess strangers cautiously and to pay particular attention to information regarding interpersonal qualities make it easier for them to maximize the emotional qualities of their social interactions, and to regulate their emotions in the face of conflicting new information.

Other than evaluating people, older adults also show a bias for emotional information when they evaluate messages. In one Canadian study (Ching and Fung, 2004), we randomly assigned younger and older adults to read pamphlets that promoted healthy eating with identical factual information but emphasizing different goals. Findings showed that health messages that emphasized eating healthily to protect the ones we love, but not those that emphasized eating healthily for personal achievement, were rated as more persuasive, evaluated more positively and better remembered by older adults, whereas younger adults did not show this bias.

Such a focus on emotions influences decision-making. Two American studies have shown that, compared with younger adults, older adults are more likely to show choice-supportive memory, i.e., to attribute more positive and fewer negative features to an option that they had previously chosen than to an option that they had rejected (Mather and Johnson, 2000). This type of memory maximizes the satisfaction that older adults derive from their choices and minimizes regrets, contributing to emotional regulation.

Sometimes, even not making a decision can serve emotional regulatory purposes. Curley, Eraker, and Yates (1984) asked younger and older participants to evaluate a medical treatment and to decide whether they would undergo the treatment. They measured whether participants decided not to make the choice at all, and let the doctor decide whether they would have the treatment. Compared with their younger counterparts, a higher percentage of older participants deferred the choice to the doctor. Although deferring judgement to others may be a passive decision making strategy, it can provide the individuals with proxy control over the decision, assuming that the individuals can choose the doctors who make the decision for them. Moreover, it can free the individuals from taking responsibility for any negative consequences of the decision – they can blame the doctor if anything goes wrong. By being more likely than younger adults to use this strategy, older adults protect themselves from the distress of the decision making process.

Age differences have also been found in how people process information. Memory is not simply a process of retrieval, but an elaborative process by which current goals influence constructions of the past (Johnson and Sherman, 1990). A focus of emotional meaningful goals leads older adults to pay more attention to, process more deeply, and consequently remember emotional information better than other types of information. Young adults do not show such biases. Carstensen and Turk-Charles (1994) asked Americans aged 20-83 years to read a narrative drawn from a popular novel and later incidentally recall as much as they could from the passage. Of what people remembered, the proportion of recalled emotional information, as opposed to neutral information, increased with each successively older age group. Moreover, when describing a past vacation, older couples provided more information on the subjective aspects of the experience, such as descriptions of people, and less information on the factual aspects, such as itineraries, than did younger couples (Gould and

Dixon, 1993). In a test of source memory, older adults recalled a greater number of feelings and evaluative statements about imagined and real experiences while younger adults recalled more sensory and perceptual details (Hashtroudi, Johnson, and Chrosniak, 1990). In terms of memory for music, older adults rated songs from their youth as more emotional and remembered those songs better than did younger adults (Schulkind, Hennis, and Rubin, 1999). Older people were also more likely to remember advertisements with emotional slogans, like "Capture those special moments," than those with information-related slogans, like "Capture the unexplored world," relative to their younger counterparts (Fung and Carstensen, 2003).

Furthermore, the type of emotional information that older adults remember is disproportionately positive. When recalling previously presented positive, negative and neutral images, the proportion of correctly recognized and recalled negative images declines linearly with age across younger, middle-aged, and older adults (Charles, Mather, and Carstensen, 2003). In recalling past events, older adults tend to underestimate the intensity of sadness experienced in the past (Levine and Bluck, 1997). They are also more likely to cite a positive episode when asked to recall the single most important experience in their moral development than are adolescents and young adults (Quackenbush and Barnett, 2001). When asked to recall their childhood at different points in their lives, people recall more positive memories with age (Field, 1981). A 14-year longitudinal study of autobiographic memory also found that while older nuns showed a tendency to remember the past more positively, younger nuns tended to remember the past more negatively (Kennedy, Mather, and Carstensen, 2004). Moreover, a study that examined age differences in attention to and memory of positive (happy), negative (sad or angry) and neutral images further found that older adults attended to negative images the least, and remembered positive images better than negative images relative to younger adults (Mather and Carstensen, 2003).

In summary, compared with younger adults, older adults are more likely to pay attention to and remember emotional, particularly positive, information. Such selective attention and memory optimize emotional experiences by avoiding antecedents that may lead to negative affect, and focusing on those that are likely to give rise to positive affect.

Western Empirical Findings on Age Differences in Response-Focused Emotional Regulation

Sometimes, antecedents that are associated with negative affect cannot be completely avoided. In those cases, people can still minimize the impact of the negative affect on themselves and others by modulating how they cope with the problems and control their emotions. These modulations are called "response-focused emotion regulation." Findings from North America and Europe again suggest that older adults seem to use this type of emotional regulation more often and are better at it than do younger adults.

Age Differences in Coping Strategies

Heckhausen and Schulz (1995) identified two important types of coping strategies for dealing with life events, namely, primary and secondary control. Primary control involves behaviors that enable individuals to shape their external environment to fit with their own needs and developmental potential. Primary control strategies are of great adaptive value to individuals and thus are usually preferred. Secondary control involves behaviors that aim at changing the individuals inwardly to accommodate environmental challenges. As individuals grow older, they become more susceptible to a variety of chronic and even life-threatening illnesses. These biological constraints limit individuals' capabilities to exert changes on the immediate environments, which prompt them to rely more on secondary control strategies (Heckhausen and Schulz, 1995). Such strategies include increased use of emotion-focused coping, mature cognitive appraisals (some call "reappraisals") of undesirable or stressful situations, flexible goal adjustments and downward comparisons.

Older people are likely to face situations (e.g., health problems) over which they have little control. Such uncontrollable situations prompt them to reduce the use of problem-focused coping – strategies that aim at solving the problem one and for all – but increase the use of emotion-focused coping – strategies that make one feel better about the problem but do not solve it (Blanchard-Fields and Irion, 1988). Indeed, Folkman, Lazarus, Pimley, and Novacek (1987) found that younger individuals identified more problems in financial and work domains than in other domains, and they resorted to more active, problem-focused forms of coping, such as confrontative coping, seeking social support, and planful problem solving, to solve them. In contrast, older individuals identified more problems in the domains of environmental and social issues, home maintenance, and health, and used more passive, intrapersonal emotion-focused forms of coping, such as distancing, acceptance of responsibility and positive reappraisal to solve them. Schulz and Decker (1985) demonstrated that older adults with spinal-cord injuries emphasized what they already have, for example, "brain", in defining the quality of their lives, instead of focusing on their losses, such as "brawn". When dealing with important challenges in life, older adults were also shown to identify religious coping as an effective means in regulating their well being (Koenig, George, and Siegler, 1988). All these emotion-focused coping strategies enable older people to minimize the negative affect associated with stressful situations, thereby achieving emotional regulation.

Other than using emotion-focused coping more often, individuals also become increasingly more mature in their coping behaviors as they grow older. Young people might engage in relatively immature defense strategies, such as repression and dissociation, more often while middle-aged adults used more altruism, humor, anticipation, and sublimation to cope with aversive life events (Vaillant, 1977). In the face of social problems, older adults demonstrated a larger repertoire of coping strategies and used them flexibly depending on the contexts (Blanchard-Fields and Camp, 1990; Blanchard-Fields, Jahnke, and Camp, 1995). Other studies showed that with maturity, there was more conscious appraisal of problem situations based on internally regulated standards (Labouvie-Vief, Hakim-Larson, and Hobart, 1987). With increasing age and emotional maturity, individuals engaged in more mature social reasoning (e.g., increased relativistic thinking) in emotionally laden situations (Blanchard-Fields, 1986). In addition, older adults made more relativistic causal attributions in problem situations that were high in emotional salience than did younger adults

(Blanchard-Fields and Norris, 1994). In fact, an age-related increase in flexibility is emerging as one of the most stable findings of the literature on coping processes in adulthood (e.g., Cytrybaum, Blum, Partick, Stein, Wadner, and Wilk, 1980; Folkman et al., 1987; Haan, 1977; Hauser, 1976; Loevinger, 1976; McCrae and Costa, 1984). Such flexibility makes it possible for older adults to view their problems from different perspectives and reduce the negative impact these problems have on their emotional well being.

Moreover, older people are more likely than their younger counterparts to adjust their goals when they encounter obstacles in life. Brandtstädter and colleagues (Brandtstädter and Greve, 1994; Brandtstädter and Rothermund, 2002) propose a dual-process framework to describe how aging individuals reduce discrepancies between their current and ideal situations. According to this framework, one group of strategies to reduce the discrepancies is known as the assimilative mode, which involves "intentional efforts to modify the actual situation in accordance with personal goals" (Brandtstädter and Rothermund, 2002, p. 117). The other group of strategies is known as the accommodative mode, which adjusts personal goals to make them consistent with situational constraints and limited resources. Age-related declines and the resulting losses in resources lead people to favor accommodative processes over assimilative ones as they age. Indeed, empirical findings confirm that older adults have fewer tenacious goal pursuits (assimilative processes) and more flexible goal adjustment (accommodative processes) when coping with crises and life transitions (Brandtstädter and Renner, 1990). Although more recent data did not reveal any age differences in tenacious goal pursuits, they still demonstrated an increase in flexibility in goal adjustment from young to old age (Heckhausen, 1994; Heckhausen and Schulz, 1994). Indeed, although older people often possess a less promising outlook of their future, they are more likely than younger adults to downwardly adjust their ideal self and to view their past in more positive ways (Ryff, 1991).

When we examine the specific goals that people set across adulthood, we also see evidences suggesting that aging is associated with adjustments that make goals easier to achieve. Buhler, Brind, and Horner (1968) asked people aged 17 to 60 to rate how relevant each of 86 life goals were to them. The authors identified 12 factors, equally divided into four overarching categories of goals: need satisfaction (necessities of life/pleasure, love and family, and sexual satisfaction), self-limiting adaptation (accepting limitations/caution, submissiveness, and avoidance of hardships), creative expansion (self-development, being a leader/achieving fame and power, and role in public life), and upholding the internal order (moral values, social values, and having success). Compared with younger people, older adults scored higher on the three factors indicating self-limiting adaptation, and lower on "self development," "role in public life," and "having success." Dittmann-Kohli and Westerhof (1997) asked participants to complete sentences starting with, "In the coming years ...." They found that while younger adults focused more on improving domains like education, career, family building and finances, older adults were more concerned with maintaining current levels of functioning and satisfaction. Further, evidences for goal adjustment with age can be found indirectly in lay formulations of psychological well being. Ryff (1989a) interviewed middle-aged and older adults about their conceptions of psychological well being. While middle-aged adults stressed being confident and assertive, older adults emphasized self-acceptance. Furthermore, in answering an open-ended question about what they would like to change in their life "given the chance," the most frequent response for older adults was "nothing" while that for middle-aged participants was "active self-improvement" (Ryff,

1989b). Older adults rated themselves lower on personal growth — "see [ing] oneself as growing and expanding" (Ryff, 1989b, 1991) — and goal seeking — "the desire to achieve new goals, to search for new and different experiences, and to be on the move" — than middle-aged and young adults. Given that beliefs about what leads to well being are related to what people strive for, these findings suggest that older people focus less on improving their lives and more on maximizing self-acceptance in the present. Having such modest goals is likely to help older adults to maintain their emotion well being in the face of the challenges in late life.

Apart from adjusting their goals, people can regulate their emotions by self-enhancing social comparisons. For example, if I have an illness that renders me unable to walk without a stick, I may feel very sad and angry about the situation. However, if I compare myself with others who have to use wheelchairs, I may find my situation more acceptable. Once again, older adults use this strategy more often than do younger adults. Schulz and Fritz (1988), and Harris and Associates (1975, 1981) showed that most older adults considered their own well-being as better than that of "most other people". Older people also perceive fewer declines in themselves when comparing themselves with similar age peers (Heckhausen and Krueger, 1993). In addition, O'Gorman (1980) found that as older adults identified a problem as more serious, they were more likely to perceive the problem to be serous for the majority of people of similar ages. Heckhausen and Krueger (1993) further showed that old respondents reported larger favorable self-other discrepancies than did young respondents. In other words, they are more likely than their younger counterparts to think that they are better than other people are. The benefits of self-enhancing social comparison were also demonstrated among elderly women facing health-threatening situations (Heidrich and Ryff, 1993) and older adults suffering from a progressively worsening condition such as arthritis (Schulz, Heckhausen, and O'Brien, 1994; Verbrugge and Jette, 1994).

In summary, the above findings on age differences in coping suggest that when bad things are avoidable, older people are more likely to use coping strategies that aim at reducing their negative affect than are younger people. Given that such strategies do not directly solve the problems, they may have negative consequences for the individual in the long run. However, in terms of emotional regulation, such strategies enable older adults to maintain their emotional well being in the face of declines and losses associated with aging. In this sense, these strategies are adaptive.

Age Differences in Emotional Control

Even when coping fails, older adults can still maintain their emotional well being by controlling their negative affect internally (e.g., by diffusing negative affect with positive affect) or by controlling the external expression of the affect (e.g., by not expressing certain emotions in certain situations). Empirical findings from North America and Europe suggest that older adults are better at both of these types of emotional control than are younger adults. Gross and colleagues (Gross et al., 1997) examined self-reported internal and external control of positive and negative emotions across several diverse samples, including African-Americans, Chinese-Americans, European-Americans Norwegians, and American nuns. Across the different samples, older adults reported greater emotional control than did younger adults. Another study found that older adults were more likely than younger adults to endorse statements suggesting increased internal emotion control, such as "I try hard to stay in a neutral state and to avoid emotional situations" (Lawton, Kleban, Rajagopal, and Dean, 1992). In terms of external expression, studies revealed that the emotion expression style of older adults was different from that of middle-aged and younger adults in problem solving situations (Felton and Revenson, 1987; Weiner and Graham, 1989). Older adults were less emotional expressive and reported less anger and hostility when attributing a problem. In general, older adults are better copers in situations eliciting negative emotions and they express fewer negative emotions in those situations (Lawton, Kleban, and Dean, 1993).

Most of the research described above is based on laboratory-based studies in which participants make global evaluations or engage in hypothetical scenarios. To assess emotional regulation in everyday life, Carstensen and colleagues (2000) used an experience-sampling paradigm in a study involving participants aged 18 – 94 years. Participants carried electronic pagers and were paged at random times five times daily for one week. Each time they were paged, participants indicated the extent to which they felt positive and negative emotions. Carstensen and colleagues found that older adults experienced greater stability of positive emotional states than did younger adults, suggesting that older adults are better able to maintain positive emotions once elicited. Although the intensity of negative emotion experienced was similar across age, once a negative mood state was experienced, older adults were quicker to return to more positive states than were younger people (Carstensen et al., 2000).

In addition, an observational study of older married couples sheds some light on possible emotional-regulatory strategies older people use to reduce negative experience. When discussing a conflict in their relationship, older couples, as compared to their middle-aged counterparts exhibited less physiological reactivity (Levenson, Carstensen, and Gottman, 1994) and expressed less anger, belligerence, disgust, and more affection with one another (Carstensen, Gottman, and Levenson, 1995). This was true for both happily and unhappily married couples, and the effect remained even after controlling for severity of the conflict discussed. These findings suggest that older people are more skilled at managing emotions.

However, it should be noted that old age is not characterized entirely by rosy happiness. Instead, a sense that each good-bye kiss may be the last may have made emotional experience in old age more complex, poignant, and deeply gratifying. Carstensen and colleagues (2000) found that age was positively associated with emotional complexity, i.e., the number of factors that accounts for an emotional experience, and emotional poignancy, i.e., the correlation between positive and negative emotions at each time point. These findings suggest that as we age, we are more likely to experience complex and bittersweet emotions. It may be this emotional richness that makes the emotional profile in old age positive and meaningful.

In short, even when negative affect is unavoidable, older adults can deploy their emotional regulatory skills to maintain emotional states that are on average positive. They can also control the expression of emotions and avoid expressing hostility and anger even in situations that elicit them. Younger adults are either not as good as older adults at using these strategies or use them less often. Moreover, old age is associated with greater emotional complexity and poignancy that make life rich and meaningful. These age-related gains allow older people to remain satisfied with their life despite undeniable losses in other domains of life.

Generalizing Western findings on Age Differences in Emotional Regulation to the East

In the above sections, we reviewed Western findings on age differences in antecedent-focused and response-focused emotional regulation. These findings suggest that with age, people maintain their emotional well being in the face of age-related challenges by selecting situations that are likely to elicit positive emotions and avoiding those that may give rise to negative emotions. They can also do so mentally by focusing their attention on the aspects of life that elicit positive emotions by displaying selective attention and memory. When bad events are unavoidable, they can minimize the negative impact of these events by coping with the events or controlling their own emotions. Below we examine whether these age differences in emotional regulation are generalizable to the East. As mentioned at the beginning of this chapter, we focus our discussion on findings obtained from the Greater China, including Mainland China, Taiwan and Hong Kong.

There are reasons to believe that Western findings on age-related emotional regulation may not be generalizable to Easten cultures. Culture is defined as "shared set of beliefs, attitudes, norms, values, and behavior organized around a central theme and found among speakers of one language, in one time period, and in one geographic region" (Triandis, 1997, p.443). Frija and Mesquita (1995) argue that emotional regulation is influenced by the culture in which people are embedded. Through the socialization processes (Saarni, 2000; Ulich and Mayring, 1992), members from different cultures internalize the normative beliefs of their cultures and gradually develop different concepts about who they are and their relationships with other people. Such self-construal and social norms affect how people experience and regulate emotions.

Antecedent-Focused Emotional Regulation

As we mentioned above, Western empirical findings suggest that compared with younger adults, older adults are more likely to practice antecedent-focused emotional regulation by limiting their social partners to the handful who are the most emotionally significant to them. These social partners are more likely to provide predictable, and usually positive, social interactions than are unfamiliar social partners, enabling older adults to avoid negative affect. In fact, even during the unlikely occasions when the interactions are not pleasant, the emotionally significance of the relationships still makes the interactions worthwhile. For example, while it is not always pleasant to interact with a rebellious child, such an interaction is certainly more emotionally reinforcing than interacting with an annoying stranger. There are reasons to believe that in the East, most people regardless of age may select emotionally close social partners over peripheral ones, making age differences in this form of antecedent-focused emotional regulation less likely to occur. A number of studies have found that familism – defined as emphasis placed on emotionally close social partners, particularly family members (Szalay, Strohl, Fu, and Lao, 1994; Yang, 1988), is practiced more in the East than in the West. In particular, Chinese are found to emphasize interpersonal relatedness to a greater degree than do North Americans and Europeans (Ho, 1991; Oyserman, Coon, and Kemmelmeier, 2002). In other to maintain a harmony relationship with others and be a good member of their culture, Chinese people, regardless of age, are expected to care for their familial members and relatives, to fulfill their obligations, and to express their positive emotional feelings to their social partners (Zhang and Yang, 1998). This general emphasis on emotionally close social partners may leave no room for age differences in social selection to occur.

In addition, there are also reasons to believe that Easterners and Westerners may differ on another form of age-related antecedent-focused emotional regulation: showing selective attention and memory for positive information. As described in previous sections of this chapter, older adults from the West are found to be more likely to show this type of bias than are their younger counterparts. Yet, the literature on cultural differences in self construal suggests that older adults from the East may show the reverse bias, i.e., they may display selective attention and memory for negative information more so than younger adults from the same culture.

Cross-cultural studies have repeatedly found that while North Americans and some Europeans are more likely to have an independent self-construal, East Asians particularly Chinese are more likely to have interdependent self-construal (Garner, Gabriel, and Lee, 1999; Markus and Kitayama, 1991; Triandis, 1989). Within an independent culture, i.e., a culture that values individuals' independence and autonomy, individuals' self is made primarily in reference to a set of internal attributes that are unique to the individuals. People are motivated to search for and identify positively valued internal characteristics of the self, and to think as well as act in a way that enables them to maintain and increase their self-esteem. Hence, these individuals may be especially attuned to positive information regarding themselves (Frey and Stahlberg, 1986; Herzog, Franks, Markus, and Holmberg, 1998), including emotions. In contrast, in cultures where a dominant interdependent self is encouraged, these positivity biases are largely attenuated or reversed (e.g., Heine and Lehman, 1995; Kitayama and Markus, 1995; Kitayama, Markus, and Matsumoto, 1995; Kitayama, Markus, Matsumoto, and Norasakkunkit, 1997). Since an interdependent cultural system is organized to foster the interpersonal relationship and embeddedness of the self within surrounding social units, attention to negative self-relevant information is necessary to avoid mistakes and future social mishaps (Azuma, 1994; Kitayama and Karasawa, 1995; Lewis, 1995; White and LeVine, 1986). As a consequence, individuals living in these cultures are socialized (Falbo, Poston, Triscari, and Zhang, 1997) to focus on negative information regarding themselves, so as not to violate the social norms and to become a better participating part of the social unit (Kitayama et al., 1997).

To the extent that people regulate their emotions by paying selective attention to the type of emotions that is important in their cultures as they age, these cultural differences in self-construal may lead to differences in age-related antecedent-focused emotional regulation across cultures. People in Western independent cultures should pay more attention to and thus show better memory for positive information as they age, as the empirical findings we reviewed above have demonstrated. But people in Eastern interdependent cultures may show such cognitive biases for negative information instead, as they grow older.

Response-Focused Emotional Regulation

Several ethnographic studies have provided evidences for the strong cultural differences in the social consequences of emotions, especially in how the expression of emotions is valued (Briggs, 1970; Mesquita and Frijda, 1992; Scheiffelin, 1983). These differences are likely to affect whether Easterners increase their emotion-focused coping and emotional control as they age, in the same way as their Western counterparts do.

The Chinese culture has a strong Confucian heritage that stresses the importance of "the fundamental moral idea of moderation, balance and subtleness" (deBary, Chan, and Watson, 1960, p.117). This heritage leads Chinese to hold stronger beliefs than Westerners that it is important to control both their internal and external emotional states (Chiu and Kosinski, 1994; Koo, 1976; Leung and Lind, 1986; Potter, 1988; Russell and Yik, 1996; Sue and Sue, 1991; Wu and Tseng, 1985; Zheng and Berry, 1991). Dire consequences for both the individual per se and the social units would result if people fail to moderate their emotions. On an individual level, the failure to regulate one's emotions is regarded as detrimental to one's physical and mental health, "the mentally healthy person was one who did not get into explosive fits of anger, get excessively happy, or become easily irritated" (Koo, 1976, p.33). On an interpersonal level, the inability to control and regulate one's emotions may threaten and disrupt the stability and harmony of social relationships, which is strongly undesirable in a collectivistic society, such as China (Bond and Hwang, 1986; Chiu and Kosinski, 1994; Markus and Kitayama, 1994). As a result, Chinese people are "more emotionally reserved, introverted, fond of tranquility, and habituated to self-restraint" compared to Westerners (Song, 1985, p.53). This cross-cultural difference emerges at very young age. Children raised in the Chinese culture are socialized to control their impulses (Ho, 1994). Cross-cultural studies revealed that Chinese babies were less active, less happily vocal, and less exploratory than European-American and European babies (Freedman, 1974; Freedman and Freedman, 1969; Kagan, Kearsley, and Zelazo, 1978). Given that an increased emphasis on internal and external control of emotions occurs at such a young age in the Chinese culture, there is not much room for age differences in these forms of response-focused emotional regulation to occur. Hence, there are reasons to expect an age-related increase in emotional control to emerge at a reduced level, or even not emerge at all, among the Chinese than among Westerners. Such a pattern is also likely to show up for coping strategies that focus on emotions.

In addition, another Confusion heritage, the principle of *holism*, may also contribute to cultural differences in age-related response-focused emotional regulation. Under the influence of Aristotelian logic, individuals in Western cultures tend to reject the coexistence of opposite concepts, such as, positive and negative emotions. The three primary propositions in Aristotelian logic (i.e., *the law of identity*: things are what they are and nothing else; *the law of contradiction*: no statement can be both true and false; *the law of the excluded middle*: no middle ground) discourage individuals who live in this culture to think in a dialectical way. In contrast, under the influence of the philosophical guiding principle of *holism*, members in the Chinese culture do not regard opposites as contradictory (Bagozzi, Wong, and Yi, 1999; Peng and Nisbett, 1999). Holism refers to the concept that everything must be interpreted in relation to everything else, and that although different systems can be in opposition to another, they can be connected together and perceived as a whole. In a content analysis of proverbs, dialectical proverbs were found four times more often in Chinese books than in

American books (Peng and Nisbett, 1999). Moreover, Chinese individuals were found to prefer dialectical proverbs to nondialectical ones, whereas the reverse was true for Americans (Peng and Nisbett, 1999; see also Briley, Morris, and Simonson, 2000). This cross-cultural difference in the acceptance of duality may lead to a high level of relativistic thinking among the Chinese culture as a whole, regardless of age.

Further, this cultural difference also influences the emotional experiences of individuals living in these cultures. For example, whereas American love songs appear to relate love either exclusively with positive or with negative emotions, Chinese love songs are more likely to associate love with both positive and negative emotions (Shaver, Wu, and Schwartz, 1992). Bagozzi et al. (1999) found that correlation between reports of pleasant and unpleasant emotions was less negative in the Asian samples than in the Western sample. As mentioned above, Carstensen et al. (2000) found among Americans that emotional poignancy, i.e., the coexistence of positive and negative emotions, increased with age. With the influence of the dialectical logic on individuals' cognition, this type of emotional poignancy may be evident among the Chinese as a whole, attenuating the age differences in this area.

In summary, cross-cultural findings on differences in social norms and self-construal between the East and the West lead one to expect that the age differences in antecedent-focused and response-focused emotional regulation found in the West may not be generalizable to the East. In particular, given the high base rates of social selection, emotion-focused coping and emotional control among the Chinese, one has reasons to believe that the Chinese are less likely to show age-related increases in these emotional regulatory strategies, compared with their Western counterparts. Moreover, while attention to positive emotions is important in Western independent cultures, attention to negative emotions is important in Eastern interdependent cultures. This may limit the generalizability of the Western finding on age differences in selective attention and memory to China. While Westerners regulate their emotions by showing attention and memory biases for positive information as they age, Chinese may achieve the same purpose by showing biases for negative information. Below we review the handful of empirical studies that examined age differences in emotional regulation in Eastern, particularly Chinese, cultures. Because the studies are very few in number, we have included findings from conference presentations, unpublished theses in addition to published articles to maximize coverage.

Eastern Empirical Findings on Age Differences in Antecedent-Focused Emotional Regulation

As mentioned above, Western findings suggest that age differences in antecedent-focused emotional regulation are evident in situation selection and cognitive processing. In terms of situation selection, the patterns of age differences do not seem to differ across cultures. Empirical studies conducted in Hong Kong, Mainland China and Taiwan suggest that like their Western counterparts, Chinese people increase their preference for emotionally close social partners as they age (Fung et al., 1999, Study 2 and 4; Fung et al., 2001). In each of these studies, participants were asked to imagine that they had 30-min of free time and would like to interact with someone. They were given the choice of an emotionally close social partner and two novel social partners. Results suggest that similar to Westerners, older

Chinese adults in Hong Kong (Fung et al., 1999), Taiwan and Mainland China (Fung et al., 2001) consistently prefer spending time with emotionally close social partners to novel partners, whereas such pattern of social preference is not found among younger Chinese adults.

However, in the area of cognitive processing, there may be evidences for cultural differences in age-related emotional regulation. Fung and Tang (2005) presented younger and older Chinese in Hong Kong with a TV health announcement that had either positive, negative or neutral background music. She found that older adults remembered the most information from the negative version. Younger adults did not show such differences. These findings suggest that Chinese adults seem to show greater memory bias for negative stimuli in their social world as they grow older, which is in direct contrast to their Western counterparts who show memory bias for positive stimuli. Nevertheless, should it be the case that negative information is more important to Easterners who value interdependence while positive information is more important to Westerners who emphasize independence, these cultural differences in age-related cognitive processing may reflect the same emotional regulatory strategy. It may be the case that in both Western and Eastern cultures, individuals, with age, show greater selective memory for information that is more consistent with their self construal. This strategy is likely to minimize conflicts and negative emotions, contributing to better emotional regulation.

EASTERN EMPIRICAL FINDINGS ON AGE DIFFERENCES IN RESPONSE-FOCUSED EMOTIONAL REGULATION

Age-related response-focused emotional regulation does not show much cultural difference either. In terms of coping, an age-related increase in emotion-focused coping strategies are evident in the East as it is in the West. Cheng (2004) examined the use of goal adjustment – minimizing discrepancy between one's current state and one's aspiration – among young, middle-aged and older Chinese adults in Hong Kong. He found that goal discrepancies in the areas of relationship and other life domains decreased with age while those in the area of health increased with age. Because goal discrepancies in the health domain had smaller effects on subjective well being than those in the relationship and other life domains, the net effect of all age-related changes in goal discrepancies on subjective well being was positive. In other words, with age, Hong Kong Chinese seem to use this form of emotion-focused coping strategy more often and this strategy is effective in helping them to maintain or improve their emotion well being.

Not only do Easterners increase their use of emotion-focused coping strategies with age, as their Western counterparts do, but they also demonstrate better control of their emotions. Ching and Fung (2004) examined age differences in emotional functioning among two large samples (N=1505 for each sample) of Chinese participants from various Mainland Chinese provinces. Despite the high base rate of emotional control among the Chinese, older Chinese showed greater levels of both internal and external control of emotions than did their younger counterparts. Perhaps as a result of these age differences in emotional control, older people enjoyed a more positive emotional profile, with similar levels of positive emotions and lowered levels of negative emotions, than did younger people. These patterns of age differences are consistent with findings obtained in the West (Carstensen, et al., 2003; Gross et al., 1997; Lawton et al., 1992), suggesting that people from both Eastern and Western cultures are better able to control the subjective feelings and outward expression of their emotions as they age. These strategies minimize the effects of negative emotions should they occur, and enable aging individuals to maintain a high level of emotion well being.

In summary, the handful of empirical studies on age differences in emotional regulation conducted in the East generally found the same results as those conducted in the West. At least in the areas of social selection, coping and emotional control, people from Eastern and Western cultures show age-related increase in emotional regulation in similar manners. In the area of cognitive processing, evidences suggest that Westerners and Easterners may show the same mechanisms of age-related emotional regulation even though their overt behaviors are different. Older adults in the West show cognitive bias for positive information whereas those in the East exhibit biases for negative information. Yet, these behaviors may both represent selective attention and memory toward the type of information that is valued in the specific culture.

Discussion and Directions for Future Research

What we have reviewed above suggests that with age, people maintain or even improve their emotional well being despite undeniable declines in physical and cognitive areas. This is the case, at least in part, because goals change with age. While younger people focus on expanding their horizons and gaining new information, older people give top priority to regulating their emotions. This focus on emotional goals motivates older people to pursue social situations that are more likely to provide emotionally meaningful social experiences, and to show biases in cognitive processing that result in better emotional regulation. It also leads older people to engage in coping strategies that aim at regulating emotional states, and to display greater emotional control. Younger adults, who on average do not prioritize emotional goals, do not show these preferences. These age differences in emotional regulation are found in both Western and Eastern cultures, despite pre-existing cultural differences in social norms and social cognition that are believed to have influences on emotional regulation.

Such cultural similarities in age-related emotional regulation may suggest that emotional regulation follows universal developmental trajectories. When personality researchers found that patterns of age differences in personality were similar across cultures (McCrae et al., 1999; Yang, McCrae, and Costa, 1998), they argued that the finding supported the universality of personality maturation (e.g., McCrae et al., 1999). We make the same claim for emotional regulation. We argue that because Eastern and Western cultures differ in their history, social norms, customs and traditions, the fact that similar patterns of age differences in emotional regulation are found across cultures may suggest that the patterns reflect actual human development in adulthood, rather than cohort or cultural effects. People, across cultures, place greater emphasis on emotions and adopt better emotional regulatory strategies as they age. This age-related gain compensates for declines and losses associated with aging in other areas, enabling psychological well being to remain stable, or even increase, in the second half of life.

However, even though the general mechanisms for developmental changes in emotional regulation may be universal, their manifestations can differ across cultures. For example, as described above, although people in all cultures employ selective memory to regulate their emotions with age, differences in social cognition across cultures may determine the type of emotions that gets remembered. Specifically, Westerners who value independence show better memory for positive information with age, whereas Easterners who treasure interdependence display better memory for negative information as they grow older. Both groups regulate their emotions by focusing on the type of emotions that matters; yet the manifestations of their preferences differ. Future cross-cultural studies on age-related emotional regulation should go beyond comparing general emotional regulatory strategies to comparing their culture-specific manifestations. In particular, it seems to be a good research strategy to first find out the characteristics that each culture values and then examine how people from each culture regulate their emotions in ways that enhance these characteristics as they grow older. For instance, the emphasis on dialectical thinking among the Chinese (e.g., Peng and Nisbett, 1999) may make them more likely to exhibit complex and poignant emotions as they age, relative to their Western counterparts.

Last but not least, the role of cognitive functioning in age-related emotional regulation should not be ignored. Park, Nisbett, and Hedden (1999) argue that the relationships between aging and cognition may differ across cultures in predictable ways. Cognitive abilities that are relatively more knowledge-based may show greater cultural differences with age, as individuals acquire more culture-specific knowledge with the passage of time. In contrast, cognitive abilities that rely more on basic cognitive resources may show smaller cultural differences with age. This is the case because basic cognitive resources tend to decline uniformly across cultures when people get older, reducing the room for cultural differences in associated functioning. Since cognitive functioning is at the root of many emotional regulatory strategies, this model may also be applicable to age-related emotional regulation across cultures. Cultural differences in emotional regulation across adulthood may be the most evident for emotional regulatory strategies that require a great deal of culture-specific knowledge, such as situation selection or external emotional control. But such cultural differences may be the least evident for emotional regulatory strategies that require high levels of basic cognitive resources, such as memory. Although the few Eastern empirical studies that we reviewed above do not seem to support these predictions, the jury is still out. More cross-cultural studies on age-related emotional regulation, particularly those that involve both Western and Eastern cultures, are needed to test these predictions.

In conclusion, unlike the downward trajectories that characterize physical and cognitive functioning with age, emotional functioning seems to be relatively well preserved across adulthood. Compared with younger adults, older adults from both Eastern and Western cultures are better able to regulate their emotions, through a wide variety of strategies ranging from selecting social partners to controlling emotional expressions. Future cross-cultural studies should examine the different manifestations of these strategies across cultures. Such studies hold promises for revealing the mechanisms underlying developmental changes in emotional regulation.

AUTHORS' NOTE

Helene H. Fung, Bob H. Ching, and Dannii Y. Yeung, Department of Psychology, Chinese University of Hong Kong.

Work by the first author was supported by two Direct Grants for Research from Chinese University of Hong Kong, and an Earmarked Research Grant, CUHK4256/03H, from Research Grants Council, Hong Kong.

REFERENCES

Ajrouch, K. J., Antonucci, T. C., and Janevic, M. R. (2001). Social networks among Blacks and Whites: The interaction between race and age. *Journal of Gerontology: Social Sciences, 56B,* S112-S118.

Antonucci, T. C., Lansford, J. E., Schaberg, L., Smith, J., Baltes, M., Akiyama, H., Takahashi, K., and Fuhrer, R. (2001). Widowhood and illness: A comparison of social network characteristics in France, Germany, Japan, and the United States. *Psychology and Aging, 16,* 655-665.

Aspinwall, L. G., and Taylor, S. E. (1997). A stitch in time: Self-regulation and proactive coping. *Psychological Bulletin*, 121, 417–436.

Azuma, H. (1994). Two modes of cognitive socialization in Japan and the United States. In P. M. Greenfield and R. Cocking (Eds.), *Cross-cultural roots of minority child development* (pp. 275-284). Hilsdale, NJ, England: Lawrence Erlbaum Associates.

Bagozzi, R. P., Wong , N., and Yi, Y. (1999). The role of culture and gender in the relationship between positive and negative affect. *Cognition and Emotion, 13,* 641-672.

Blanchard-Fields, F. (1986). Reasoning on social dilemmas varying in emotional saliency: An adult developmental perspective. *Psychology and Aging, 1,* 325-333.

Blanchard-Fields, F., and Camp, C. J. (1990). Affect, individual differences, and real world problem solving across the adult life span. In T. Hess (Ed.), *Aging and cognition,: Knowledge organization and utilization* (pp. 461-497). Amsterdam: North-Holland.

Blanchard-Fields, F., and Irion, J. C. (1988). Coping strategies from the perspective of two developmental markers: Age and social reasoning. *Journal of Genetic Psychology, 149,* 141-151.

Blanchard-Fields, F., Jahnke, H., and Camp, C. (1995). Age differences in problem solving style: The role of emotional salience. *Psychology and Aging, 10,* 173-180.Bond, M. H., and Hwang, K. K. (1986). The social psychology of the Chinese people. In M. H. Bond (Ed.), *The psychology of the Chinese people.* New York: Oxford University Press.

Blanchard-Fields, F., and Norris, L. (1994). Causal attributions from adolescence through adulthood: Age differences, ego level, and generalized response style. *Aging and Cognition, 1,* 67-86.

Bond, M. H., and Hwang, K. (1986). The social psychology of Chinese people. In M. H. Bond (Ed.), *The psychology of the Chinese people* (pp. 213-266). New York, US: Oxford University Press.

Brandtstädter, J., and Greve, W. (1994). The aging self: Stabilizing and protective processes. *Developmental Review, 14,* 52-80.

Brandtstädter, J., and Renner, G. (1990). Tenacious goal pursuit and flexible goal adjustment: Explication and age-related analysis of assimilative and accommodation strategies of coping. *Psychological and Aging, 5,* 58-67.

Brandtstädter, J., and Rothermund, K. (2002). The life-course dynamics of goal pursuit and goal adjustment: A two-process framework. *Developmental Review, 22,* 117-150.

Briggs, J. L. (1970). *Never in anger: Portrait of an Eskimo family.* Cambridge, MA: Harvard University Press.

Briley, D., Morris, M. W., and Simonson, I. (2000). Reasons as carriers of culture: Dynamic vs. dispositional models of cultural influence on decision making? *Journal of Consumer Research, 27,* 157-178.

Buhler, C., Brind, A., and Horner, A. (1968). Old age as a phase of human life: Questionnaire Study. *Human Development, 11,* 53-63.

Carstensen, L. L. (1992). Social and emotional patterns in adulthood: Support for socioemotional selectivity theory. *Psychology and Aging, 7,* 331-338.

Carstensen, L. L. (1995). Evidence for a life-span theory of socioemotional selectivity. *Current Directions in Psychological Science, 4(5),* 151-156.

Carstensen, L. L. (1998). A life-span approach to social motivation. In J. Heckhausen and C. S. Dweck (Eds.), *Motivation and self-regulation across the life span* (pp. 341-364). New York, US: Cambridge University Press.

Carstensen, L. L., Fung, H. H., and Charles, S. T. (2003). Socioemotional selectivity theory and the regulation of emotion in the second half of life. *Motivation and Emotion, 27,* 103-123.

Carstense, L. L., Gottman, J. M., and Levenson, R. W. (1995). Emotional behavior in long-term marriage. *Psychology and Aging, 10,* 140-149.

Carstensen, L. L., Gross, J. J., and Fung, H. H. (1997). The social context of emotional experience. *Annual Review of Gerontology and Geriatrics, 17,* 325-352.

Carstensen, L. L., Issacowitz, D. M., and Charles, S. T. (1999). Taking time seriously: A theory of socioemotional selectivity. *American Psychologist, 54(3),* 165-181.

Carstensen, L. L., Pasupathi, M., Mayr, U., and Nesselroade, J. R. (2000). Emotional experience in everyday life across the adult life span. *Journal of Personality and Social Psychology, 79(4),* 644-655.

Carstensen, L. L., and Turk-Charles, S. (1994). The salience of emotion across the adult life span. *Psychology and Aging, 9(2),* 259-264.

Charles, S., Mather, M., and Carstensen, L. L. (2003). Aging and emotional memory: The forgettable nature of negative images for older adults. *Journal of Experimental Psychology: General, 132(2),* 310-324.

Cheng, S-T. (2004). Age and subjective well-being revisited: A discrepancy perspective. *Psychology and Aging, 19,* 409-415.

Ching, B. H., and Fung, H. H. (2004, July). *Age Differences in Goals: Its Implications for Health Promotion.* Poster presented at the XVIIIth Biennial meeting of the International Society for the Study of Behavioral Development, Ghent, Belgium.

Chiu, R. K., and Kosinski, F. A. (1994). Is Chinese conflict-handling behavior influenced by Chinese values? *Social Behavior and Personality, 22,* 81-90.

Curley, S. P., Eraker, S. A., and Yates, J. F. (1984). An investigation of patients' reactions to therapeutic uncertainly. *Medical Decision Making,* 4, 501-511.

Cytrynbaum, S., Blum, L., Partick, R., Stein, J., Wadner, D., and Wilk, C. (1980). Midlife development: A personality and social systems perspective. In L. W. Poon (Ed.), *Aging in the 1980s: Psychological issues* (pp. 463-474). Washington, DC: American Psychological Association.

deBary, W. T., Chan, W. T., and Watson, B. (1960). The mean. In W. T. deBary (Ed.), *Introduction to Oriental civilizations: Sources of Chinese tradition* (Vol. 1, pp.117-121). New York: Columbia University Press.

Diamond, L. M., and Aspinwall, L. G. (2003). Emotion regulation across the life span: An integrative perspective emphasizing self-Regulation, positive affect, and dyadic processes. *Motivation and Emotion, 27,* 125-156.

Diener, E., and Suh, E. (1997). Measuring quality of life: Economic, social, and subjective indicators. *Social Indicators Research, 40(1-2),* 189-216.

Dittmann-Kohli., F., and Westerhof, G. J. (1997). The SELE-Sentence Completion Questionnaire: A new instrument for the assessment of personal meanings in aging research. *Anuario de Psciologia, 73(2),* 7-18.

Falbo, T., Poston, D. L., Jr., Triscari, . S., and Zhang, X. (1997). Self-enhancing illusions among Chinese school children. *Journal of Cross Cultural Psychology, 28,* 172-191.

Felton, B. J., and Revenson, T. A. (1987). Age differences in coping with chronic illness. *Psychology and Aging, 2,* 164-170.

Field, D., and Minkler, M. (1988). Continuity and change in social support between young-old and old-old or very-old age. *Journal of Gerontology: Psychological Sciences, 43,* P100-106.

Field, T. (1981). Infant arousal attention and affect during early interactions. *Advances in Infancy Research, 1,* 57-100.

Fingerman, K. L., and Birditt, K. S. (2003). Do age differences in close and problematic family ties reflect the pool of available relatives? *Journal of Gerontology: Psychological Sciences, 58B,* P80-P87.

Folkman, S., Lazarus, R. S., Pimley, S., and Novacek, J. (1987). Age differences in stress and coping processes. *Psychology and Aging, 2,* 171-184.

Fredrickson, B. L., and Carstensen, L. L. (1990). Choosing social partners: How age and anticipated endings make people more selective. *Psychology and Aging, 5,* 335-347.

Freedman, D. G. (1974). *Human infancy: An evolutionary perspective.* Hillsdale, NJ: Lawrence Erlbaum Associates.

Freedman, D. G., and Freedman, N. C. (1969). Behavioral differences between Chinese-American and European-American newborns. *Nature, 224,* 1227.

Frey, D., and Stahlberg, D. (1986). Selection of information after receiving more or less reliable self-threatening information. *Personality and Social Psychology Bulletin, 12,* 434-441.

Frija, N. H., and Mesquita, B. (1995). The social roles and functions of emotions. In S. Kitayama and H. R. Markus (Eds.), *Emotion and culture: Empirical studies of mutual influence* (pp. 51-87). Washington, DC: American Psychological Association.

Fung, H. H., and Carstensen, L. L. (2003). Sending memorable messages to the old: Age differences in preferences and memory for advertisements. *Journal of Personality and Social Psychology, 85(1),* 163-178.

Fung, H. H., Carstensen, L. L., and Lang, F. R. (2001). Age-related patterns in social networks among European Americans and African Americans: Implications for socioemotional selectivity across the life span. *International Journal of Aging and Human Development, 52,* 185-206.

Fung, H. H., Carstensen, L. L., and Lutz, A. M. (1999). Influence of time on social preferences: Implications for life-span development. *Psychology and Aging, 14,* 595-604.

Fung, H. H., Lai, P., and Ng, R. (2001). Age differences in social preferences among Taiwanese and Mainland Chinese: The role of perceived time. *Psychology and Aging, 16,* 351-356.

Fung, H. H., and Tang, L. Y. T. (2005). Age differences in memory for emotional messages: Do older people always remember the positive better? *Ageing International, 30*, 123-146.

Gardner, W. L., Gabriel, S., and Lee, A. (1999). "I" value freedom, but "we" value relationships: Self-construal priming mirrors cultural differences in judgment. *Psychological Science, 10*, 321-326.

Gould, O. N., and Dixon, R. A. (1993). How we spent our vacation: Collaborative storytelling by young and old adults. *Psychology and Aging, 8,* 10-17.

Gross, J. J. (1998). Antecedent- and response-focused emotion regulation: Divergent consequences for experience, expression, and physiology. *Journal of Personality and Social Psychology,* 74, 224–237.

Gross, J. J., Carstensen, L. C., Pasupathi, M., Tsai, J., Gotestam-Skorpen, K., and Hsu, A. Y. C. (1997). Emotion and aging: Experience, expression, and control. *Psychology and Aging, 12,* 590-599.

Haan, N. (1977). *Coping and defending: Processes of self-environment organization.* New York: Academic Press.

Harris, L., and Associates (1975). *The myth and reality of aging in America.* Washington, DC: National Council on the Aging.

Harris, L., and Associates (1981). *Aging in the eighties: American in transition.* Washington, DC: National Council on the Aging.

Hashtroudi, S., Johnson, M. K., and Chroniak, L. D. (1990). Aging and qualitative characteristics of memories for perceived and imagined complex events. *Psychology and Aging, 5,* 119-126.

Hauser, S. T. (1976). Loevinger's model and measure of ego development: A critical review. *Psychological Bulletin, 83,* 928-955.

Heckhausen, J. (1994). *Developmental regulation in East- and West- Berliners, Primary and secondary control of aging-related and sociohistorical challenges.* Unpublished manuscript, Max Planck Institute for Human Development and Education, Berlin, Germany.

Heckhausen, J. and Krueger, J. (1993). Developmental expectations for the self and "most other people": Age-grading in three functions of social comparison. *Developmental Psychology, 29,* 539-548.

Heckhausen, J., and Schulz, R. (1995). A Life-span Theory of Control. *Psychological Review, 102*, 284-304.

Heidrich, S. M., and Ryff, C. D. (1993). The role of social comparison processes in the psychological adaptation of elderly adults. *Journal of Gerontology: Psychological Sciences, 48,* 127-136.

Heine, S., and Lehman, D. (1995). The cultural construction of self-enhancement: An examination of group-serving bias. *Journal of Personality and Social Psychology, 68,* 603-618.

Herzog, A. R., Franks, M. M., Markus, H. R., and Holmberg, D. (1998). Activities and well-being in older age: Effects of self-concept and educational attainment. *Psychology and Aging, 13*, 179-185.

Hess, T. M., Bolstad, C. A., Woodburn, S. M., and Auman, C. (1999). Trait diagnosticity versus behavioral consistency as determinants of impression change in adulthood. *Psychology and Aging, 14,* 77-89.

Hess, T. M., and Pullen, S. M. (1994). Adult age differences in impression change processes. *Psychology and Aging, 9,* 237-250.

Ho, D. Y. F. (1991). Relational orientation and methodological relationalism. *Bulletin of the Hong Kong Psychological Society, 26-27,* 81-95.

Ho, D. Y. F. (1994). Cognitive socialization in Confucian cultures. In P. M. Greenfield and R. R. Cocking (Eds.), *Cross-cultural roots of minority child development.* Hillsdale, NJ: Lawrence Erlbaum.

Johnson, M. K., and Sherman, S. J. (1990). Constructing and reconstructing the past and the future in the present. In E. T. Higgins and R. M. Sorrentino (Eds.), *Handbook of motivation and cognition: Foundations of social behavior*, Vol. 2 (pp. 482-526). New York, US: Guilford Press.

Kagan, J., Kearsley, R. B., and Zelazo, P. R. (1978). *Infancy: Its place in human development.* Cambridge, MA: Harvard University Press.

Kennedy, Q., Mather, M., and Carstensen, L.L. (2004) The role of motivation in the age-related positive bias in autobiographical memory. *Psychological Science, 15(3),* 208-214.

Kitayama, S., and Karasawa, M. (1995). Self: A cultural psychological perspective. *Japanese Journal of Experimental Social Psychology, 35*, 133-163.

Kitayama, S., and Markus, H. R. (1995). Culture and self: Implications for internationalizing psychology. In N. R. Goldberger and J. B. Veroff (Eds.), *The culture and psychology reader* (pp. 366-383). New York, US: New York University Press.

Kitayama, S., Markus, H. R., and Matsumoto, H. (1995). Culture, self, and emotion: A cultural perspective on "self-conscious" emotions. In J. P. Tangney and K. W. Fischer (Eds.), *Self-conscious emotions: The psychology of shame, guilt, embarrassment, and pride* (pp. 439-464). New York, US: Guilford Press.

Kitayama, S., Markus, H. R., Matsumoto, H., and Norasakkunkit, V. (1997). Individual and collective processes in the construction of the self: Self-enhancement in the United States and self-criticism in Japan. *Journal of Personality and Social Psychology, 72,* 1245-1267.

Koenig, H. G., George, L. K., and Siegler, I. C. (1988). The use of religion and other emotion-regulating coping strategies among older adults. *Gerontologist, 28,* 303-310.

Koo, L.C.L. (1976). *Nourishment of life:* The culture of health in traditional Chinese society. Unpublished dissertation thesis, University of California, Berkeley.

LaBouvie-Vief, G., Hakim-Larson, J., and Hobart, C. J. (1987). Age, ego level, and the life-span development of coping and defense processes. *Psychology and Aging, 2,* 286-293.

Lang, F. R. (2000). Endings and continuity of social relationships: Maximizing intrinsic benefits within personal networks when feeling near to death. *Journal of Social and Personal Relationships, 17,* 155-182.

Lang, F. R., and Carstensen, L. L. (1994). Close emotional relationships in late life: Further support for proactive aging in the social domain. *Psychology and Aging, 9,* 315-324.

Lang, F. R., Staudinger, U. M., and Carstensen, L. L. (1998). Perspectives on socioemotional selectivity in late life: How personality and social context do (and do not) make a difference. *Journal of Gerontology: Psychological Sciences, 53B,* P21-P30.

Lansford, J. E., Sherman, A. M., and Antonucci, T. C. (1998). Satisfaction with social networks: An examination of socioemotional selectivity theory across cohorts. *Psychology and Aging, 13,* 544-552.

Lawton, M. P., Kleban, M. H., and Dean, J. (1993). Affect and age: Cross-sectional comparisons of structure and prevalence. *Psychology and Aging, 8,* 165-175.

Lawton, M. P., Kleban, M. H., Rajagopal, D., and Dean, J. (1992). The dimensions of affective experiences in three age groups. *Psychology and Aging, 7,* 171-184.

Leung, K., and Lind, E. A. (1986). Procedural justice and culture: Effects of culture, gender, and investigator status on procedural preferences. *Journal of Personality and Social Psychology, 50,* 1134-1140.

Levenson, R. W., Carstensen, L. L., and Gottman, J. M. (1994). Influence of age and gender on affect, physiology, and their intercorrelations: A study of long-term marriages. *Journal of Personality and Social Psychology, 67*, 56-68.

Levine, L. J., and Bluck, S. (1997). Experienced and remembered emotional intensity in older adults. *Psychology and Aging, 12,* 514-523.

Lewis, M. (1995). Embarrassment: The emotion of self-exposure and evaluation. In J. P. Tangney and K. W. Fischer (Eds.), *Self-conscious emotions: The psychology of shame, guilt, embarrassment, and pride* (pp. 198-218). New York, US: Guilford Press.

Loevinger, J. (1976). Origins of conscience. *Psychological Issues, 9*, 265-297.

Markus, H. R., and Kitayama, S. (1991). Culture and the self: Implications for cognition, emotion, and motivation. *Psychological Review, 98,* 224-253.

Markus, H. R., and Kitayama, S. (1994). The cultural construction of self and emotion: Implications for social behavior. In S. Kitayama and H. R. Markus (Eds.), *Emotion and culture: Empirical studies of mutual influence* (pp. 89-132). Washington, DC: American Psychological Association.

Mather, M., and Carstensen, L. L. (2003). Aging and attentional biases for emotional faces. *Psychological Science, 14,* 409-415.

Mather, M., and Johnson, M.K. (2000). Choice-supportive source monitoring: Do our decisions seem better to us as we age? *Psychology and Aging, 15,* 596-606.

McCrae, R. R., and Costa, P. T. (1984). *Emerging lives, enduring dispositions: Personality in adulthood.* Boston: Little, Brown.

McCrae, R. R., Costa, P. T. Jr., Ostendorf, F., Angleitner, A., Caprara, G.. V., Barbaranelli, C., Lima, M. P. D., Simoes, A., Marusic, I., Bratko, D., Chae, J-H., and Piedmont, R. L. (1999). Age Differences in Personality Across the Adult Life Span: Parallels in Five Cultures. *Developmental Psychology, 35,* 466-477.

Mesquita, B., and Frija, N. H. (1992). Cultural variations in emotions: A review. *Psychological Bulletin, 112,* 179-204.

Morgan, D. L. (1988). Age differences in social network participation. *Journal of Gerontology: Social Sciences, 43,* S129-137.

Mroczek, D. K. (2001). Age and emotion in adulthood. *Current Directions in Psychological Sciences, 10*, 87-90.

O'Gormann, H. J. (1980). False consciousness of kind: Pluralistic ignorance among the aged. *Research on Aging, 2,* 105-128.

Oyserman, D., Coon, H. M., and Kemmelmeier, M. (2002). Rethinking individualism and collectivism: Evaluation of theoretical assumptions and meta-analyses. *Psychological Bulletin, 128,* 3-72.

Park, D. C., Nisbett, R., and Hedden, T. (1999). Aging, culture, and cognition. *Journal of Gerontology: Psychological sciences, 54B,* P75-P84.

Peng, K., and Nisbett, R. E. (1999). Dialectical responses to questions about dialectical thinking. *American Psychologist, 55*, 1067-1068.

Potter, S. H. (1988). The cultural construction of emotion in rural Chinese social life. *Ethos, 16*, 181-208.

Quackenbush, S. W., and Barnett, M. A. (2001). Recollection and evaluation of critical experiences in moral development: A cross-sectional examination. *Basic and Applied Social Psychology, 23(1),* 55-64.

Russell, J. A., and Yik, M. S. M. (1996). Emotion among the Chinese. In M. H. Bond (Ed.), *The handbook of Chinese psychology* (pp. 166-188). Hong Kong: Oxford University Press.

Ryff, C. D. (1989a). Happiness is everything, or is it? Explorations on the meaning of psychological well-being. *Journal of Personality and Social Psychology, 57(6),* 1069-1081.

Ryff, C. D. (1989b). In the eye of the beholder: Views of psychological well-being among middle aged and older adults. *Psychology and Aging, 4(2),* 195-210.

Ryff, C. D. (1991). Possible selves in adulthood and old age: A tale of shifting horizons. *Psychology and Aging, 6,* 286-295.

Saarni, C. (2000). Emotional competence: Developmental perspective. In R. Bar-On and J. D. A. Parker (2000). *The handbook of emotional intelligence: Theory, development, assessment, and application at home, school, and in the workplace* (pp. 68-91). San Francisco, CA, US: Jossey-Bass.

Schieffelin, E. D. (1983). Anger and shame in the tropical forest: An affect as a cultural system in Paua New Guinea. *Ethos, 11,* 181-191.

Schulkind, M. D., Hennis, L. K., and Rubin, D. C. (1999). Music, emotion, and autobiographic memory: They're playing your song. *Memory and Cognition, 27(6),* 948-955.

Schulz, R., and Decker, S. (1985). Long-term adjustment to physical disability: The role of social support, perceived control, and self-blame. *Journal of Personality and Social Psychology, 48,* 1162-1172.

Schulz, R., and Fritz, S. (1988). Origins of stereotypes of the elderly: An experimental study of the self-other discrepancy. *Experimental Aging Research, 13,* 189-195.

Schulz, R., Heckhausen, J., and O'Brien, A. T. (1994) Control and the disablement process in the elderly. *Journal of Social Behavior and Personality, 9,* 139-152.

Shaver, P. R., Wu, S., and Schwartz, J. C. (1992). Cross-cultural similarities and differences in emotion and its representation? In Clark, M. S. (Eds.), *Emotion.* Newbury Park, CA: Sage, 175-212.

Song, W. (1985). A preliminary study of the character traits of the Chinese. In W. S. Tseng and D. Y. H. Wu (Eds.), *Chinese culture and mental health* (pp.47-55). Orlando, FL: Academic Press.

Sue, D., and Sue, D. (1991). *Counseling the culturally different: Theory and Practice.* New York: John Wiley.

Szalay, L. B., Strohl, J. B., Fu, L., and Lao, P-S. (1994). American and Chinese perceptions and belief systems: A People's Republic of China-Taiwanese comparison. New York: Plenum Press.

Triandis, H. (1989). The self and social behavior in differing cultural contexts. *Psychological Review, 96,* 506-520.

Triandis, H. (1997). Cross-cultural perspectives on personality. In R. Hogan, J. Johnson, and S. R. Briggs (Eds.), *Handbook of personality psychology* (pp. 439-464). San Diego, CA: Academic Press.

Ulich, D., and Mayring, P. (1992). *Psychologie der Emotionen* [Psychology of emotions]. Stuttgart, Germany: Kohlhammer.

Vaillant, G. E. (1977). *Adaptation to life. Boston*: Little, Brown.

van Tilburg, T. (1998). Losing and gaining in old age: Changes in personal network size and social support in a four-year longitudinal study. *Journal of Gerontology: Social Sciences, 53B,* S313-S323.

Verbrugge, L. M., and Jette, A. M. (1994). The disablement process. *Social Science and Medicine, 38,* 1-14.

Weiner, B., and Graham, S. (1989). Understanding the motivational role of affect: Lifespan research from an attributional perspective. *Cognition and Emotion, 3*, 401-419.

White, M. I., and LeVine, R. A. (1986). What is an "ii ko" (good child)? In H. W. Stevenson, H. Azuma, and K. Hakuta (Eds.), *Child development and education in Japan* (pp. 55-62). New York, US: W H Freeman.

Wu, D. Y. H., and Tseng, W. S. (1985). Introduction: The characteristics of Chinese culture. In W. S. Tseng and D. Y. H. Wu (Eds.), *Chinese culture and mental health* (pp. 29-42). Orlando, FL: Academic Press.

Yang, C F. (1988). Familism and development: An examination of the role of family in contemporary China mainland, Hong Kong and Taiwan. In D. Sinha and H. S. R. Kao (Eds.). *Social values and development: Asian perspectives.* New Delhi: Sage Publications.

Yang, J., McCrae, R. R., and Costa, P. T. Jr. (1998). Adult age differences in personality traits in the United States and the People's Republic of China. *Journal of Gerontology: Psychological Sciences, 53B,* 375-383.

Zhang, Z., and Yang, C. F. (1998). Beyond distributive Justine: The reasonableness norm in Chinese reward allocation. *Asian Journal of Social Psychology, 1,* 253-269.

Zheng, X., and Berry, J. W. (1991). Psychological adaptation of Chinese sojourners in Canada. *International Journal of Psychology, 26,* 451-470.

In: Aging and the Elderly: Psychology, Sociology and Health ISBN 1-60021-190-9
Editor: L. O. Randall, pp. 89-114

Chapter 4

ENVIRONMENTAL COMPLEXITY AND INTELLECTUAL FUNCTIONING IN OLDER PEOPLE: RESEARCH FINDINGS AND IMPLICATIONS

Mesfin Samuel Mulatu
The MayaTech Corporation, Atlanta, Georgia, USA
Carmi Schooler
National Institute of Mental Health, Bethesda, Maryland, USA

ABSTRACT

In this chapter we review the research examining the effects of the complexity of paid work and leisure time activities on older people's intellectual functioning. We find that much of the research does not take sufficient account of the possibility that correlations found between intellectual functioning and the complexity of paid work and leisure time activities may reflect the possibility that having a high level of intellectual functioning increases the likelihood that an individual may want to, or be in a position where they are expected to, engage in cognitively demanding tasks. Nevertheless, this research evidence is at least congruent with the possibility that carrying out intellectually demanding activities positively effects older individuals' intellectual functioning. We find stronger evidence for the positive effects of cognitively complex activities on older people's intellectual functioning in studies that employ statistics permitting the separation of the effects of complex activities on individuals' intellectual functioning from the effects of individuals' intellectual functioning on their likelihood carrying out complex intellectually demanding activities at work or at leisure. The tenor of findings from relevant animal and human experimental studies, as well as the outcomes of intervention studies with both normal individuals and those suffering from dementia, provide further support for the positive effects of cognitively complex activities on the intellectual functioning of the elderly. We conclude by discussing the theoretical and practical implications of the evidence that environmental complexity has a positive effect on the intellectual functioning of older people.

General Background and Theory

In this chapter, we examine the effects of complexity of paid work and leisure time activities on older peoples' intellectual functioning. In doing so we provide evidence that even late in the life course carrying out intellectually demanding tasks both on and off of the job positively affects intellectual functioning. Establishing the existence of such a cognitive effect of occupational and non-occupational conditions is clearly of direct interest to those concerned with understanding how the environment affects the psychological functioning of older people. At a theoretical level, gaining such an understanding is obviously important for what it would tell us about the nature of the human condition and life course. At a more practical level, such knowledge would also provide necessary insights into designing programs and environments that would improve the life experience of the elderly.

Plausible, yet contradictory, hypotheses exist about the effects of intellectually demanding activities on the cognitive functioning of normal older adults. On the one hand, there are reasons to believe that older individuals would be more adversely affected than younger ones by intellectually demanding environmental conditions. If cognitive speed (Salthouse, 1991) and/or working memory (Baddeley, 1986) decline with age, one might predict that older workers would react particularly poorly to such demanding environmental conditions. On the other hand, it could be argued that the very existence of such deficits might make it more important for older than for younger individuals to be in environments that demand that they continue to practice and develop their intellectual skills (see Schooler, Caplan, & Oates, 1998, for an overview of the psychological literature relevant to issues of aging and work).

As we shall see there is a fair amount of evidence demonstrating the existence of a correlation between elderly individuals' levels of intellectual functioning and the intellectual demandingness of the tasks they perform. The core problem is discerning the direction of causal effects that underlie this correlation. Any given correlation between relatively high levels of cognitive function and participation in a particular cognitively demanding activity can be, on the one hand, the result of dealing with the cognitive demands imposed by that activity. On the other hand, such a correlation may be the result of having characteristics that increase the likelihood of selecting, or being selected, to engage in and stay engaged that activity. At its most basic level, the question is how much is such a correlation the result of the effect of the characteristics of the environment on the characteristics of the person and how much of the correlation is the result of the plausible reciprocal effect of the characteristics of the person on the environment.

There are really only two basic ways of dealing with this issue: 1) experimentation or 2) complex statistical modeling of longitudinal data (e.g., structural equation modeling) – neither of which is perfect. Experiments, in which subjects are randomly assigned to relevant experimental conditions, are almost invariably limited in: a) types and numbers of participants that can be used, and b) the power, length and encompassingness of the manipulations. Statistical modeling, in turn, is limited by: a) the inability to completely rule out the possibility that some variable not included in the model is at work either in terms of selecting individuals into particular environments or because a given set of environmental conditions may have different effects on different types of individuals, and b) the intractability of certain types and distributions of data to appropriate statistical manipulation.

We believe that, given the limitations of both types of approach, at present the best estimates of the effects of environmental conditions on the intellectual functioning of elderly individuals in the real world is provided by statistical modeling of longitudinal data. The original findings based on the latter approach come from the Kohn-Schooler research program on the psychological effects of occupational conditions carried out on a representative sample of US workers by the Laboratory of Socio-Environmental Studies of the National Institute of Mental Health.

In what follows we will 1) describe these early Kohn-Schooler US studies and tests of the generalizability of their findings in other industrial societies, 2) discuss other relatively recent relevant studies that do not directly face the issue of plausible reciprocal effects, including studies on normal and clinically significant cognitive decline, 3) detail our own more recent studies based on the original Kohn-Schooler sample that extend the earlier findings outside of the work place and along the life course, and 4) discuss some experimental studies that lend further support to the findings and provide some insight into relevant cognitive and neuropsychobiological mechanisms.

Earlier Kohn-Schooler Studies of Environmental Complexity and Intellectual Functioning

The early Kohn-Schooler studies (Kohn & Schooler, 1978, 1983) explored the potential reciprocal and/or cross-lagged effects of environmental complexity and intellectual functioning. The research program was carried out in the Laboratory of Socioenvironmental Studies of the National Institute of Mental Health. It used structural equation model (SEM) based analyses of longitudinal survey data collected from a representative sample of American men in 1964 and a representative sub-sample of those men re-interviewed in 1974. In terms of cognitive functioning, its central hypothesis was that cognitively complex environmental conditions (e.g., paid work, leisure activities) have a positive effect, and cognitively simple environmental conditions have a negative effect on overall intellectual functioning of individuals exposed to them. The program also hypothesized that individuals' levels of intellectual functioning reciprocally affected the cognitive demandingness of their environments because individuals would be relatively more likely to choose to, to be chosen to, and to continue to participate in activities whose cognitive demands matched their intellectual capacities. In most of these studies, the use of SEM permitted the estimation of non-recursive reciprocal effects models that tested the degree to which the correlation found between an environmental condition and a psychological characteristic reflected the effect of the environmental condition on that psychological characteristic-- as compared to the degree to which having that characteristic leads to choosing or keeping that environmental condition.

Job Complexity and Intellectual Functioning

The most extensively studied environmental complexity factor in the Kohn-Schooler research program is the substantive complexity of paid work. In terms of its effect on intellectual functioning, the program's central longitudinal finding is that job conditions offering challenge and opportunity for doing self-directed substantively complex work increase men's intellectual flexibility. Work conditions that limit intellectual challenge and self-direction on the job decrease men's intellectual flexibility (Kohn & Schooler, 1983). Kohn and Schooler also found a significant lagged effect of earlier intellectual functioning on the subsequent substantive complexity of men's paid work, suggesting a reciprocal relationship over time between complexity of work done and psychological functioning.

Several other non-longitudinal studies from the Kohn-Schooler research program provided further support for the hypothesized casual connection between complex, cognitively-demanding work conditions and intellectual functioning. These included studies of U.S. women's paid work (J. Miller, Kohn, Schooler, & K. Miller, 1979; Kohn & Schooler, 1983, chap. 8), as well as studies of paid work in a variety of cross-cultural settings including Japan (A. Naoi & Schooler, 1985; M. Naoi & Schooler, 1990; Schooler & M. Naoi, 1988), Poland (Kohn & Slomczynski, 1990), and Ukraine (Kohn, et al., 1997). The same relationship between substantively complex work and intellectual flexibility had also been found in other types of work, such as school work (K. Miller, Kohn, & Schooler, 1986) and women's housework (Schooler, J. Miller, K. Miller, & Richtand, 1984; Kohn & Schooler, 1983, chap. 10; for fuller reviews and discussions of these various extensions of the Kohn-Schooler occupational findings see Schooler, 1990, 1996).

Another important finding comes from Miller, Slomczynski, and Kohn's (1985) analyses of the causal connection between substantively complex work and intellectual flexibility in different age cohorts in both the United States and Poland. Using SEM to estimate reciprocal effects models with the data from the Kohn-Schooler US survey and its Polish replication, Miller, Slomczynski, and Kohn found that in both countries, substantively complex work increases intellectual flexibility in both younger and older cohorts. Taking into account the overall pattern of their findings, particularly with their US sample (i.e., the 1964-1974 Kohn-Schooler sample), Miller, Slomczynski, and Kohn suggest that "the reciprocal effects of the substantive complexity and ideational flexibility are not only as strong for older as for younger men but may even be stronger for older men" (p. 609). What clearly differed among the cohorts was the substantive complexity of the work done. In both countries, older workers did less substantively complex work.

The Kohn-Schooler research program also provided evidence that the intellectual demandingness of occupational conditions can affect the intellectual demandingness of off-the-job experiences. Using data from the Kohn-Schooler occupational study, K. Miller and Kohn (1983) compared the degree to which doing substantively complex work on the job increases the intellectual complexity of leisure time activities to the degree to which having intellectually complex leisure time activities increases the substantive complexity of work done on the job. They found both reciprocal causal paths to be significant. As expected, given the greater control that individuals would seem to have over the nature of their leisure time activities than of their jobs, the path from the substantive complexity of individuals' leisure time activities to the substantive complexity of their work was significantly smaller than it's reciprocal. These conclusions hold true even when individuals' levels of intellectual functioning are controlled.

Leisure Activities and Intellectual Functioning

Although the above studies did not directly link leisure time activity to intellectual functioning, a recent study that has its historical origins in the Kohn-Schooler research program has provided evidence suggesting that the complexity of leisure activities has a positive effect on intellectual functioning. Based on research carried out in Eastern Europe, Kohn and colleagues (2000) found that the complexity of activities outside, as well as in, paid employment is linked to intellectual flexibility. Kohn et al. find this empirical connection to exist even under the conditions of radical social change typifying Poland as it moved from a socialist to a capitalist economy in the winter of 1992. They uncover very specific empirical links, not only between intellectual flexibility and the substantive complexity of men's and women's paid employment and women's housework, but also between intellectual flexibility and the complexity of both male and female pensioners' activities. The absence of longitudinal data in their East-European study deterred Kohn et al. from using SEM to estimate reciprocal effects models that would assess the causal patterns underlying these relationships. In the absence of such analyses, Kohn et al. make the case that the consonance of their findings with those of longitudinal and simulated longitudinal analyses of past studies strongly suggests that these relationships, too, are reciprocal.

In sum, the Kohn-Schooler research program provides clear evidence for the existence of reciprocal effects between the substantive complexity of paid work and intellectual functioning of individuals in various societies. Related cross-cultural studies have also provided evidence that substantive complexity of work and leisure time activities are clearly related to better intellectual functioning. More generally, the results from earlier Kohn-Schooler occupational studies are consistent with a large body of research from a wide range of disciplines including cognitive aging and animal-based neurobiology studies which strongly suggests that exposure to complex environments increases intellectual functioning throughout the life course and across species. A detailed review of the earlier psychological evidence is presented in Schooler (1984, 1990), which also presents a rough-hewn theory of the psychological mechanisms underlying such effects. Mohammed et al. (2002) provide a quite complete up-to-date review of relevant animal studies demonstrating the neuroplastic changes in the brains of both young and old mammals in response to environmental enrichment. In a later section of this chapter, we will describe some examples of such research. In the following section, we review relatively recent studies from other research groups aimed at investigating the relationship between environmental complexity and cognitive functioning in older people.

Other Studies Linking Environmental Complexity and Intellectual Functioning

Interest in the effects of environmental factors on aging has sparked a great deal of research directed at the correlates or determinants of cognitive functioning among older people with or without dementia or other degenerative diseases. Although the findings from these studies are not completely consistent, the preponderance of the evidence is quite consistent with the hypothesis that exposure to enriched or intellectually challenging environments has a positive effect on intellectual functioning among older people. There is, however, a caveat that hinders our fully accepting their findings as proof of this hypothesis. Although sometimes longitudinal, these studies tend to employ research approaches that focus on testing for the existence of relationships between environmental conditions and cognitive functioning, while controlling for the effects of other potentially relevant factors (e.g., education). The research approaches they employ, however, do not directly explore the potential reciprocal relationships between environmental complexity and intellectual functioning. Consequently, they do not rule out the possibility that the relationships that they find are due to the greater likelihood that relatively intelligent individuals will be selected into, and selectively stay in, relatively intellectually demanding environments.

Environmental Complexity and Normal Cognitive Functioning

Job Complexity and Normal Cognitive Functioning

Using non-longitudinal data collected by the U.S. Employment Service, Avolio and Waldman examined the relationship between the cognitive demandingness of jobs and intellectual functioning across the life span. In their first paper, they found a significant positive correlation between the intellectual functioning of workers and job complexity (Avolio & Waldman, 1990). In their second paper (Avolio & Waldman, 1994) they found a positive relationship between worker intellectual functioning and a fairly rough measure of the cognitive demands of their occupations, even when age, race and gender and education are taken into account. In neither paper was there a significant interaction among age, cognitive demandingness of their job and intellectual functioning. The absence of such an interaction suggests that the relationships between cognitive functioning and the cognitive demands of job conditions as Avolio and Waldman index them do not vary with age. More generally, Avolio and Waldman (1994) conclude that their findings suggest that there "may be unique factors in the work context that affect the maintenance or abilities, the decline of abilities or both across the life span" (p. 438).

In a prospective study, Bosma and colleagues (2003) explored the relationships between mental workload, educational attainment, and cognitive functioning among 708 Dutch men and women aged 50 to 80. The authors coded the self-reported description of the study participants' current or most recent job using a scheme similar to the U.S. Dictionary of Occupational Titles. A mental workload score was then assigned to each job category depending on responses to questions that asked whether or not the job was mentally demanding and requires strong concentration, great precision, and working under time pressure. The study revealed two important findings: 1) lower levels of educational attainment and cognitive workload at baseline were significantly associated with stronger decline in longitudinal cognitive functioning, measured by differences in scores on processing speed, memory and a general cognitive status examination; 2) cognitive workload accounted for 42% of the effect of educational attainment on cognitive functioning. The authors concluded that providing work-related cognitive stimuli and challenges for poorly educated people might help in reducing the age-related gap in cognitive decline between poorly and highly educated people.

Leisure Activities and Normal Cognitive Functioning

Bosma and colleagues (2002) provided some evidence for the potential reciprocal effects between leisure time activities and cognitive functioning among 830 non-demented middle and old-aged men and women in The Netherlands. In this 3-year longitudinal study, the authors estimated two separate regression models. In the first model, level of leisure activities at baseline was related to follow-up cognitive functioning, even when age, sex, educational level, and baseline cognitive functioning were controlled. In the second model, cognitive functioning at baseline was related to follow-up leisure activities, controlling for baseline age, sex, educational level, and leisure activities. The authors thus found a converse positive relationship between leisure activities and cognitive functioning, and suggested that stimulating individuals to participate in leisure activities may prevent the development of adverse cognitive functioning which in turn would affect participation in leisure activities. Although the authors did not test the reciprocal effects in the same model simultaneously, their findings are congruent with the hypothesis (Schooler, 1984, 1990) that environmental complexity has a positive effect on intellectual functioning throughout the life span.

Two other papers based on longitudinal data sets unrelated to the Kohn- Schooler studies report having tested the Schooler environmental complexity hypothesis with apparently conflicting results: supported vs. not supported. Pushkar Gold, Andres, Etezadi, Arbuckle, Schwartzman, and Chaikelson (1995) see their analyses of data from the Canadian Army Veterans Study as supporting the hypothesis by demonstrating that an engaged life-style, which they specifically link to exposure to complex environments, has a positive effect on intellectual functioning late in life. Hultsch, Hertzog, Small, and Dixon (1999), using data from the Victoria Longitudinal Study, view their analyses as not providing a strong support to the environmental complexity hypothesis. They reach their conclusion because a model in which exposure to environmental complexity increases intellectual functioning fits their data no better than a model in which the reverse effect of high levels of intellectual functioning increase exposure to complex environments. In addition, Hultsch et al. (1999) reanalyzed the Pushkar Gold et al. (1995) Canadian Veterans' data and conclude that when properly analyzed this data set also supports their conclusion that the levels of intellectual functioning has a stronger effect on participation in complex lifestyle activities than the reverse effect Pushkar Gold et al. (1995) reported. These conclusions led to a round of conflicting comments by the two sets of authors (Hertzog, Hultsch, & Dixon, 1999; Pushkar, Etezadi, Andres, Arbuckle, Schwartzman, & Chaikelson, 1999) with each side staunchly defending its position. Although both studies' findings are congruent with the existence of a reciprocal causal connection between exposure to complex environments and relatively high level intellectual functioning, neither study directly evaluated this possibility.

In a recent cross-sectional study that explored the relationship between cognitive stimulation and cognitive functioning among adults aged 20 to 80, Salthouse, Berish, and Miles (2002) claim to have found no evidence that engaging in cognitively stimulating activities and cognitive functioning are related and, therefore, no support for the hypothesis that cognitive stimulation preserves or enhances functioning that would otherwise decline with age. Their findings are in sharp contrast with the growing evidence that supports the positive effects of engaging in complex environments on cognitive functioning. By the authors' admission, the cross-sectional nature of the study and the fact that the study participants were relatively highly educated and healthy may have underestimated the relationships between cognitive stimulation and cognitive functioning. Of at least equal concern, is that their measure of cognitive stimulation was a subjective one – based on the respondents' own judgment of the cognitive demandingness of the activities in which they participate. It seems more than plausible that this subjectivity may have seriously affected their results, since there is every reason to believe that individuals' ratings of the cognitive demandingness of a given activity would be affected by their level of cognitive functioning.

In sum, with the exception of Salthouse et al. (2002), the studies reviewed in this section provide support to, or are at least congruent with, the environmental complexity and/or the cognitive reserve hypothesis. Nevertheless, despite some efforts at estimating separate models to test each hypothesis, none of these studies deals forthrightly with the question of the degree to which correlations found between levels of environmental complexity and intellectual functioning reflect the psychological effects of complex environments or the degree to which individuals who function well intellectually select or are selected into such environments.

Environmental Complexity and Clinical Cognitive Decline

Job Complexity and Clinical Cognitive Decline

An indirect support for the positive effects of occupational complexity on intellectual functioning is provided by studies that linked occupational categories with the incidence of clinically significant cognitive decline among older people. In a longitudinal Swedish study that followed 913 non-demented older people (aged 75 or more) for more than six years, Qiu et al. (2003) found the longest held occupational position to be one of the predictors of the risk of Alzheimer's disease. Specifically, the authors found that having manual work as the longest held occupational position, particularly work involving goods production, was associated with greater risk for Alzheimer's disease and all types of dementia than having a non-manual work. Although the authors speculated that exposure to multi-toxic work environment, poor socio-economic conditions and lifestyle, and lower initial intelligence as potential mechanisms underlying the association between manual work and the risk of Alzheimer's disease and dementia, other occupational mechanisms, such as the routineness and cognitively less challenging nature of manual work, cannot be ruled out.

Several other studies from the United States and other industrialized societies have also found a link between occupational conditions or categories and dementia among older populations. In the United States, Stern et al. (1994) followed 593 non-demented individuals 60 years or older for one to four years. They found that the risk of incident dementia was significantly higher among individuals with lower occupational attainment and education, and concluded that a deficit in these factors may contribute to lower cognitive reserve that potentially delays the manifestation of dementia. In a longitudinal study in France, Dartigues and colleagues (1992) analyzed their baseline data from a large community sample (N=3777) of people aged 65 and older. The authors found that, after controlling for age, sex, educational level, and other covariates, farm workers, domestic service employees, and blue-collar workers had higher risk of cognitive impairment than did participants who had an "intellectual occupation". In a longitudinal analysis using the same sample, they found that women farmers had a higher risk of dementia compared to men and women professionals and managers (Helmer, et al., 2001). No difference was found in the risk of Alzheimer's disease by occupation.

Although the above studies provide evidence that links occupational conditions to declining cognitive functioning among older people, they generally do not seem to have estimated the degree to which their findings reflect the relationship between levels of cognitive performance and the likelihood of getting and keeping a job characterized by a given level of cognitive demand. Consequently, the direction of the causal connection underlying the observed correlations remains unknown. In addition, when the cognitive demandingness of the work environment is estimated through the use of broad occupational categories, the level of occupational complexity is not directly measured, but only assumed.

Leisure Activities and Clinical Cognitive Decline

Relevant studies also generally report a positive relationship between participation in leisure time activities, particularly cognitively demanding ones, and non-demented cognitive functioning among older people. For instance, Wilson et al. (2002) tested the hypothesis that frequent participation in cognitive activities is associated with a reduced risk of Alzheimer disease, using data from a sample of 801 Catholic nuns, priests, and brothers in the United States. The authors found that a unit of cognitive activity score, measured by seven common activities such as reading newspaper, listening to radio, and reading books, at baseline was associated with a 33% reduction in risk of Alzheimer disease approximately four years later at follow-up. In addition, controlling for age, gender, education, and baseline cognitive functioning, a unit of increase in cognitive activity was associated with reduced general cognitive aging by 47%, working memory by 60%, and perceptual speed by 30%.

Similarly, Verghese and colleagues (2003) followed 469 older people in New York aged 75 years or above for about five years, and examined the effects of the effects of leisure time activities and the risk of dementia. The authors found participation in leisure activities to be associated with a reduced risk of dementia, even after controlling for base-line cognitive status, age, sex, educational level, and chronic medical illnesses. More importantly, the study revealed that it was participation in cognitively demanding leisure activities (e.g., reading, playing board games, and playing musical instruments), rather than participation in physical leisure activities, that had a positive effect on cognitive functioning.

Similar results have also been reported by studies from other industrial nations. Using data from 776 participants (aged 75 years and older) in a longitudinal population study in Stockholm, Sweden, Wang, et al. (2002) examined whether engagement in various leisure activities more than six years before the diagnosis of dementia was related to increased or decreased risk of the incidence of dementia. Wang et al. found that frequent engagement in mental, social, or productive activities at baseline was inversely associated with the incidence of dementia. Not unlike the Verghese et al. study, the results of this study suggest that the participation of older people in socially and intellectually stimulating activities may be relevant in the preservation of their cognitive functioning. Another Swedish study has also found that greater participation in overall leisure time activities, that included intellectual-cultural, self-empowering, and domestic activities, was associated with lower levels of risk for Alzheimer's disease and dementia twenty years later (Crowe et al. 2003). Interestingly, in this study greater participation in intellectual-cultural activities reduced the risk of Alzheimer's disease among female more than male participants.

Friedland and colleagues (2001) have also established that, compared to healthy case-controls, patients with Alzheimer's disease show reduced diversity of overall activities and intensity of intellectual activities at least five years prior to the onset of the disease. Healthy controls were found to be more active than Alzheimer's disease patients during their early adulthood (ages 20-39) as well as mid-adulthood (ages 40-50) in all activity categories, including passive, social, and intellectual activities, even when age, gender, education, and income adequacy were taken into account. The findings for middle adulthood also held true when early adult leisure activity level is controlled. The fact that spending relatively little leisure time in intellectually demanding activities in middle adulthood is predictive of Alzheimer's disease, even when the percent of leisure time spent in such activities in early adulthood is controlled, decreases the likelihood that the lower level of intellectual leisure time activities in middle adulthood characteristic of those who later develop AD is a function of some type of early-adulthood pre-symptomatic cognitive dysfunction such as described in the Nun Study (Snowden et al., 1996).

All in all, the findings of the studies described here, which are generally representative of those in the literature, are strikingly congruent with the possibility that participating in relatively intellectually demanding leisure time activities acts to decrease the likelihood of senile dementia. Carrying out such activities may have such an effect through increasing cognitive reserve that "may buffer the underlying damage associated with the early stages of dementia, thereby delaying the onset of symptoms" (Coyle, 2000, p. 2490), and/or by promoting "plastic changes in the brain that circumvent the pathology underlying the symptoms of dementia" (Coyle, 2002, p. 2490).

Recent Findings from the Section on Socioenvironmental Studies on Environmental Complexity and Intellectual Functioning

Several relatively recent papers from our NIMH Section of Socio-Environmental Studies (SSES) have specifically tested the possibility of reciprocal effects between environmental complexity and intellectual studies in older individuals (Schooler, Mulatu & Oates 1999, Schooler & Mulatu 2001, Schooler, Mulatu & Oates 2004). In these papers we expanded the earlier Kohn-Schooler studies by examining the reciprocal relationships between the complexity of paid work (Schooler, Mulatu, & Oates, 1999) or leisure time activities (Schooler & Mulatu, 2001) and intellectual functioning using data collected in 1974 and in 1994/1995, when the original participants had aged by about 20 years. In order to provide the context to our discussion, we briefly describe: 1) the sample from which the longitudinal data for these studies were derived; 2) our measures of environmental complexity and intellectual functioning, and 3) our mode of data analysis and major findings.

Characteristics of the Longitudinal Sample

The first wave data collection for the Kohn-Schooler study of the psychological effects of occupational conditions began in 1964, during which a national representative sample (N= 3101) of employed men were interviewed in 1964. The sample was an area probability sample drawn by the National Opinion Research Center (NORC) of males over 16 years of age then currently employed at least 25 hours per week in non-military occupations. In 1974,

NORC interviewed a representative sub-sample of approximately one-fourth of the 1964 respondents who were less than 65 years old at that time. Of the 883 men who were randomly selected for the follow-up study, 820 (93%) were located. Of the 785 men who were still alive, 687 (88%) were interviewed. In addition, in the 1974 study we also interviewed the wife of every male respondent who was then married. Interviews were conducted with 555 women, 90% of the 617 eligible. They ranged in age from 26 to 65 years. In the 1994/1995 follow-up, we succeeded in locating 95% (650) of the 687 households that took part in the 1974 survey. Of the 1242 men and women interviewed in 1974, 707 (352 men and 355 women) were re-interviewed in 1994/1995; others were not located, had died, or did not complete the interview because of illness or refusal.

In our study examining the reciprocal effects of substantive complexity of paid work and intellectual functioning (Schooler, Mulatu, & Oates, 1999), we focused only on those people who worked both in 1974 and 1994/1995. There were 244 men and women who worked in both times, of which 11 did not provide work-related data and were subsequently excluded. Thus, the effective sample size for this study was 233, of which 160 were males and 73 were females. Age of the participants ranged from 41 to 83; their median age was 57. Fourteen respondents were African Americans and the rest were European Americans. Their median level of education was high school graduate with some technical schooling.

In our analysis examining the reciprocal effects of cognitively demanding leisure time activities and intellectual functioning (Schooler & Mulatu, 2001), we focused on all those that provided data on their leisure time activities and intellectual functioning. Seventy two out of the 707 participants were excluded because they completed only a shortened telephone version of the survey that did not contain necessary questions about leisure time activities. Thus, the effective sample size for this study was 635: 315 men and 320 women. The respondents ranged in age from 41 to 88 years with a mean of 64.5 (SD = 9.6). There were 595 European Americans, 33 African Americans, and 7 respondents from other racial or ethnic origins. Their median level of education was high school graduate with some technical schooling. During the 1994/1995 follow-up interview, 265 (41.7%) were working for pay.

All in all, the differences we found between those we did and did not re-interview suggest that we may want to temper the generalizations we make with the acknowledgment that female, older, unemployed, less educated people, and African Americans may be slightly underrepresented in our 1994 sample. Nevertheless, unless there are some unknown interactions involving these variables biasing who among the located respondents was re-interviewed, and the relationships among our variables of central concern (i.e., intellectual functioning and the cognitive complexity of work and leisure activities), the findings we report are probably generalizable. Our results are not likely to be unduly influenced by differences between the characteristics of those who were and who were not reinterviewed. This is so, not only because the characteristics identified as affecting the likelihood of being reinterviewed were statistically controlled, but also because the individual, in a sense, serves as his/her own control since our analyses essentially involve an examination of how each individual's work or leisure time activity affects and is affected by his/her own intellectual functioning over time.

Measurement of Environmental Complexity

Substantive Complexity of Work

We defined substantively complex work as work that in its very substance requires thought and independent judgment (Kohn & Schooler, 1983, p. 106). Indices for the latent concept of substantive complexity of work are derived from detailed open- and closed-ended questions about the participants' work with things, data (or ideas) and people. For the 1974 and 1994/1995 jobs, these questions provided the basis for seven ratings: appraisals of complexity of work with things, with data and with people based on those of the Dictionary of Occupational Titles ([DOT]; U.S. Department of Labor, 1965), the respondents' estimates of the amount of time they spent working at each type of activity and an appraisal of the overall complexity of work. Each index of complexity of work was rated on Likert type scales. For example, complexity of work with data was rated on a 1 to 9 scale: 1 = no significant work with data to 9 = synthesizing. Hours of work with things ranged from 0 to 90 and were recorded as given.

Complexity of Leisure Activities

We defined the cognitive complexity of leisure time activities in similar terms as we defined the complexity of paid work, except that the term refers to activities that are not done as part of paid work or housework. Our *Cognitive Leisure Activities* latent factor was measured by six items that were included in both the 1974 and 1994/1995 surveys. These were: 1) the number of books read within the past six months; 2) the number of magazines read regularly; 2) the intellectual level of the magazines read, rated from low to high intellectuality on a five point scale; 4) the frequency of visits to fine art institutions or events including museums, concerts, and plays within the past six months; 5) the number of special interests, hobbies, and activities; and 6) the number of hours spent on special interests, hobbies, and activities in a month.

Measurement of Intellectual Functioning

We define *intellectual flexibility*, our measure of intellectual functioning, as cognitive flexibility in coping with the intellectual demands of a complex situation (see Kohn & Schooler, 1983, p. 112). Indices for this factor included the following: 1) a summary score for performance on a portion of the Embedded Figures Test (Witkin, Dyk, Faterson, Goodenough, & Karp, 1962); 2) the interviewer's appraisal of the participant's intelligence made on the basis of the interviewer's impression during the interview session, rated on a five point scale (from 1 = dull or uncomprehending to 5 = much above average intelligence); 3) the frequency with which the respondent agreed when asked the many agree-disagree questions included in the interview (because some of the questions included in the battery were stated positively and others negatively, an overall tendency to agree suggested that the participant was not thinking carefully about and was less differentiating among the questions); 4) a rating of the degree to which the answer to the question "What are all of the arguments you can think of for or against allowing cigarette commercials on TV?" provided reasons for both sides of the argument; and 5) a rating of the adequacy of the answer to a hypothetical question about how the respondent would decide between two alternate locations for a hamburger stand (adequacy being judged by a concern with potential costs, with potential sales and with the understanding that profits result from the difference between the

Data Analysis and Major Findings

In each of our studies, we first established the soundness of the measurement properties of the environmental complexity and intellectual functioning measures. We then examined whether or not previous findings of reciprocal effects between environmental complexity and intellectual functioning can be extended, even after our respondents have aged by 20 years. Our general model showing the hypothesized reciprocal relationships between environmental complexity and intellectual functioning are shown in Figure 1.

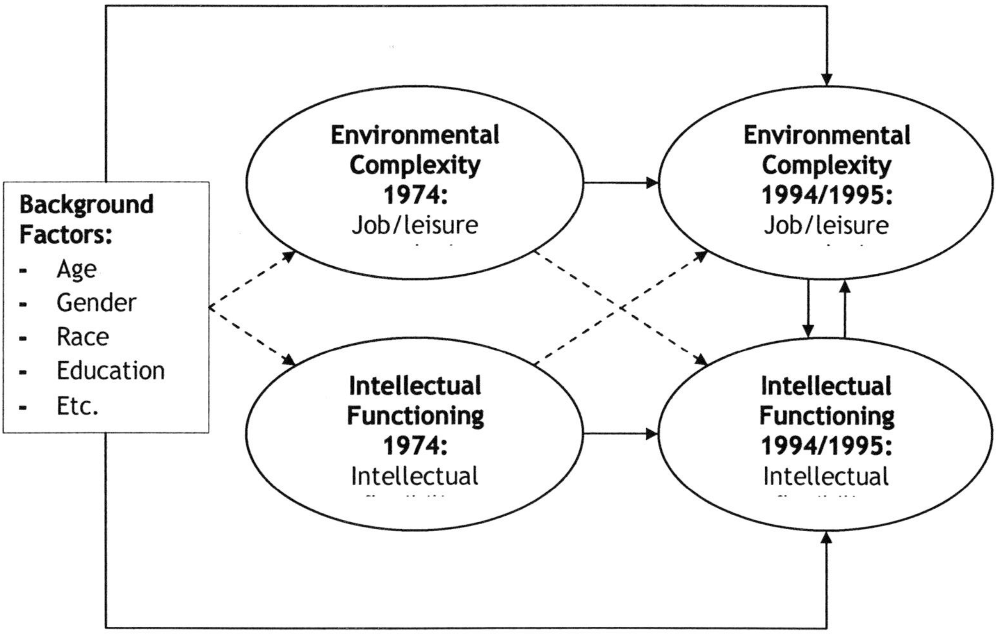

Figure 1. General model of environmental complexity and intellectual functioning.

We chose to model the relationships of the work and leisure time environmental complexity latent factors to intellectual functioning separately. We did so because we had leisure time activity measures on the non-working as well as the working members of our sample and were therefore able to carry out the leisure analyses on a larger sample and avoid the complexities of modeling the combined effects leisure and work activities on a relatively small sized sample.

Adequacy of the Core Longitudinal Measures

Using SEM, we tested the appropriateness of our measures for substantive complexity of work, cognitive leisure activities, and intellectual flexibility. In testing our measurement models, we constrained the factor loadings (λs) for the same observed indicators to be equal across time (i.e., 1974 vs. 1994/1995) and across groups (e.g., younger vs. older) in analyses that involved multiple groups. In each case, we did, however, examine the modification indices to see whether these constraints significantly distorted the model. There were only minor group or overtime differences, and we allowed these differences to be incorporated in the models by relaxing the constraints.

Table 1. Completely standardized factor loadings of the core 1974 -1994/1995 measures of environmental complexity and intellectual functioning factors

Observed Indictors	Standardized Loadings
Substantive Complexity of Work Factor	
1. Complexity of work with data	.77[a]
2. Complexity of work with things	.17**
3. Complexity of work with people	.62***
4. Overall complexity of work	.67***
5. Hours of work with things	-.41***
6. Hours of work with data	.44***
7. Hours of work with people	.37***
χ^2/df	1.62
RMSEA	.07
CFI	.87
Cognitive Leisure Activities Factor	
1. Number of magazines read	.78[a]
2. Number of books read	.22***
3. Intellectual level of magazines read	.77***
4. Frequency of visits to arts	.35***
5. Number of hobbies/ interests	.45***
6. Hours spent on hobbies/ interests	.31***
χ^2/df	2.26
RMSEA	.06
CFI	.95
Intellectual Flexibility Factor	
1. Interviewer's estimate of intelligence	.48[a]
2. Embedded Figures Test	.32***
3. 'Agree' score on agree-disagree question	-.45***
4. 'Cigarette Commercial' question	.28***
5. 'Hamburger Stand' question	.21***
χ^2/df	2.57
RMSEA	.07
CFI	.90

Note: ** $p < .01$; *** $p < .001$; [a] = reference variables whose t-values can not be computed. In all analyses, indicators of concepts are constrained to be invariant across groups (i.e., younger = older or Working = Non-working) and across time (i.e., 1974 = 1994/1995). Number of observations for the substantive complexity model was 233; for cognitive leisure activity model it was 635.

As shown in Table 1, our measurement models fit the data very well, with most of the fit indices being well within the acceptable range and the specific parameter indices showing that the indicators as significant indices of the latent factors. Thus, the meaning of the latent concepts as defined by the factor loadings is invariant across time and groups in our analyses.

We have also confirmed that our two measures, namely Cognitive Leisure Activities and Intellectual Flexibility, are also strongly correlated with standard measures used elsewhere. We did this by correlating these factors with corresponding factors created with data available only in 1994/1995. Leisure activity measures in 1994/1995 included the six items used to indicate our longitudinal Cognitive Leisure Activity factor as well as five ratings of the complexity leisure time activities with people and data and the hours spent on these activities -- parallel measure to the substantive complexity of paid work. The correlation between Cognitive Leisure Activities and the new factor, Complexity of Leisure Activities in 1994/1995, was quite high (r = .89 p < .0001) suggesting that our longitudinally available measure indeed taps both the complexity and intellectuality of leisure time activities. Similarly, our Intellectual Flexibility measure was highly correlated (r = .86, p < .0001) with newly available factor, Psychometric Intellectual Functioning, which was based on scores of standard cognitive tests, including immediate recall, category fluency, number series, verbal meaning, identical pictures, and different uses tests. Thus, we confirmed that our survey based intellectual functioning measures was as good a measure as the standard cognitive measures available in the field.

Job Complexity and Intellectual Functioning

In order to deal with the small sample size we have for this analysis (N=233), we followed a two-stage causal modeling approach. Initially, the measurement model was developed and estimated. The covariances between the latent factors from these measurement models were then saved and used as input data in the subsequent causal modeling. The model specifications were as follows: reciprocal effects between 1994/1995 Substantive Complexity of Work and 1994/1995 Intellectual Flexibility, paths from 1974 Substantive Complexity of Work and from 1974 Intellectual Flexibility to their to corresponding 1994/1995 endogenous factors; and paths to these endogenous factors from all socio-demographic characteristics, including age, gender, education, and others demographic characteristics were included as statistical controls.

Given our interest in age related differences and similarities, we tested this model in an age-based multigroup analysis by splitting the sample in to two age groups using the median age of 57. In testing this causal model, only the error and residual variances and covariances were allowed to vary across groups, and modification indices were inspected to determine the presence or absence of significant causal parameters that needed relaxing. In subsequent re-estimations of the model, we also dropped insignificant structural paths.

Our model fit the data very well (χ^2 [df= 218, N=233]=142.20, p = 1.00; RMSEA = .00; CFI = 1.00) and that the hypothesized relationships were actually confirmed (see Figure 2 below). First, we found significant paths from 1994/1995 Substantive Complexity of Work and 1994/1995 Intellectual Flexibility as well as a significant reverse path from 1994/1995 Intellectual Flexibility to 1994/1995 Substantive Complexity of Work – thus confirming the existence of reciprocal relationships. Second, we found a significant age group difference in the path from 1994/1995 Substantive Complexity of Work to 1994/1995 Intellectual Flexibility, showing that the impact of Substantive Complexity on Intellectual Flexibility is about twice as great in the older group (β = .50, t = 14.87) than in the younger group (β = .26, t = 3.47). Third, although there was no age group difference in the reverse path from 1994/1995 Intellectual Flexibility to 1994/1995 Substantive Complexity of Work, the relative magnitude of this path (β = .25) compared to its reciprocal (the path from 1994/1995 Substantive Complexity to 1994/1995 Intellectual Flexibility) was different for the two groups. For the younger group it is about the same size as the reciprocal effect of Substantive Complexity on Intellectual Flexibility; for the older group, it is about half the size. Finally, background sociodemographic characteristics have important direct and indirect effects on Substantive Complexity of Work as well as Intellectual Flexibility.

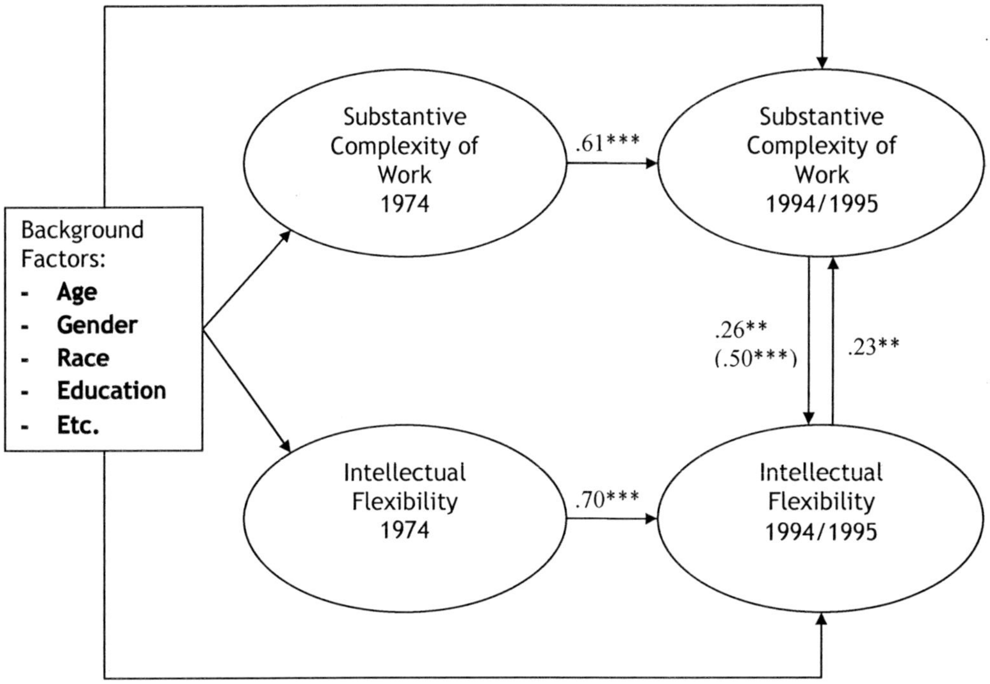

Note. Chi-sqaure= 142.20, p = 1.00; chi-square/d.f. = .65; RMSEA = .00; CFI = 1.00.
Numbers in the figure are completely standardized coefficients. * p < .05; ** p < .01; *** p < .001. Paths from background variables to substantive complexity and intellectual flexibility and intercorrelations of the exogenous variables are also not shown. When two coefficients are provided for a path, the one within the bracket is for the older group and the other for the younger group.

Figure 2. Longitudinal reciprocal relationships between substantive complexity of paid work and intellectual flexibility among younger and older workers.

Leisure Complexity and Intellectual Functioning

Unlike our analyses involving substantive complexity of paid work and intellectual flexibility, we used full-information modeling approach in our analysis of the relationship between leisure time activities and intellectual flexibility. Here again, the major decisive factor was the relatively large sample size (N= 635) we have to handle our complex model. We also chose to compare the 1994/1995 working vs. not working group, primarily because we believed that the nature and complexity of leisure time activities is significantly associated with whether or not the individuals are working.

Having confirmed the validity of an invariant measurement model for our latent factors among working and non-working groups and across the two time periods, we proposed the following causal parameters: reciprocal effects between 1994/1995 Cognitive Leisure Activities and 1994/1995 Intellectual Flexibility and, paths from 1974 Cognitive Leisure Activities and 1974 Intellectual Flexibility to corresponding 1994/1995 endogenous factors; and paths to these endogenous factors from all socio-demographic characteristics. In this model, only the error and residual variances and covariances were allowed to vary across groups, and modification indices were inspected to determine the presence or absence of significant causal parameters that needed relaxing. In subsequent re-estimations of the model, we also dropped insignificant structural paths.

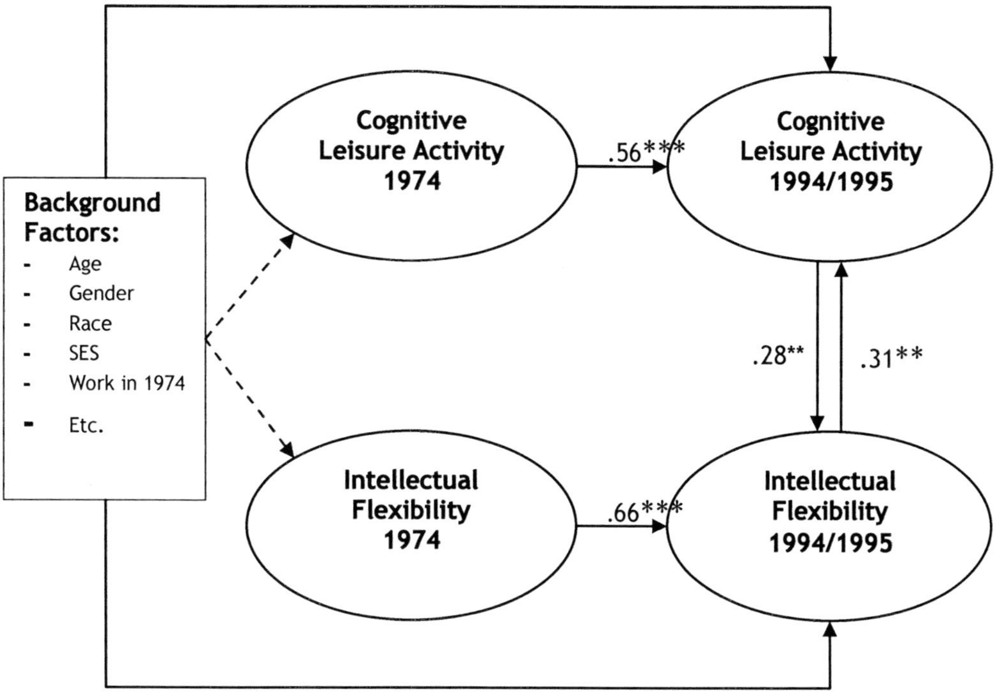

Note. Chi-square = 938.10; p < .001; chi-square/d.f. = 1.53; RMSEA = .04; CFI = .93. Numbers in the figure are completely standardized coefficients. * p < .05; ** p < .01; *** p < .001. Paths from background variables to cognitive leisure activity and intellectual flexibility and intercorrelations of the exogenous variables are also not shown.

Figure 3. Longitudinal reciprocal relationships between cognitive leisure activity and intellectual flexibility among working and non-working older people.

Our final model showed very good fit to the data (χ^2 [614, N = 635] = 1080.41; $p < .001$; RMSEA = .05; CFI = .91), and also indicates that there were significant reciprocal effects between 1994/1995 Cognitive Leisure Activities and 1994/1995 Intellectual Flexibility (see Figure 3 below). Being intellectually flexible resulted in carrying out relatively complex leisure activities (β = .34, $\underline{p} \leq .001$). Conversely, carrying out relatively complex leisure activities resulted in higher levels of intellectual functioning ($\beta = .26$, $p < .05$). The effect of level of intellectual functioning on complexity of leisure time activities was, in fact, slightly greater than the reciprocal effect. In this model, as in our model involving substantive complexity, background factors such as age, race, and socio-economic status had both direct and indirect effects on Cognitive Leisure Activities and Intellectual Flexibility. This reciprocal relationship between cognitive leisure activities and intellectual functioning remained even after employment status and levels of health were accounted for in the model.

Significance and Implications of Recent SSES Findings

The central findings of our two recent studies provide evidence that the substantive complexity of paid work and leisure time activities of middle aged and older adults affects their intellectual functioning. Doing more complex work and leisure time activities increases intellectual functioning; doing less complex work or leisure activities decreases intellectual functioning. As we have seen, this causal pattern holds true when we compare the effects of complex paid work on older and younger workers and of complex leisure time activities on older and younger individuals. The effects of complex leisure time activities are also the same for those who work for pay with those who do not. We have also found evidence that the reciprocal effect exists. Having higher levels of intellectual functioning leads people to carry out more complex paid work as well as more intellectually demanding leisure time activities. Although these reciprocal effects we found are relatively modest, they indicate that the intellectual benefits for middle-aged and older adults of doing intellectually challenging things on the job and off the job are significant and meaningful.

Our results extend earlier Kohn and Schooler's (1983) findings about the effects of substantive complexity of work on intellectual functioning when the present sample was twenty years younger. Our findings also indicate that the effects of dealing with cognitively complex environmental demands on the cognitive functioning of both the older and younger members of our sample extends beyond doing such work for pay to carrying out relatively cognitively complex leisure time tasks. Together, our findings about work and leisure time provide consistent, credibly strong evidence that even in old age, carrying out self-directed complex tasks has a positive effect on intellectual processes. They thus afford further support for the generalizability of the hypothesis (Schooler 1984, 1990) that dealing with cognitively demanding environments increases one's level of intellectual functioning throughout the life span. Within the age range of our sample (41-88 years), the effects of environmental conditions on psychological functioning are at least as strong for older as for younger adults. Indeed, in one of the studies, we have found greater effects of substantive complexity on intellectual functioning in older than younger adults, suggesting that older adults may be psychologically more affected by environmental conditions than younger ones. These findings raise the practical issues of the desirability and possibility of societal interventions to at least maintain the complexity of the environments to which older individuals are exposed.

As for the more general theoretical implications of our findings, by showing that, even late in life, social-structurally influenced environmental circumstances can have notable effects on intellectual functioning, our results provide striking evidence against sociobiological theories, such as put forth by Herrnstein and Murray (1994), that posit strong forms of genetic determinism. Using our findings on the positive cognitive effects of dealing with complex environmental demands in both work and leisure activities as relevant and important evidence, Dickens and Flynn (2001) have made a strong case that intelligence is a function of environmental and genetic factors and, importantly, the interactions between them. Our conclusions about the positive effects of doing self-directed substantively complex work on intellectual functioning also provide a clue to, at least, a partial explanation of what has been termed the "Flynn effect" (Neisser, 1998) – the trend in industrial societies, ever since testing began, for scores over a wide range of intelligence tests to rise by about 3 IQ points per decade (Flynn, 1987). If technical and economic development leads to more complex environments and to more intellectually demanding work conditions, our findings imply that such increased environmental complexity should result in higher levels of intellectual functioning. Such an increase in environmental complexity almost certainly occurred in the move from rural to urban settings and from pre-modern agricultural to commercial and manufacturing occupations. There is also evidence that the substantive complexity of work continues to increase at later levels of development (Attwell, 1987; Dickens & Flynn, 2001; Form, 1987; Penn, Rose, & Rubery, 1994). Given this increasing complexity of work demands and other aspects of life and the causal link between levels of environmental complexity and intellectual functioning, the ongoing gains in intelligence test performance that Flynn (1987) found can be seen as due, in some large part, to the way the world has become more complex. For a full discussion of the plausibility of this view of the Flynn effect, see Schooler (1998).

We have also provided evidence that individuals' levels of intellectual functioning reciprocally affect the complexity of the work they do or the leisure time activities they engage in. Our findings support the assertion of, among others, Farkas and colleagues' (1997) that individuals' levels of cognitive skill level determine their access to occupations requiring more cognitive skill. The same holds true for the intellectual demandingness of their leisure time activities. Because of the positive reciprocal relationship between environmental complexity and intellectual functioning, those with relatively low levels of intellectual functioning may be doubly disadvantaged in that the cognitive effects of the jobs they hold or the leisure activities they engage in tend to decrease their cognitive functioning even further.

All in all, our findings strongly suggest that, even if doing cross-word puzzles per se may not be effective (cf. Hambrick, Salthouse, & Meinz, 1999), doing substantively complex tasks, either at work or at leisure, is an "analog of aerobic exercises" (Hertzog, Hultsch & Dixon, 1999, p. 528). Even in old age, working out on a regimen of substantively complex tasks appears to build the capacity to deal with the intellectual challenges that complex environments provide.

Our studies, however, are primarily based on longitudinal survey data. As such they do not pretend to explicate the basic neurobiological or psychosocial mechanisms through which complex environments and intellectual functioning affect one another. We now turn to recent experimental animal studies and human intervention studies that, not only provide supporting evidence for the cognitive effects of exposure to complex environments, but also suggest potential neurobiological and psychological mechanisms through which exposure to cognitively complex environments affects intellectual functioning.

EXPERIMENTAL STUDIES ON ENVIRONMENTAL COMPLEXITY AND INTELLECTUAL FUNCTIONING

As we have just noted, further evidence for the positive effect of environmental complexity on intellectual functioning throughout the life span comes both from experimental studies involving animals and from human quasi-experimental cognitive intervention studies. In this section we present some examples of each type of study. Their findings provide examples of the available experimental and quasi-experimental evidence that brain and/or cognitive plasticity continues throughout the lifespan and that stimulating cognitively complex environments are significant elements in promoting such plasticity.

Experimental Animal Studies

Using beagle dogs, Milgram (2003) found significant age-related decline in discrimination learning task among the old test-sophisticated dogs compared to their young counterparts. However, the study found no similar difference in cognitive performance between test-naive old and young dogs, suggesting that older animals benefit significantly less from prior cognitive experience than younger animals. Focusing only on the aged beagle dogs, Milgram also tested whether a comprehensive psycho-behavioral intervention improves cognitive functioning. Beagle dogs in the intervention group received increased activity involving regular exercise, environmental enrichment involving toys, and cognitive enrichment involving neuropsychological test experiences; beagle dogs in the control group were not provided the above stimulating conditions. The study revealed no significant difference between the groups after one year of enrichment, but a significant difference was found in favor of the intervention group after two years of intervention, suggesting that a program of sustained cognitive and behavioral enrichment would be necessary to maintain cognitive functioning or prevent age-dependent cognitive decline among older animals.

In a separate study using aged female mice, Frick and Fernandez (2003) found not only a positive effect of environmental enrichment on cognitive functioning but also a potential neurobiological mechanism for this effect. In this study, Frick and Fernandez compared the levels of spatial memory acquisition and the presynaptic protein synaptophysin in the hippocampus and frontoparietal cortex areas among three groups of mice: young control, aged control, and aged enriched. "Because synaptophysin is a constituent of neurotransmitter-presynaptic vesicle membranes… an increase in synaptophysin may reflect an increase in neurotransmission" (Frick & Fernandez, 2003, p. 623,). Control mice were group-housed but did not receive enrichment, whereas enriched mice received environmental stimulation for more than three weeks in the form of rodent toys, variously shaped objects, and running wheels. Findings indicated no significant difference in spatial memory acquisition between enriched aged mice and young control mice, but a significant impairment in spatial memory acquisition among older control mice when compared to young control mice. In addition, hippocampal and cortical synaptophysin levels were also increased in aged enriched mice compared to young and old controls that received no enrichment. These findings proved that environmental enrichment improved both spatial memory acquisition and synaptic protein levels that may serve as the neurobiological basis of environmental effects on cognition.

The above two studies are just two examples of a mounting body of evidence that shows enriched environments improve cognitive functioning, including enhanced learning, memory, and problem-solving abilities. These psychological changes parallel significant neurobiological changes including increased cortical thickness, synaptic contacts and transmission, neuron size, and overall brain weight in laboratory animals (Rosenzweig & Bennett, 1996; Schrott, 1997, for an extensive review see Mohammed et al. 2002).

Human Intervention Studies

Recent cognitive intervention studies with older people using control group vs. experimental group designs have also shown that cognitive stimulation helps prevent or slow down the rate of cognitive decline associated with age or dementia. For instance, Spector and colleagues (2003) conducted a randomized controlled trial to evaluate the efficacy of an evidence-based cognitive stimulation program on cognitive functioning and quality of life of people with dementia. The intervention group received 14 sessions (45 minutes per session) of cognitive stimulation and reality orientation, focusing on such topics as using money, word games, present day, famous faces, and a range of other personal and social activities. Compared to the control group participants who did not participate in these sessions, intervention participants showed significant improvement in their cognitive functioning as well as in their quality of life. The authors noted that the magnitude of the intervention effects were comparable to those reported by clinical trials of drugs for dementia.

Ball and colleagues (2002) conducted a larger and more elaborate randomized controlled trial to evaluate the effectiveness of three forms of cognitive training interventions in improving cognitive and daily functioning in independent-living older adults. The three intervention groups received ten sessions (60-75 minutes per session) of training in verbal episodic memory, problem solving reasoning, and speed of processing respectively. The intervention sessions involved instructions on cognitive strategies with increasing difficulty levels as well as individual and group exercises to practice these strategies. Booster sessions were provided after 11 months of the initial intervention for 60% of the original participants. The study revealed that each intervention improved the targeted cognitive ability compared to the baseline and control group values both on the immediate post-training evaluation, and, to a lesser extent, on the second evaluation at 24 months. Unlike the Spector et al.'s (2003) study, Ball and colleagues did not find the positive effects of cognitive training to significantly generalize to improvement in everyday functioning.

In short, animal experimental studies and controlled human intervention studies such as those described above generally support the hypothesis that cognitively demanding environments have a positive effect on cognitive functioning across species and throughout the life-course. They can also be seen as providing hope that psychosocial interventions that provide cognitively stimulating environments may help prevent cognitive decline and perhaps increase the quality of life people with dementia.

Conclusion

Mohammed et al. (2002) summarize their recent extensive review of neurobiological research on environmental enrichment and the brain by noting that "(t)he findings of environmentally induced changes in the brains of aged organisms are compatible with the notion of 'use it or lose' it" (p.126). They conclude by asserting that "(e)nvironmental stimulation can sustain neurotrophin levels in this [i.e., basal forebrain] and other brain regions and help to maintain function by increasing neural reserve in the aged individual. The impact of environmental enrichment on the brain appears to be a universal phenomenon having been observed in many different species—from flies to philosophers" (p.127). Our survey of relevant psychological and sociological research on the effects of cognitively complex environments on human intellectual functioning provides quite consistent support for this point of view from the behavioral sciences. The results of our own SEM based reciprocal effects models demonstrate that the correlations found between levels of intellectual functioning and environmental complexity are due, at least in part, to such environmental effects. Our analyses rule out the possibility that such correlations result solely from the degree to which individuals who function well intellectually select or are selected into such environments and are more able to successfully maintain themselves in such conditions than those functioning less well intellectually.

As is often the case, psychological and sociological level phenomena add complications beyond those that arise when only neurobiological level phenomena are considered. As we have seen, our SEM based findings indicate that having higher levels of intellectual functioning results in people engaging in more complex paid work as well as more intellectually demanding leisure time activities. Consequently, those with relatively low levels of intellectual functioning are doubly disadvantaged in that the cognitive effects of the jobs they hold and the leisure time activities they carry out act over time to increase their comparative disadvantage in cognitive functioning even further.

Finally, although, as we have seen, both our own and others' findings quite consistently support the hypotheses that engaging in cognitively demanding activities, both on and off of the job, has a positive effect on intellectual functioning, at present we have, at best, an only rudimentary idea of the psychological and neurobiological processes underlying such an effect. Furthermore, we have no real idea of what the limits of such environmental effects on cognitive functioning are and how such limits may change during different stages of the life course. Nevertheless, everything we know points to the fact that the intellectual functioning of older individuals benefits from their dealing with the cognitive challenges presented by relatively complex environments. Using it helps, at least some, in not losing it.

References

Attwell, P. (1987). The deskilling controversy. *Work and Occupations, 14*, 323-346.

Avolio, B., & Waldman, D. (1994). Variations in cognitive, perceptual, and psychomotor abilities across the working life span: Examining the effects of race, sex, experience, education, and occupational type. *Psychology and Aging, 9*, 430-442.

Avolio, B. J., & Waldman, D. A. (1990). An examination of age and cognitive test performance across job complexity and occupational types. *Journal of Applied Psychology, 75*, 43-50.

Baddeley, A. (1986). *Working Memory*. Oxford, England: Clarendon Press.

Ball, K., Berch, D. B., Helmers, K. F., Jobe, J. B., Leveck, M. D., Marsiske, M., et al. (2002). Effects od cognitive training interventions with older adults. A randomized controlled trial. *Journal of American Medical Association, 288*(18), 2271- 2281.

Bosma, H., van Boxtel, M. P. J., Ponds, R. W. H. M., Houx, P., & Jolles, J. (2003). Education and age-related cognitive decline: The contribution of mental workload. *Educational Gerentology, 29*, 165- 173.

Bosma, H., van Boxtel, M. P. J., Ponds, R. W. H. M., Jelicic, M., Houx, P., Metesemakers, J., et al. (2002). Engaged lifestyle and cognitive function in middle and old-aged, non-demented persons: a reciprocal association? *Journal for Gerentology and Geriatrics, 35*(6), 575- 581.

Crowe, M., Andel, R., Pedersen, N. L., Johansson, B., & Gatz, M. (2003). Does participation in leisure activities lead to reduced risk of Alzheimer's Disease? *Journal of Gerontology, 58B*(5), 249- 255.

Coyle, J. T. (2003). Use it or lose it - do effortful mental activities protect against dementia? *New England Journal of Medicine, 348*, 2489-2490.

Dartigues, J. F., Gagon, M., Letenneur, L., Barberger-Gateau, P., Commenges, D., Evaldre, M., et al. (1992). Principal lifetime occupation and cognitive impairment in a French elderly cohort. *American Journal of Epidemiology, 135*(9), 981- 989.

Dickens, W. T., & Flynn, J. R. (2001). Heritability estimates versus large environmental effects: the IQ paradox resolved. *Psychol Rev, 108*(2), 346-369.

Farkas, G., England, P., Vicknair, K., & Kilbourne, B. S. (1997). Cognitive skill, skill demands of jobs, and earnings among young European American, African American, and Mexican American workers. *Social Forces, 75*(3), 913-938.

Flynn, J. R. (1987). Massive IQ gains in 14 nations: What IQ tests really measure. *Psychological Bulletin, 101*, 171-191.

Form, W. (1987). On the degradation of job skills. *Annual Review of Sociology, 13*, 29-47.

Frick, K. M., & Fernandez, S. M. (2003). Enrichment enhances spatial memory and increases synaptophysin levels in aged female mice. *Neurobiol Aging, 24*(4), 615-626.

Friedland, R. P., Fritsch, T., Smyth, K. A., Koss, E., Lerner, A. L., Chen, C. H., et al. (2001). Patients with Alzheimer's Disease have reduced activities in midlife compared with healthy control-group members. *PNAS, 98*(6), 3440- 3445.

Hambrick, D. Z., Salthouse, T. A., & Meinz, E. J. (1999). Predictors of crossword puzzle proficiency and moderators of age-cognition relations. *Journal of Experimental Psychology: General, 128*, 131- 164.

Helmer, C., Letenneur, L., Rouch, I., Richard-Harston, S., Barberger-Gateau, P., Fabrigoule, C., et al. (2001). Occupation during life and risk of dementia in French elderly community residents. *Journal of Neurological Neurosurgery Psychiatry, 71*, 303- 309.

Herrnstein, R. J., & Murray, C. A. (1994). *The bell curve : intelligence and class structure in American life*. New York: Free Press.

Hertzog, C., Hultsch, D. F., & Dixon, R. A. (1999). On the problem of detecting effects of lifestyle on cognitive change in adulthood. *Psychology & Aging., 14*, 528-534.

Hultsch, D. F., Hertzog, C., Small, B. J., & Dixon, R. A. (1999). Use it or lose it: Engaged lifestyle as a buffer of cognitive decline in aging? *Psychology & Aging., 14*, 245- 263.

Kohn, M. L., & Schooler, C. (1978). The reciprocal effects of the substantive complexity of work and intellectual flexibility: A longitudinal assessment. *American Journal of Sociology, 84*, 24-52.

Kohn, M. L., & Schooler, C. (1983). *Work and personality: An inquiry into the impact of social stratification*. Norwood, New Jersey: Ablex Publishing Co.

Kohn, M. L., Slomczynski, K. M., Janicka, K., Khmelko, V., & et al. (1997). Social structure and personality under conditions of radical social change: A comparative analysis of Poland and Ukraine. *American Sociological Review, 62*(4), 614-638.

Kohn, M. L., & Slomczyski, K. M. (1990). *Social Structure and Self-direction: A comparative analysis of the United States and Poland*. Oxford: Basil Blackwell.

Kohn, M. L., Zaborowski, W., Janicka, K., Mach, B. W., Khmelko, V., Slomczynski, K. M., et al. (2000). Complexity of activities and personality under conditions of radical social change: A comparative analysis of Poland and Ukraine. *Social Psychology Quarterly, 63*(3), 187-207.

Milgram, N. W. (2003). Cognitive experience and its effect on age-dependent cognitive decline in beagle dogs. *Neurochem Res, 28*(11), 1677-1682.

Miller, J., Schooler, C., Kohn, M. L., & Miller, K. A. (1979). Women and work: The psychological effects of occupational conditions. *American Journal of Sociology, 85*, 66-94.

Miller, J., Slomczynski, K. M., & Kohn, M. L. (1985). Continuity of learning-generalization: The effect of job on men's intellective process in the United States and Poland. *American Journal of Sociology, 91*, 593-615.

Miller, K. A., & Kohn, M. L. (1983). "The reciprocal effects of job conditions and the intellectuality of leisure-time activities." In M. L. Kohn & C. Schooler (Eds.), *Work and Personality: An Inquiry into the Impact of Social Stratification* (pp. 217-241). Norwood, NJ: Ablex Publishing Co.

Miller, K. A., Kohn, M. L., & Schooler, C. (1986). Educational self-direction and personality. *American Sociological Review, 51*, 372-390.

Mohammed, A. H., Zhu, S. W., Darmopil, S., Hjerling-Leffler, J., Ernfors, P., Winblad, B., et al. (2002). Environmental enrichment and the brain. *Progress in the Brain Research, 138*, 109- 133.

Naoi, A., & Schooler, C. (1985). Occupational conditions and psychological functioning in Japan. *American Journal of Sociology, 90*, 729-752.

Naoi, M., & Schooler, C. (1990). Psychological consequences of occupational conditions among Japanese wives. *Social Psychology Quarterly, 58*, 100-116.

Neisser, U. (1998). Introduction: Rising Test Scores and What They Mean. In U. Neisser (Ed.), *The Rising Curve: Long-Term Gains in IQ and Related Measures* (pp. 3-22). Washington, DC: American Psychological Association.

Penn, R., Rose, M., & Rubery, J. (Eds.). (1994). *Skill and Occupational Change*. Oxford: Oxford University Press.

Pushkar, D., Etezadi, J., Andres, D., Arbuckle, T., Schwartzman, A. E., & Chaikelson, J. (1999). Models of intelligence in late life: Comment on Hultsch et al. *Psychology and Aging, 14*, 520-527.

Pushkar-Gold, D., Andres, D., Etezadi, J., Arbuckle, T., Schwartzman, A., & Chaikelson, J. (1995). Structural equation model of intellectual change and continuity and predictors of intelligence in older men. *Psychol Aging, 10*(2), 294-303.

Qiu, C., Karp, A., von Strauss, E., Winblad, B., Fratiglioni, L., & Bellander, T. (2003). Lifetime princepal occupation and risk of Alzheimer's Disease in the Kungsholmen Project. *American Journal of Industrial Medicine, 43*, 204- 211.

Rosenzweig, M. R., & Bennett, E. L. (1996). Psychobiology of plasticity: effects of training and experience on brain and behavior. *Behav Brain Res, 78*(1), 57-65.

Salthouse, T. A. (1991). Mediation of adult age differences in cognition by reductions in working memory and speed of processing. *Psychological Science, 2*, 179-183.

Salthouse, T. A., Berish, D. E., & Miles, J. D. (2002). The role of cognitive stimulation on the relations between age and cognitive functioning. *Psychology & Aging., 17*(4), 548- 557.

Schooler, C. (1984). Psychological effects of complex environments during the life span: A review and theory. *Intelligence, 8*, 259-281.

Schooler, C. (1990). Psychosocial factors and effective cognitive functioning through the life span. In J. E. Birren & K. W. Schaie (Eds.), *Handbook of the psychology of aging* (pp. 347-358). Orlando, Florida: Academic Press.

Schooler, C. (1998). Environmental complexity and the Flynn effect. In U. Neisser (Ed.), *The Rising Curve: Long-Term Gains in IQ and Related Measures* (pp. 67-79). Washington, DC: American Psychological Association.

Schooler, C., Caplan, L. J., & Oates, G. (1998). Aging and work: An overview. In K. W. Schaie & C. Schooler (Eds.), *Impact of Work on Older Adults* (pp. 1-19). New York, NY: Springer.

Schooler, C., Neumann, E., Caplan, L. J., & Roberts, B. R. (1997). Continued inhibitory capacity throughout adulthood: conceptual negative priming in younger and older adults. *Psychol Aging, 12*(4), 667-674.

Schooler, C., Neumann, E., Caplan, L. J., & Roberts, B. R. (1997). A time course analysis of Stroop interference and facilitation: comparing normal individuals and individuals with schizophrenia. *J Exp Psychol Gen, 126*(1), 19-36.

Schooler, C., Miller, J., Miller, K. A., & Richtand, C. N. (1984). Work for the household: Its nature and consequences for husbands and wives. *American Journal of Sociology, 90*, 97-124.

Schooler, C., & Mulatu, M. S. (2001). The reciprocal effects of leisure time activities and intellectual functioning in older people: A longitudinal analysis. *Psychology and Aging, 16*, 466-482.

Schooler, C., Mulatu, M. S., & Oates, G. (1999). The continuing effects of substantively complex work on the intellectual functioning of older workers. *Psychology and Aging, 14*(3), 483-506.

Schooler, C., Mulatu, M. S., & Oates, G. (2004). Effects of occupational self-direction on the intellectual functioning and self-directed orientations of older workers: Findings and implications for individuals and societies. *American Journal of Sociology, 110 (1)*, 161-197.

Schooler, C., & Naoi, M. (1988). The psychological effects of traditional and of economically peripheral job settings in Japan. *American Journal of Sociology, 94*(2), 335-355.

Schrott, L. M. (1997). Effect of training and environment on brain morphology and behavior. *Acta Paediatr Suppl, 422*, 45-47.

Snowden, D. A., Kemper, S. J., Mortimer, J. T., Greiner, L. H., Wekstein, D. R., & Marksbery, W. R. (1996). Linguistic ability in early life and cognitive function and Alzheimers disease in late life. *Journal of the American Medical Association, 275*, 528-532.

Spector, A., Thorgrimsen, L., Woods, B., Royan, L., Davies, S., Butterworth, M., et al. (2003). Efficacy of an evidence-based cognitive stimulation therapy programme for people with dementia. *British Journal of Psychiatry, 183*, 248- 254.

Stern, Y., Gurland, B., Tatemichi, T. K., Tang, M. X., Wilder, D., & Mayeux, R. (1994). Influence of education and occupation on the incidence of Alzheimer's Disease. *Journal of American Medical Association, 272*(18), 1405-1406.

United States Department Of Labor. (1965). *Dictionary of occupational titles* (Third Edition ed.). Washington, D.C.: U.S. Government Printing Office.

Verghese, J., Lipton, R. B., Katz, M. J., Hall, C. B., Derby, C. A., Kuslansky, G., et al. (2003). Leisure activities and the risk of dementia in the eldery. *The New England Journal of Medicine, 348*, 2508- 2516.

Wang, H.-X., Karp, A., Winblad, B., & Fratiglioni, L. (2002). Late-life engagement in social and leisure activities is associated with a decreased risk of dementia: A longitudinal study from the Kungsholmen Project. *American Journal of Epidemiology, 155*, 1081- 1087.

Willis, S. L., & Schaie, K. W. (1986). Training the elderly on the ability factors of spatial orientation and inductive reasoning. *Psychology and Aging, 1*, 239-247.

Wilson, R. S., Mendes de Leon, C. F., Barnes, L. L., Schneider, J. A., Bienias, J. L., Evans, D. A., et al. (2002). Participation in cognitively stimulating activities and risk of incident Alzhiemer's Disease. *Journal of American Medical Association, 287*, 742- 748.

Witkin, H. A., Dyk, R. B., Faterson, H. F., Goodenough, D. R., & Karp, S. A. (1962). *Psychological differentiation: Studies of Development*. New York: John Wiley.

In: Aging and the Elderly: Psychology, Sociology and Health ISBN 1-60021-190-9
Editor: L. O. Randall, pp. 115-137

Chapter 5

SOCIAL SUPPORT AND AGING

Regan A. R. Gurung* and Dean Von Dras
University of Wisconsin, Green Bay, WI, USA

ABSTRACT

The numbers of older adults is increasing every year (U.S Census Bureau, 2004). As the population grows older and life expectancy increases, it becomes even more important to identify factors that reduce the incidence of chronic illnesses of middle and later adulthood and aid in coping (Smith, Kendall, & Keefe, 2002; Siegler, Bashan, Steffens, Bosworth, & Costa, 2002). One of the most critical factors is social support and social networks which have positive effects on the health and well-being of adults of all ages (Antonucci & Jackson, 1987; Bowling, 1994; Fratiglioni, Wang, Ericsson, Mayten, & Wimblad, 2000; Gotlib & Whiffen, 1992; Helgeson & Cohen, 1996; House, Umberson, & Landis, 1988; Kriegsman, Pennix, & Van Eijk, 1995; Reifman, 1995; Sarason, Sarason & Gurung, 2001; Schwarzer & Leppin, 1992).

In this chapter we first, following Bruner's (1990) call for understanding behavior within the context in which occurs, expand on ecological frameworks used to illuminate causes of behavior (e.g., Bronfenbrenner, 1986; Revenson, 1990, 1994), positing a contextually oriented framework as an analytic structure for describing and explicating social support processes. In a selective review of the literature, influences of intra- and interpersonal characteristics as well as cultural factors that mediate perceptions of social support and influence behavior are discussed. Next, we describe a longitudinal study of changes in social support that illustrates the utility of a contextual approach.

The results of Gurung et al., (2003) illustrate the dynamic nature of social support in a healthy aging cohort over time and across different sources. More broadly, it also highlights the utility of factoring in different contexts. The MacArthur Study data nicely capture people operating different independent and overlapping contexts: an intrapersonal context, an interpersonal context, and a temporal context. Clearly, each context overlaps

* Correspondence should be addressed to Regan A. R. Gurung gurungr@uwgb.edu or to Regan A. R. Gurung at Human Development and Psychology, MAC-314C, University of Wisconsin, Green Bay, 2420 Nicolet Drive, Green Bay, WI 54311.

with others and all influence behavior. Further studies of support and efforts to provide it might be especially attuned to the different contexts that social support is transacted in.

INTRODUCTION

The numbers of older adults is increasing every year (U.S Census Bureau, 2004). As the population grows older and life expectancy increases, it becomes even more important to identify factors that reduce the incidence of chronic illnesses of middle and later adulthood and aid in coping (Smith, Kendall, & Keefe, 2002; Siegler, Bashan, Steffens, Bosworth, & Costa, 2002). One of the most critical factors is social support and social networks which have positive effects on the health and well-being of adults of all ages (Antonucci & Jackson, 1987; Bowling, 1994; Fratiglioni, Wang, Ericsson, Mayten, & Wimblad, 2000; Gotlib & Whiffen, 1992; Helgeson & Cohen, 1996; House, Umberson, & Landis, 1988; Kriegsman, Pennix, & Van Eijk, 1995; Reifman, 1995; Sarason, Sarason & Gurung, 2001; Schwarzer & Leppin, 1992). Increases in life expectancy, coupled with changing needs that may require social support, highlight the importance of understanding the social networks of older adults, the factors that influence social support receipt, and the factors that may threaten the availability of this important resource. In this chapter we first, following Bruner's (1990) call for understanding behavior within the context in which occurs, expand on ecological frameworks used to illuminate causes of behavior (e.g., Bronfenbrenner, 1986; Revenson, 1990, 1994), positing a contextually oriented framework as an analytic structure for describing and explicating social support processes. In a selective review of the literature, influences of intra- and interpersonal characteristics as well as cultural factors that mediate perceptions of social support and influence behavior are discussed. Next, we describe a longitudinal study of changes in social support that illustrates the utility of a contextual approach.

SOCIAL SUPPORT AND CONTEXT

Social support has been described as the communication of being loved, respected, valued, and esteemed, as well as the mutual obligation of participating in an interpersonal network that provides assistance and aid to its members (Pines, Ben-Ari, Utasi, & Larson, 2002). Indeed, as Mutran, Reed, and Sudha (2002) note, "social support implies that something is given to another who receives it (p. 70)." As a result there is an enhancement of the receiver's well-being, health, and ability to operate more successfully in various domains of life (Mutran et al., 2002). To understand the microsocial and macrosocial aspects of supportive relationships (House, Umberson, & Landis, 1988), a contextually oriented framework that recognizes the overlap of intra- and interpersonal, and sociocultural influences on social support processes is most useful. Conceptually, this contextual orientation, much like the narrative of one's life story, "presupposes an ongoing texture of multiple, elaborated events, each being influenced by collateral episodes and by the efforts of multiple agents (Hermans, 1992, p. 362)." Thus following Revenson's (1990, 1994) operationalism, in this framework there are three primary assumptions and various strata of social influence to consider.

The first assumption is that people operate within many independent and overlapping contexts: an intrapersonal context, an interpersonal context, a sociocultural context, a situational context, and temporal context. Each context overlaps with others and all may influence behavior. For example, social support (the interpersonal context) received by a person striving to attain the athletic goal of a running a sub-5-minute mile may enhance self-esteem and confidence in one's ability (the intrapersonal context), but perhaps is more of an enhancement for men (the sociocultural context), and only during young adulthood (the temporal context) when physical fitness is highlighted as key for entry into particular performance areas such as being a member of a running club (the situational context).

With regard for the intraindividual strata, research directed at understanding self-regulation processes highlight a variety of person-situation interactions that influence one's attitudes (e.g., Tesser, 2002), personal control beliefs (e.g., Baumeister, Heatherton & Tice, 1994; Carver & Scheier, 1998), motivation (e.g., Andersen, Reznick, & Chen, 1997; Higgins, 1996), characterization and knowledge of self (e.g., Steele, 1988; Mischel & Shoda, 1995), as well as behavior (e.g., Cantor, 1994; Snyder & Cantor, 1998). Similarly, intrapersonal characteristics are suggested to filter perceptions as well as influence interpersonal behaviors. For example, across the assessment periods of young, middle, and older adulthood, extraversion has been shown to be positively associated with perceived social support (e.g., Costa, Zonderman, & McCrae, 1985; Cutrona & Russell, 1987) as well as social activity and seeking of support (VonDras & Siegler, 1997). The double-edged sword of personal characteristics that influence social perceptions as well as behavior is also found in research that suggests perceptions of plentiful social support to be significantly associated with high self-esteem (e.g., Sarason, Levine, Basham, & Sarason, 1983; VonDras, Williams, Kaplan, & Siegler, 1996), as well as low levels of hostility (e.g., VonDras, Siegler, Barefoot, Williams, & Mark, 1999), neuroticism (e.g., Costa et al., 1985; Hooker et al., 1998; Cutrona & Russell, 1987), loneliness (e.g., Jones, 1985; Sarason, Sarason, Hacker, & Basham,1985) and depression (e.g., Cohen, 1991; Frasure-Smith, Lesperance, & Talajic, 1995; Jones, 1985; Roberts, Kaplan, Shema, & Strawbridge, 1997). Other research has suggests mediating influences of intrapersonal characteristics. For example, research involving independently functioning adults ranging in age from 60 to 96 years that examined the mediating influence of perceived control on aspects of social support (Bisconti & Bergeman, 1999) report high personal control to be positively related to the perceived quantity of support provided by family and friends, as well as satisfaction with support. Moreover, personal control was observed to mediate relationships between these aspects of support and depression (Bisconti & Bergeman, 1999). Research examining the psychosocial dimensions of role identity in pre-retirement adults suggested high friendship identity to be positively related with commitment to friends and satisfaction with life (Siebert, Mutran & Reitzes, 1999). Further, aspects of one's identity are suggested to affect the support provided by family members and friends, with receipt of these supportive behaviors in turn acting to sustain a continuity of identity and activity into later life (Roper, Molnar, & Wrisberg, 2003). Thus not only do one's intrapersonal characteristics filter perceptions, they also direct actions that elicit responses from others that sustain identity, reinforce social norms and attitudes, and facilitate adaptive behaviors throughout life (Hafner & Welz, 1989).

With further consideration of the assumption that intra- and interpersonal, situational, and temporal contexts overlap, it is noted that age or "timing of life events" is one of the underlying dimensions by which social interactions are thought to be regulated (Neugarten, Moore, & Lowe, 1965). For example, classic research investigating age norms that operate in American society noted "a prescriptive timetable for the ordering of major life events: a time in the life span when men and women are expected to marry, a time to raise children, a time to retire (Neugarten et al., 1965, p. 711)." Thus, the marital relationship is one domain where the timing of life events and functioning of interpersonal relationships have been suggested to be of paramount importance (Neugarten et al., 1965; Schulz & Rau, 1985). In many cultures, the marital vow designates the interdependency of husband and wife, as well as explicit promises to provide support and care. With regard to the temporal context then, one's spouse is generally presumed to be a primary source of social support and caregiving for the married individual across the life course (Bolger, Foster, Vinokur, & Ng, 1996; Hess & Soldo, 1985; Longino & Lipman, 1985, Revenson, 1994). With advancing age, however, significant changes in marital relationships (e.g., Gilford, 1984; Longino & Lipman, 1985; Pineo, 1961) and social roles (e.g., Moen, Robison, & Fields, 1994; Robison, Moen, Dempster-McClain, 1995) are noted. For example, declines in intimacy and marital satisfaction have been noted concomitants of advancing age for some marital couples (Gilford, 1984; Pineo, 1961). Furthermore, while spouses, and especially wives, occupy a primary caregiving role for an ill partner, with advancing age one is more likely to experience worry concerning spouse's illness, recovery, disability, and threat to life while tending to an ill partner (Farkas & Himes, 1998; Revenson, 1994). Similarly, research involving spouses of Alzheimer Disease patients suggest that spouses experience greater caregiver burden in terms of stress and negative affect, and thus are more likely to perceive an inadequate level of social support (Clipp & George, 1990), suggesting an overlap between interpersonal and temporal contexts. Moreover, younger caregivers of patients with dementia were found to be lonelier and more resentful of their roles than older caregivers (Fitting, Rabins, Lucas, & Eastham, 1986), again suggesting a temporal dimension to influence perceptions and processes of social support. Other research has suggested that perceived support of one's romantic partner to be associated with depression and loneliness (Segrin, 2003). Moveover, age was found to interact with perceived support from partner and influence level of depression, with the strongest influence of perceived partner support on depression being found in young adults (Segrin, 2003). Therefore across the life-course, the perceptions of social support made by intimate partners in many ways may reflect the positive and negative dynamics and characteristics of their interpersonal relationships (Coyne & DeLongis, 1986) and influence other behaviors and aspects of life.

A second assumption of the contextual framework (Revenson, 1990, 1994) is that each person is involved in reciprocal relationships with members of their social network. Indeed, one's interpersonal relationships are seen to dynamically influence the individual's conceptualizations of self (e.g., Chen & Andersen, 1999; Andersen, Chen, & Miranda, 2002; Hinkely & Andersen, 1996) as well as the social support they provide (e.g., Fiske, Coyne, & Smith, 1991; Frank, Campbell, & Shields, 1992; Frazier, Port, & Hoff, 1996; Krantz & Moos, 1987; Michella, 1987; VonDras, Siegler, Barefoot, Williams, & Mark, 2000; VonDras & Madey, 2004). These reciprocal relationships exert both overt and covert influences on the individual's cognitions, emotions, and actions. For example the person aspiring to attain a particular health goal may be more successful in its attainment as a function of the positive aspects of social support and assistance provided by others (e.g., Eitel, Hatchett, Friend, Griffin, & Wadhwa, 1995; Hatchett, Friend, Symister, & Wadhwa, 1997; Oxman & Hull, 1997). Conversely, the individual receiving aid may also reciprocally influence supporting others (e.g., Bookwala & Schultz, 1996; Coyne & Smith, 1991; Coyne et al., 1987; Tower & Kassel, 1996). The reciprocal nature of one's relationships and caregiving responsibilities also change across the life course and situations, with an increase in the assistance (e.g., monitoring treatment regime, attending to daily needs) provided to ill spouses, children, and other family member becoming more probable as one advances in age (Moen et al., 1994; Pavalko & Artis, 1997; Robison et al., 1995). Other research has suggested that with advancing age there is an aging of and decline in the number of one's social network members, as well as a decline in the individual's frequency of contact with network members (Antonucci & Akiyama, 1987; Bosse, Aldwin, Levenson, Workman-Daniels, & Ekerdt, 1990; Lang, Staudinger, & Carstensen, 1998; van Tilburg, 1998). Despite the decline in contact frequency, however, longitudinal research suggests increased instrumental and emotional support (van Tilburg, 1998). Other research has suggested that with increasing age there is a decline in the perceived demandingness of one's relationships with family and friends, and an increase in the perceived support received from one's children (Lynch, 1998). Thus while later life is more likely to bring illness, disability, and greater need for assistance (Coe, 1983) as well as greater situational demands on caregiving (e.g., Moen et al., 1994; Robison et al., 1995), "older needy persons receive more various (types of) support from fewer network members (Antonucci & Akiyama, 1987, p. 524)."

Research involving medical populations has provided key support for the assumption of reciprocal effects and their link to other behaviors and outcomes. Importantly, they again highlight the marital dyad and family as moderators of social support processes and other behavioral outcomes. For example, greater rates of hospital remission were observed in depressed patients as a function of their spouse's report of social and family problems (Krantz & Moos, 1987). In a similar fashion, greater psychological distress has been observed among spouses or significant others of hospitalized depressed patients than of non-hospitalized depressed patients (Coyne et al., 1987), suggesting that clinical depression is often reflective of "a more generally distressed interpersonal context (Coyne et al., 1987, p. 351)." Longitudinal investigation has also indicated significant associations between spouses' levels of depression and depressive symptomologies (Tower & Kasl, 1997); also suggesting that characteristics of one spouse influences the psychological well-being of the other. Taken together, these investigations illustrate that the psychological characteristics of family and friends may interact and moderate social support processes. Indeed, reciprocal effects of receiving and providing social support have been noted in family and friends who care for people who endure chronic health problems (e.g., Antonucci, 1991; Cohen, 1991; Schulz, Tompkins, Wood, & Decker, 1987; Tompkins, Schulz, & Rau, 1988.). Research in this area suggests that social support can be both a benefit to the patient, buffering stress and improving the probability of survival (Lewis, Rook, & Schwarzer, 1994; Vogt, 1992), while at the same time a source of burden for the care provider who may experience increasing emotional, physical, and financial strain over time (Hansson & Carpenter, 1994). Especially with regard to physical illness, caregivers, while providing support and assistance may themselves lack assistance and support. For example, research investigating cancer patients and their caregiving spouses indicated that caregivers were significantly more likely to worry about the patient's future, and reported receiving significantly lower levels of emotional support, family assistance, help in taking action, and help in getting proper treatment than did the patient (Davis-Ali, Chesler, & Chesney, 1993). Similarly, research involving kidney transplant patients and their caregiving spouses suggested that caregivers who are high in stress are likely to report more depressive symptoms, lower marital satisfaction, and offer less helpful and more unhelpful support to the patient (Frazier, Davis-Ali, & Dahl, 1995; Frazier, Port, & Hoff, 1996). Further, noting the reciprocal nature of interpersonal relationships, longitudinal research investigating the provision and receipt of support and disregard in fertile and infertile married couples indicated positive association between spouses' receipt and provision of support to their partner (Abbey, Andrews, & Halman, 1995). While various aspects of social support are usually undifferentiated using traditional measurement techniques (cf. House & Kahn, 1985; Kessler & McLeod, 1985), however research by VonDras and Madey (2004) allude to the dynamic and reciprocal effects that occur in interpersonal relationships; showing that individuals who express low satisfaction with social relationships because of poor quality or receipt of negative feedback, report greater desire to seek support from other network members. Further, receipt of instrumental support was found to be a unique predictor of the individual's intention to pursue important health goals (VonDras & Madey, 2004). Overall, these investigations support the interdependent and reciprocal relationship assumption of the contextual framework, and underscore the many different ways social support enhances health and well-being.

A third assumption of the contextual framework is that there are levels of analysis that range from the individual to the dyad, to group, network, and culture. Therefore a systems level analysis, one that includes network and cultural levels of analysis is crucial to understanding behavior from a contextual perspective. For example, the behavior and activities of the individual who pursues a health goal also produces a rearrangement of the activities and routines of other network members. Thus when there are changes in the individual's social behavior, there may also be changes in the receipt and exchange of resources and activities of social network members (e.g., Cantor, 1994; Clip & George, 1990; Fitting, Rabins, Lucas, & Eastman, 1986; Lynch, 1998; Snyder & Cantor, 1998). As pointed out by Pines et al. (2002), social support, as defined by the functions of listening and sharing a social reality, along with providing technical and emotional support is a universal need for all people in all cultures. However, as Nemoto (1989) notes, "cultural norms which may influence the expression of need for social support, social support activities, satisfaction with social ties, and social support networks have been ignored in the social support research (p. 56)." This is especially true with regard to cross-cultural social support research that involves older adults. Nevertheless, available research using young adults suggests important cultural orientations may be part of the interpretation and expression of social support within various settings. For example cross-cultural investigation revealed differences on the dimension of individualism/collectivism, with Arab-Israeli student, members of a collectivist culture, reporting greater availability of support functions than did American students, members of an individualistic culture (Pines et al., 2002). Indeed, collectivistic values are suggested to lead to greater cooperation, where as individualistic values is suggested to foster competition (Tjosvold, Law, & Sun, 2003). Research by Goodwin and Giles (2003) suggested that while members of collectivist (Indonesia) and individualistic (Britain) cultures are just as likely to provide various types of social support to a friend, members of a collectivistic culture are more willing to offer support to strangers than members of an individualistic culture. Thus while social support is an important facet of everyone's life, however its receipt and provision may vary within different cultures. Western culture is oriented towards ideals of personal control and independence, thus the provision of support may be constrained so as to foster individual autonomy. In contrast, eastern culture focuses on values of harmony within the group and interdependence, thus provision of support may be more liberal so as to underscore the collective (Triandis, 1995). Research in a college student population by Triandis, Leung, Villareal, and Clack (1985, Study 3) indicated that individuals with a collectivistic orientation (allocentric) expressed greater satisfaction and availability of social support, i.e., satisfaction with being listened to, being important to others lives, others being dependable when help is needed , counting on others to help, availability of others who listen openly and uncritically. Further, Triandis et al. (1985, Study 3), report that individuals with an individualistic orientation (idiocentric) reported greater loneliness and were higher in independence than collectivists; in contrast, collectivists reported greater association in roles with parents and siblings, and greater respect in the foreman-worker and worker-foreman roles. Morever, collectivists were found to express greater cooperation than individualists. Other research (Triandis, Bontempo, Villareal, Asai, & Lucca, 1988, Study 3) suggests that in comparison to individualisitic oriented individuals, collectivists perceive greater and a higher quality of social support. With further consideration of association with other personal dimensions, collectivism has been shown to be associated with greater sociability, emotional closeness to one's in-group, and family integrity, where as individualism is related to greater competition and self-reliance (Triandis & Gelfand, 1998, Study 3). Similarly, research by Scott, Ciarrochi, and Deane (2004) indicates that college students high in individualistic orientation report smaller and less satisfying social support networks, lower emotional competence and less likely to seek help in times of need (distress). Research involving Japanese and U.S. adults ranging in age from 19 to 70 years suggested important nuances in social relationships that reflect cultural roles and social expectations of young, midlife and older adults (VonDras, Malcore, Pouliot, & Iwahashi, 2004). These data suggested that the perceptions of equality in relationships reflect underlying individual and interdependent orientations of both cultures, as well as generational influences, with U.S. and Japanese older adults reporting giving more to family relationships (VonDras et al., 2004). While these modest findings suggesting ways in which culture may moderate perceptions of the support and interpersonal behaviors, there is yet a great need to understand social support processes in within different cultural settings.

A Focus on Temporal Context: Changes in Social Support

The question of whether and how available social support may change is of particular importance for older adults because the networks of the elderly are at greater risk for changes in membership. Age-specific experiences such as retirement, adult children leaving the home, health declines that make socializing more difficult, the loss of a spouse or close friends, and relocation to institutional facilities have led laypersons and scientists alike to hypothesize that older adults are vulnerable to a loss of social support (Bosse, Aldwin, Levenson, Spiro, & Mroczek, 1993; Miller & Cavanaugh, 1990; Morgan, 1989). Several theoretical frameworks have been developed to understand the social networks of older adults including the Hierarchical-Compensatory Model (Cantor, 1979), Socioemotional Selectivity Theory (Carstensen, 1987), Activity Theory (Cummings & Henry, 1961), Disengagement theory

(Havighurst & Albrecht, 1953), the Social Convoy Model (Kahn & Antonucci, 1980), the Task-Specific Model (Litwak, 1985), and the Functional-Specificity Model (Weiss, 1974). Some are especially relevant to age-related change (e.g., Carstensen, 1987, Kahn & Antonucci, 1980) while others inform a focus on sources and types of support (e.g., Litwak, 1985; Simons, 1983/84; Weiss, 1974).

Theories of Change

The Social Convoy Model (Antonucci, 1991; Kahn & Antonucci, 1980) provides a conceptual framework for studying age-related changes in structural and compositional characteristics of social networks. It postulates that people are motivated to maintain their social network sizes as they age, although there may be changes in the composition of the networks. Individuals construct and maintain social relationships while becoming increasingly aware of specific strengths and weaknesses of particular members. This knowledge allows them to select different network members for different functions (e.g., certain people are relied on for emotional support, others for instrumental support) and possibly avoid those members who are not supportive. Empirical support for the model (Kahn & Antonucci, 1984) clearly identifies the importance of simultaneously looking at different sources when studying changes in age-related social support. Although specific non-supportive network members may drop out over time, the Social Convoy Model suggests that general levels of support will be constant or even increase, given that social support is coordinated to optimize support receipt.

Socioemotional Selectivity Theory (Carstensen, 1987,1991) proposes that people prune their social networks to maintain a desired emotional state depending on the extent to which time is perceived as limited. Basic functions of social interaction, such as regulating desired emotional states, differ in respect to their relative importance for determining social preferences across the lifespan. Emphasis in old age is placed on achieving short-term emotional goals. Correspondingly, whereas older adults' social networks may be smaller than those of younger adults, the numbers of close relationships are comparable (Lang & Carstensen, 1998). For example, Lang and Carstensen (1994) examined the interrelationships among age, network composition, and social support in a representative sample of 156 community dwelling and institutionalized adults aged 70-104 yrs and found that the social networks of older people were only half as large as those of younger people, but the number of very close relationships did not differ across age groups.

Both theories have received some support (Antonucci & Akiyama, 1995; Carstensen, Isaacowitz, & Charles, 1999; Lansford, Sherman, & Antonucci, 1998), with evidence indicating that it is not necessarily the size, membership, or particular structure of the network, but the quality of transactions (i.e., perceived and received social support) that is critical to mental and physical health. The present study builds on empirical tests of these theories to examine changes in functional social support. Even though network size may decrease (e.g., due to Socioemotional Selectivity) and membership may change (e.g., according to the Social Convoy Model), both theories lead us to the hypotheses that the quality of support in networks of the elderly remain the same or actually increase over time and that this will be true especially of emotional support.

Differentiating Support by Type and Source

Two major theoretical models suggest that different sources of support serve different support functions. In his Task-Specific Model, Litwak (1985) reported that different sources of support (e.g. friends versus spouse) typically provided different types of support (e.g. companionship versus housecleaning). A review by Crohan and Antonucci (1989) found that family members more often provide instrumental support, and friends more often provide emotional support and companionship.

A related theory, Weiss's (1974) Functional-Specificity Model, suggested that individuals' requirements for specific forms of support can only be met within certain relationships. Even when the same type of support is provided by different sources, its impact may not be the same. In support of this theory, Simons (1983/84) found that only elderly participants' relationships with their spouses and children, but not with other individuals, were related to feelings of security. Felton and Berry (1992) found that informational support to older adults contributed more to well-being when provided by kin than when provided by nonkin, whereas emotional support contributed more to well-being when provided by nonkin than when provided by kin. Thus, alterations in the composition of social networks over time could alter the relative availability and efficiency of different types of support due to changes in the availability of certain types of ties (Connidis & Davies, 1990; Peters, Hoyt, Babchuk, Kaiser, & Iijima, 1987; Seeman & Berkman, 1988; Simons, 1983/1984).

An Empirical Example of the Contextual Approach

Using a contextual analysis to study social support involves factoring in intra-individual factors such as psychological factors (e.g., mastery and self-efficacy), inter-individual factors (e.g., a relationship such as marriage and reciprocity between partners), and temporal changes (e.g., support receipt over time). Few studies incorporate all these different aspects. One notable example is provided by Gurung, Taylor, and Seeman (2003) who used data from the MacArthur Successful Aging Study (MSAS), a longitudinal study of relatively high functioning men and women aged 70-79. This next section summarizes the main results of this study as an exemplar of the contextual approach.

The MSAS was originally designed to examine a broad range of factors hypothesized to be associated with "successful aging" (Rowe & Kahn, 1987). Participants were sampled on the basis of age and both physical and cognitive functioning from three community-based cohorts of the National Institute on Aging's Established Populations for Epidemiologic Studies of the Elderly (EPESE) in Durham, North Carolina; East Boston, Massachusetts; and New Haven, Connecticut (Cornoni-Huntley, Brock, Ostfeld, Taylor, & Wallace, 1986).

Age-eligible men and women (N = 4030) were screened using four criteria of physical functioning and two criteria of cognitive functioning to identify those functioning in the top third of the age group. The selection criteria included: 1) no reported disability on the 7-item Activities of Daily Living (ADL) scale (Katz, Ford, Moskowitz, Jackson, & Jaffe, 1963); 2) no more than one reported mild disability on 8 items tapping gross mobility and range of motion (Nagi, 1976; Rosow, & Breslau, 1966); 3) ability to hold a semi-tandem balance for at least 10 seconds; 4) ability to stand from a seated position 5 times within 20 seconds; 5) scores of 6 or more correct on the 9-item Short Portable Mental Status Questionnaire (Pfeiffer, 1975); and 6) ability to remember 3 or more of 6 elements on a delayed recall of a short story (see Gurung, et al., 2003 for details).

The MacArthur battery included assessments of frequency of receipt of emotional and instrumental support, as well as the frequency of negative interactions involving conflict or excessive demands, from 3 sources (spouse, children, and friends and family). Psychological predictors included measures of social ties, self efficacy, mastery, and depression. Separate tests of physical ability (timed measures of gait, balance, chair stands, foot taps, and manual ability), was used to assess physical functioning, and cognitive performance was assessed with 5 tasks as first developed by Inouye, Albert, Mohs, Sun, and Berkman, (1993, see for additional details on total score construction and psychometric properties). A 12-item somatization subscale from the Hopkins Symptom Checklist (Derogatis, Lipman, Rickels, Uhlenhuth, & Covi, 1974) was also included in the analyses.

Main Findings

One-way analyses of variance revealed significant gender differences on several of the psychological variables. Women reported higher levels of depression, F (1,436) = 12.66, $p <$ .001, lower levels of emotional support from their spouses, F (1,436) = 6.57, $p < .05$, and lower levels of instrumental support from their spouses, F (1,436) = 10.61, $p < .001$. Men reported higher levels of mastery, F (1,438) = 4.21, $p < .05$, self-efficacy, F (1,438) = 7.92, $p < .01$, and physical functioning, F (1,438) = 27.59, $p < .001$ at baseline. At Time 2, women reported lower levels of emotional support from their spouses, F (1,438) = 14.71, $p < .001$) and lower levels of instrumental support from their spouses, F (1,438)= 21.61, $p < .001$.

Associations between Different Types of Support

In general, different types of reported social support correlated moderately both within and across sources. For the 1988/89 data, emotional and instrumental support consistently showed the highest correlations with each other within each source, ranging from $r = .29$ ($p < .01$) for support from friends and relatives to $r = .41$ ($p < .01$) for support from the spouse. Negative behaviors were significantly negatively correlated with emotional and instrumental support with moderate to low magnitude except in the case of emotional support from the spouse, where it was higher ($r = -.33$, $p < .01$), and in the case of emotional support from friends and relatives where negative behaviors were not significantly correlated. When comparing support across sources, each of the three types of social behaviors showed significant intercorrelations, with associations for negative behaviors showing the highest magnitude. For example, participants who reported high levels of negative behaviors from their children also reported high levels of negative behaviors from their friends and relatives, $r = .43$ ($p < .01$). The magnitude and patterns of correlations across social relationship measures were similar for both the 1988/89 and the 1991 data collection points.

A mixed ANOVA with one between subjects variable (gender of participant) and three within subjects variables (source of social support: spouse, children, friends/relatives; type of social behavior: emotional support, instrumental support, negative behavior; and time: time1, time2) was conducted to compare the different types of social behavior across gender and source over time.

As expected, the ANOVA showed significant within-subjects main effects for source $F(2, 436) = 203.49$, $p <.001$, type $F(2, 436) = 1180.51$, $p <.001$, and time $F(1, 436) = 19.96$, $p <.001$, and a significant between-subject main effect for gender, $F(1, 436) = 6.51$, $p <.05$, qualified by a significant gender by source interaction, $F(2, 436) = 10.33$, $p <.001$, a time by source interaction, $F(2, 436) = 10.33$, $p <.001$ and a significant source by type of support interaction, $F(4, 434) = 68.06$, $p <.001$. Finally, there was also a significant three-way source by type by gender interaction, $F(4, 434) = 4.05$, $p <.01$. Overall, the directions of the effects were consistent with predictions. The data pattern showed that, whereas men received the most emotional support from their wives, the women in the sample said they received the most emotional support from their children and from friends and relatives, at both time points. Both men and women received the highest levels of instrumental support and negative behaviors from their spouses followed by their children, followed by their friends and relatives. The men's social support increased over time for all types of support from all sources. The women's social support increased over time for all types of support from their children and friends and relatives, but not from their spouses.

Gurung et al., (2003) used hierarchical multiple regression analysis to predict changes over time in the types of social support from each of the three sources using demographic and psychological data. Emotional support showed moderate levels of stability with prior levels (i.e., 1988/89) accounting for 29% (from spouse), 10% (from children), and 10% (from friends/relatives) of the variance in later (i.e., 1991) levels when entered in the first step. Gender accounted for significant portions of additional variance in emotional support from the friends/relatives, $F\ (3,433) = 5.28$, $p < .01$, but not from either the spouse or children; specifically, women but not men reported getting more support from friends/relatives over time. The step controlling for physical and cognitive functioning was not significant for emotional support from any source. As predicted, results from the psychological predictors indicated that the people in better psychological condition at Time 1 were those who got more support over time, especially support from friends and relatives. Specifically, participants who had more social ties and who were less depressed at Time 1 reported greater increases in emotional support from friends and relatives at Time 2, $F\ (5,432) = 3.74$, $p < .01$.

Instrumental support was more variable over time than emotional support with prior levels (i.e., 1988/89) accounting for 16% (from spouse), 17% (from friends/relatives) and 10% (from children) of the variance in later (i.e., 1991) levels when entered in the first step. The sociodemographics variables again showed limited predictive power in regard to changes in instrumental support and accounted only for significant portions of additional variance for support from the spouse, $F\ (3,434) = 5.02$, $p < .01$, but not from either the friends/relatives or children. The step controlling for physical and cognitive levels was not significant for instrumental support from any source. As hypothesized, the psychosocial measures entered in the final step significantly predicted additional variance in instrumental support from friends and family, $F\ (4,433) = 3.66$, $p < .01$, and from children, $F(4,433) = 2.39$, $p < .05$, with social ties being the significant predictor. Those with a greater number of social ties reported greater increases in instrumental support from their children and from their friends and relatives at time 2, controlling for time 1 levels.

Prior levels (i.e., 1988/89) of negative behaviors accounted for 31% (spouse), 24% (children) 19% (friends/relatives) of the variance in later (i.e., 1991) levels when entered in the first step. The sociodemographic variables predicted changes in negative behaviors of the spouse, accounting for 2% of additional variance, F (3,433) = 2.86, $p < .05$, and of friends and relatives, accounting for 2% of additional variance, F (3,433) = 2.91, $p < .05$. Women experienced greater increases in negative behaviors from their spouses over time than did men. Younger participants and those with higher income levels experienced greater increases in negative behaviors from their friends and relatives over time than did older, less affluent participants. The step controlling for physical and cognitive levels was significant in predicting changes in negative behavior only for friends/relatives, F (3,433) = 3.53, $p < .05$; specifically, participants with lower cognitive functioning reported greater increases in negative interactions. The psychosocial measures entered in the final step significantly predicted additional variance in negative behaviors from friends and relatives, F (4,432) = 3.66, $p < .01$, and from spouse, F (4,432) = 3.10, $p < .05$. As predicted, participants who were more depressed at Time 1 experienced greater increases in negative behaviors from their spouses and friends and families.

Implications

As shown by Gurung et al. (2003), social support is a dynamic process that ebbs and flows well into later years of adult development. In providing a richly detailed picture of intricacies of support receipt, the results highlight the importance of focusing on both the source and type of support. Supportive transactions do increase over time, and that these changes vary across sources and by type of support. There were also significant gender differences indicating that men and women experience different benefits and gaps in social support.

The data reviewed here extends previous work on the dynamic nature of support (e.g., Antonucci, 1990). On the positive side, to the extent that the pruning of networks may have occurred, it did not appear to eliminate close others (cf., Carstensen, 1995) and for the most part, did not result in the loss of support. In fact, while the number of reported social ties decreased over time, the amount of emotional and instrumental support reported, for the most part, increased. These findings are consistent with the Social Convoy Model and Socioemotional Selectivity theory, in showing that older adults do not lose social support as they age (Antonucci & Akiyama, 1995; Field, 1999; Lang, 2000). The results also revealed that the size of the support network and sources of support were important to social support receipt.

Unfortunately, individuals who might have benefited most from greater social support due to their poorer baseline psychological functioning did not experience beneficial changes in support over time. Indeed, the opposite was true. Cognitively-impaired individuals at Time 1 reported more negative interactions with friends and extended family at Time 2. Depressed individuals at Time 1 reported smaller increases in emotional support and greater increases in negative interactions with the spouse and with friends and relatives at Time 2. These patterns of support suggest that poorer psychological functioning does not affect all aspects of the older adults' networks evenly or in the same ways. Friends and extended family are not as closely tied to their elderly friends as spouse and children are. They may, as a result, be less patient or tolerant of cognitive dysfunction and distress and also have more discretion to reduce their support of troubled individuals, which may be why these relationships especially suffered in the wake of distress and dysfunction. Alternatively, depressed people may withdraw from the discretionary elements of their networks—friends and relatives—whereas such withdrawal may be less practical with immediate family. For whichever reason, spouses may have to bear the brunt of a partner's emotional distress. The spouse's withdrawal of emotional and instrumental support in response to these problems may be untenable, but a spouse may nonetheless feel the need to express his or her irritation and upset to the distressed partner, thus increasing the number of negative interactions experienced over time, as was found in the present results. These findings suggest that a focus on characteristics of individuals that evoke support received from others is useful (e.g., Pierce, et al., 1997), as well as a dynamic analysis of how support obtained (or not) from one person may affect the support sought from another network member.

Source, Type of Support and Gender

The varying patterns of social support across source, type, and gender underscore the importance of using a contextual approach. In particular, the findings suggest that theories like the Functional Specificity Model and Task Specificity Model may not apply to both genders equally. Although men regarded their spouses as their major source of emotional support and reported receiving more emotional support from their wives than from other network members (e.g., Simons, 1983/1984), this was not the case for women; the women in our sample received significantly higher levels of emotional support from their children, friends and relatives than from their spouses.

Past studies have suggested that having a lot of social ties may be particularly beneficial for women (Shye, Mullooly, Freeborn, & Pope, 1995), while functional support (i.e., having supportive ties) may be especially beneficial for men (Rowe & Kahn, 1998). The present study suggests that this pattern may be an artifact of the lesser support that women receive from their husbands. Women may have to draw on children, friends and relatives to get the emotional support they need, if it is not forthcoming from the spouse. Even though the women in this sample reported fewer ties than men did, the support received from their broader social ties was greater (e.g., emotional support from children, friends, and relatives), and thus, a large number of social ties may look especially beneficial for women.

Distinguishing among different types of support is also important to a full understanding of older adult networks. As predicted, we found that emotional support showed moderate stability over time. This stability is likely beneficial because fluctuating social transactions can negatively influence the person's trust and confidence in relationships that could correspondingly negatively affect mental health (Lang, Featherman, & Nesselroade, 1997). If older adults perceive a relatively steady flow of emotional support, this assurance may contribute to better physical and psychological health (e.g., Krause, 1994; Lang & Carstensen, 1998). Although not predicted, the receipt of instrumental support also showed moderate increases over time, suggesting that well maintained networks and close others may serve a range of supportive functions.

Conclusion

The results of Gurung et al., (2003) illustrate the dynamic nature of social support in a healthy aging cohort over time and across different sources. More broadly, it also highlights the utility of factoring in different contexts. The MacArthur Study data nicely capture people operating different independent and overlapping contexts: an intrapersonal context, an interpersonal context, and a temporal context. Clearly, each context overlaps with others and all influence behavior. Further studies of support and efforts to provide it might be especially attuned to the different contexts that social support is transacted in.

Authors' Notes

The authors wish to thank Shelley Taylor and Teresa Seeman for access to the data described in this chapter. The empirical study described in this study was published by the first author, Shelley Taylor, and Teresa Seeman in *Psychology and Aging.*

References

Abbey, A., Andrews, F. M., & Halman, J. L. (1996). Provision and receipt of social support and disregard: What is their impact on the marital life quality of infertile and fertile couples? *Journal of Personality & Social Psychology, 68*, 455-469

Andersen, S. M., Chen, S., & Miranda, R. (2002). Significant others and the self. *Self and Identity, 1*, 159-168.

Andersen, S. M., Reznick, I., & Chen, S. (1997). Self in relation to others: Cognitive and motivational underpinnings. In J. G. Snodgrass & R. I. Thompson (Eds.), *The self across psychology: Self-recognition, self-awareness, and the self-concept* (pp. 233-275). New York: New York Academy of Science.

Antonucci, T. C. (1991). Attachment, social support, and coping with negative life events in mature adulthood. In E. M. Cummings, A. L. Greene, and K. H. Karraker (Eds.) Life-*span developmental psychology: Perspectives on stress and coping* (pp. 261-276). Hillsdale, NJ: Erlbaum.

Antonucci, T. C., & Akiyama, H. (1987). An examination of sex differences in social support among older men and women, *Sex Roles, 17*, 737-749.

Antonucci, T. C., & Akiyama, H. (1995). Convoys of social relations: Family and friendships within a life span context. In R. Blieszner & V. H. Bedford (Eds.), *Handbook of aging and the family* (pp. 355-371). Westport, CT: Greenwood Press.

Antonucci, T. C., & Jackson, J. S. (1987). Social support, interpersonal efficacy, and health: A life course perspective. In L. L. Carstensen & B. A. Edelstein (Eds.), *Handbook of clinical gerontology* (pp. 291-311). New York: Pergamon Press.

Baumeister, R. G., Heatherton, T. F., & Tice, D. M. (1994). *Losing control: How and why people fail at self-regulation.* San Diego, CA: Academic Press.

Berkman, L. F., Vaccarino, V., & Seeman, T. (1993). Gender differences in cardiovascular morbidity and mortality: The contribution of social networks and support. *Annals of Behavioral Medicine, 15*, 112-118.

Bisconti, T. L., & Bergeman, C. S. (1999). Perceived social control as a mediator of the relationships among social support, psychological well-being, and perceived health. *The Gerontologist, 39*, 94-103.

Blazer, D. G., Burchett, B., Service, C., & George, L.K. (1991). The association of age and depression among the elderly: An epidemiologic exploration. *Journals of Gerontology, 46*, M210-M215.

Blazer, D. G., Hughes, D. C., & George, L.K. (1992). Age and impaired subjective support: Predictors of depressive symptoms at one-year follow-up. *Journal of Nervous and Mental Disease, 180*, 172-178.

Bolger, N., Foster, M., Vinokaur, A. D., & Ng, R. (1996). Close relationships and adjustment to a life crisis: The case of breast cancer. *Journal of Personality and Social Psychology, 70*, 283-294.

Bookwala, J., & Schulz, R. (1996). Spousal similarity in subjective well-being: The Cardiovascular Health Study. *Psychology and Aging, 11*, 582-590.

Bosses, R., Aldwin, C. M., Levenson, M. R., Spiro, A. III, & Mroczek, D. K. (1993). Change in social support after retirement: Longitudinal findings from the normative aging study. *Journal of Gerontology: Psychological Sciences, 48,* P210-P217.

Bosses, R., Aldwin, C. M., Levenson, M. R., Workman-Daniels, K., & Ekerdt, D. JH. (1990). Differences in social support among retirees and workers: Findings from the normative aging study. *Psychology of Aging, 5*, 41-47.

Bowling, A. (1994). Social networks and social support among older people and implications for emotional well-being and psychiatric morbidity. *International Review of Psychiatry, 6*, 41-58.

Bronfenbrenner, U. (1986). Ecology of the family as a context for human development: Research perspectives. *Developmental Psychology, 22*, 723-742.

Bruner, J. (1990). *Acts of meaning*. Cambridge, MA: Harvard Press.

Cantor, M. H. (1979). Neighbors and friends: An overlooked resource in the informal support system. *Research on Aging, 1,* 434-463.

Cantor, N. (1994). Life task problem-solving: Situational affordances and personal needs. *Personality and Social Psychology Bulletin*, *20*, 235-243.

Carstensen, L. L. (1987). Age-related changes in social activity. In L. L. Carstensen & B. A. Edelstein (Eds.), *Handbook of clinical gerontology* (pp. 222-237). New York: Pergamon.

Carstensen, L. L. (1991). Socioemotional and selectivity theory: Social activity in life-span context. *Annual Review of Gerontology and Geriatrics, 11,* 195-217.

Carstensen, L. L. (1995). Evidence for a life-span theory of socioemotional selectivity. *Current directions in Psychological Science, 5,* 151-156.

Carstensen, L. L., Isaacowitz, D. M., & Charles, S.T. (1999). Taking time seriously: A theory of socioemotional selectivity. *American Psychologist, 54*, 165-181.

Carver, C. S., & Scheier, M. F. (1998). *On the self-regulation of behavior*. New York: Cambridge University Press.

Chen, S., & Andersen, S. M. (1999). Relationships from the past in the present: Significant-other representations and transference in interpersonal life. In M. P. Zanna (Ed.),

Advances in Experimental Social Psychology, Vol. 31 (pp. 123-190). San Diego, CA: Academic Press.

Clip, E. C., & George, L., K. (1990). Caregiver needs and patterns of social support. *Journal of Gerontology: Social Sciences, 45*, S102-111.

Coe, R. M. (1983). Social epidemiology of diseases of aging. In H. T. Blumenthal (Ed.), *Handbook of the diseases of aging* (pp. 45-70). New York: Van Nostrand Reinhold.

Cohen, S. (1991). Social support and physical health: Symptoms, health behaviors, and infectious disease. In E. M. Cummings, A. L. Greene, & K. H. Karraker (Eds.), *Life-span developmental psychology perspectives on stress and coping* (pp. 213-234). Hillsdale, NJ: Erlbaum.

Connidis, I. A. & Davies, L. (1990). Confidants and companions in alter life: The place of family and friends. *Journal of Gerontology, 45,* 141-149.

Cornoni-Huntley, J., Brock, D. B., Ostfeld, A., Taylor, J. O., & Wallace, R. B. (Eds.). (1986). *Established populations for epidemiologic studies of the elderly, resource data book.* NIH publication 86-2443. Bethesda: NIH.

Costa, P. T., Jr., Zonderman, A. B., & McCrae, R. R. (1985). Longitudinal course of social support among men in the Baltimore Longitudinal Study of Aging. In I. G., Sarason & B. R. Sarason (Eds.), *Social support: Theory, research and applications* (pp. 137-154). Bonston: Martinus Nijohoff.

Coyne, J. C., & DeLongis, A. (1986). Going beyond social support: The role of social relationships in adaptation. *Journal of Consulting and Clinical Psychology, 54*, 454-460.

Coyne, J. C., & DeLongis, A. (1986). Going beyond social support: The role of social relationships in adaptation. *Journal of Consulting and Clinical Psychology, 54,* 454-460.

Coyne, J. C., & Smith, D. A. F. (1991). Couples coping with a myocardial infarction: A contextual perspective on wives' distress. *Journal or Personality and Social Psychology*, *61*, 404-412

Coyne, J. C., Kessler, R. C., Tal, M., Turnbull, J., Wortman, C., & Greden, J. F. (1987). Living with a depressed person. *Journal of Consulting and Clinical Psychology*, *55*, 347-352.

Crohan, S. & Antonucci, T. C. (1989). Friends as a source of social support in old age. In R. G. Adams & R. Blieszner (Eds.), *Older adult friendships: Structure and process* (pp. 129-146). Newbury Park, CA: Sage.

Cummings, W. E. & Henry, J. (1961). *Growing old, the process of disengagement.* New York: Basic Books.

Cutler, S. J., & Hendricks, J. (2000). Age differences in voluntary association memberships: Fact or artifact. *Journal of Gerontology, 55B,* S98-S107.

Cutrona, C. E., & Russell, D. W. (1987). The provisions of social relationships and adaptation to stress. *Advances in Personal Relationships, 1*, 37-67.

Davis-Ali, S. H., Chesler, M. A., & Chesney, B. K. (1993). Recognizing cancer as a family disease: worries and support reported by patients and spouses. *Social Work in Health Care, 19*(2), 45-65.

Derogatis, L. R., Lipman, R.S., Rickels, K., Uhlenhuth, E. H., & Covi, L. (1974). The Hopkins Symptoms Checklist (HSCL): A self-report symptom inventory. *Behavioral Science, 19,* 1-15.

Eitel, P., Hatchett, L., Friend, R., Griffin, K. W., & Wadhwa, N. K. (1995). Burden of self-care in seriously ill patients: Impact on adjustment. *Health Psychology, 14*, 457-463.

Farkas, J. I., & Himes, C. L. (1997). The influence of caregiving and employment on the voluntary activities of midlife and older women. *Journal of Gerontology: Social Sciences, 52B*, S180-S189.

Felton, B. J. & Berry, C. A. (1992). Do the sources of the urban elderly's social support determine its psychological consequences? *Psychology and Aging, 7,* 89-97.

Field, D. (1999). A cross-cultural persepective on continutiy and change in social relations in old age: Introduction to a special issue. *International Journal of Aging and Human Development, 48,* 257-261.

Fiske, V., Coyne, J. C., & Smith, D. A. (1991). Couples coping with myocardial infarction: An empirical reconsideration of the role of overprotectiveness. *Journal of Family Psychology, 5*, 4-20.

Fitting, M., Rabins, P., Lucas, M. J., & Eastman, J. (1986). Caregivers for dementia patients: A comparison of husbands and wives. *The Gerontologist, 26*, 248-252

Flaherty, J., & Richman, J. A. (1989). Gender differences in the perception and utilization of social support: Theoretical perspectives and an empirical test. *Social Science and Medicine, 28* (12), 1221-1228.

Frank, P., Campbell, T. L., & Shields, C. G. (1992). Social relationships and health: The relative roles of family functioning and social support. *Social Science and Medicine, 34*, 779-788.

Frasure-Smith, N, Lesperance, F., & Talajic, M. (1995). The impact of negative emotions on prognosis following myocardial infarction: Is it more than depression? *Health Psychology, 14,* 388-398.

Fratiglioni, L., Wang, H. X., Ericsson, K., Mayten, M., & Wimblad, B. (2000). Influence of social network on occurrence of dementia: a community-based longitudinal study. *Lancet, 355*, 1315-1319.

Frazier, P. A., Davis-Ali, S. H., & Dahl, K. E. (1995). Stressors, social support, and adjustments in kidney transplant patients and their spouses. *Social Work in Health Care, 21*(2) 93-108.

Frazier, P. A., Port, C. L., & Hoff, P. (1996). Social support: The provider's experience. *Journal of Personal and Interpersonal Loss, 1*, 109-128.

Gilford, R. (1984). Contrasts in marital satisfaction throughout old age: An exchange theory analysis. *Journal of Gerontology, 39*, 325-333

Goodwin, R., & Giles, S. (2003). Social support provision and cultural values in Indonesian and Britain. *Journal of Cross-Cultural Psychology, 34*, 240-245.

Gotlib, I. H., & Whiffen, V. E. (1992). The interpersonal context of depression. In W. H. Jones & D. Perlman (Eds.), *Advances in personal relationships* (Vol. 3, pp. 177-206). London: Kingsley.

Gurung, R. A. R., Taylor, S. E, & Seeman, T. (2003). Accounting for changes in social support among married older adults: Insights from the MacArthur Studies of Successful Aging. *Psychology and Aging,* 18(3), 487-496.

Hafner, H., & Welz, R. (1989). Social networks and mental disorder (with special reference to the elderly). In D. Hamburg and N. Sartorius (Eds.*) Health and behavior: Selected perspectives* (pp. 150-161). New York: Cambridge University Press.

Hansson, R. O., & Carpenter, B. N. (1994). Relationships in old age: Coping with the challenge of transition. New York: Guilford Press.

Hatchet, L., Friend, R., Symister, P., & Wadhwa, N. (1997). Interpersonal expectations, social support, and adjustment to chronic illness. *Journal of Personality and Social Psychology, 73*, 560-573.

Havighurst, R. J., & Albrecht, R. E. (1953). *Older people*. New York: Longmans Green.

Helgeson, V. S., & Cohen, S. (1996). Social support and adjustment to cancer: Reconciling descriptive, correlational, and intervention research. *Health Psychology, 15,* 135-148.

Hermans, H. J. M. (1992). Telling and retelling one's self-narrative: A contextual approach to life-span development. *Human Development, 35*, 361-375.

Hess, B. B., & Soldo, B. J. (1985). Husband and wife networks. In W. J. Sauer and R. T. Coward (Eds.), *Social support networks and the care of the elderly* (pp. 67-92). New York: Springer.

Higgins, E. T. (1996). Ideals, oughts, and regulatory focus: Affect and motivation from distinct pains and pleasures. In P. M. Gollwitzer and J. A. Bargh (Eds.), *The psychology of action* (pp. 91-114). New York: Guilford.

Hinkley, K., & Andersen, S. M. (1996). The working self-concept transference: Significant-other activation and self change. *Journal of Personality and Social Psychology*, *71*, 1279-1295.

Hobfoll, S. E., London, P., & Orr, E. (1988). Mastery, intimacy, and stress resistance during war. *Journal of Community Psychology, 16* (3), 317-331.

Hooker, K., Monahan, D. J., Bowman, S. R., Frazier L. D., & Shifren, K. (1998). Personality counts for a lot: Predictors of mental and physical health of spouse caregivers in two disease groups. *Journal of Gerontology: Psychological Sciences, 53B*, P73-P85.

House, J. S., & Kahn, R. L. (1985). Measures and concepts of social support. In S. Cohen, & S. L. Syme (Eds.) *Social support and health* (pp. 83-108). New York: Academic Press.

House, J. S., Umberson, D., & Landis, K. (1988). Structures and processes of social support. *Annual Review of Sociology, 14,* 293-318.

Inouye, S. K., Albert, M. S., Mohs, R., Sun, K., & Berkman, L. F. (1993). Cognitive performance in a high-functioning community-dwelling elderly population. *Journal of Gerontology, 48,* M146-M151.

Jones, W. H. (1985). The psychology of loneliness: Some personality issues in the study of social support. In I.G. Sarason and B.R. Sarason (Eds.), *Social support: Theory , research and applications* (pp. 225-241). Boston, MA: Martinus Nijhoff.

Kahn, R. L., & Antonucci, T. C. (1980). Convoys over the life course. Attachment, roles, and social support. In P. B. Baltes & O. G. Brim (Eds.), *Life-span development and behavior* (pp. 254-283). New York: Academic Press.

Kahn, R. L., & Antonucci, T. C. (1984). Social supports of the elderly: Family/friends/professionals. *Final report to the National Institute on Aging*, #AG01632.

Kaplan, E., Goodglass, H., Weintraub, S. (1983). The Boston Naming Test and scoring booklet. In H. Goodglass, & E. Kaplan (Eds.), *The assessment of aphasia and related disorders* (2nd ed.). Philadelphia: Lea and Febiger.

Katz, S. C., Ford, A. B., Moskowitz, R. W., Jackson, B. A., & Jaffe, A. W. (1963). Studies of illness in the aged- The Index of ADL: A standardized measure of biological and psychosocial function. *Journal of the American Medical Association, 185,* 914-919.

Kessler, R. C., & McLeod, J. D. (1985). Social support and mental health in community samples. In S. Cohen, & S. L. Syme (Eds.) *Social support and health* (pp. 219-240). New York: Academic Press.

Krantz, S. E., & Moos, R. H. (1987). Functioning and life context among spouses of remitted and nonremitted depressed patients. *Journal of Consulting and Clinical Psychology, 55,* 353-360.

Krause, N. (1994). Stressors in salient social roles and well-being in later life. *Journal of Gerontology: Psychological Sciences, 49,* P137-148.

Kriegsman, D. M. W., Pennix, B. W. H. J., & Van Eijk, J. T. M. (1995). A criterion-based literature survey of the relationship between family support and incidence and course of chronic disease in the elderly. *Family Systems Medicine, 13,* 39-68.

Lang, F. R. (2000). Endings and continuity of social relationships : Maximizing intrinsic benefits within personal networks when feeling near death. *Journal of Social and Personal Relationships, 17,* 155-182.

Lang, F. R., & Carstensen, L. L. (1994). Close emotional relationships in late life: Further support for proactive aging in the social domain. *Psychology and Aging, 9,* 315-324.

Lang, F. R., & Carstensen, L. L. (1998). Social relationships and adaptation in later life. In A. S. Bellack & M. Hersen (Eds.), *Comprehensive Clinical Psychology,* (pp.55-72). Oxford: Permagon.

Lang, F. R., Featherman, D. L., & Nesselroade, J. R. (1997). Social self efficacy and short-term variability in personal relationships: The MacArthur Successful Aging Studies. *Psychology and Aging,* 12, 657-666.

Lang, F. R., Staudinger, U. M., & Cartensen, L. L. (1998). Perspectives on socioemotional selectivity in late life: How personality and social context do (and do not) make a difference. *Journal of Gerontology: Psychological Sciences, 53B,* P21-P30.

Lansford, J. E., Sherman, A. M., & Antonucci, T. C. (1998). Satisfaction with social networks: An examination of socioemotional selectivity theory across cohorts. *Psychology and Aging, 13,* 544-552.

Lewis, M. A., Rook, K. S., & Schwarzer, R. (1994). Social support, social control, and health among the elderly. In G. N. Penny, P. Bennett, and M. Herbert (Eds.) *Health psychology: A lifespan perspective* (pp. 191-211). Chur, Switzerland: Harwood.

Litwak, E. (1985). *Helping the elderly: The complementary roles of informal networks and formal systems.* New York: Guilford Press.

Longino, C. F., & Lipman, A. (1985). The support systems of women. In W. J. Sauer and R. T., Coward (Eds.), *Social support networks and the care of the elderly* (pp. 219-233). New York: Springer.

Lynch, S. A. (1998). Who supports whom? How age and gender affect the perceived quality of support from family and friends. *The Gerontologist, 38,* 231-238.

Michella, J. L. (1987). Interpersonal and individual impacts of a husband's heart attack. In A. Baum and J. E. Singer (Eds.), *Handbook of Psychology of Health* (Vol. 5, pp. 255-301). Hillsdale, NJ: Erlbaum.

Miller, S. S., & Cavanaugh, J. C. (1990). The meaning of grandparenthood and its relationship to demographic, relationship, and social participation variables. *Journals of Gerontology: Psychological Sciences, 45,* P244-P246.

Mischel, W. & Shoda, Y. (1995). A cognitive-affective system theory of personality: Reconceptualizing situations, dispositions, dynamics, and invariance in personality structure. *Psychological Review, 102*, 246-268.

Moen, P., Robison, J., & Fields, V. (1994). Women's work and caregiving roles: A life course approach. *Journal of Gerontology: Social Sciences, 49*, S176-S186.

Morgan, D. L. (1989). Adjusting to widowhood: Do social networks really make it easier? *The Gerontologist, 29,* 101-107.

Mutran, E. J., Reed, P. S., & Sudha, S. (2002). Social support: Clarifying the construct with applications for minority populations. In J. H. Skinner, J. A., Teresi, D. Holmes, S. M. Stahl, and A. L. Stewart (Eds.), *Multicultural measurement in older populations* (pp. 69-82). New York, Springer.

Nagi, S. Z. (1976). An epidemiology of disability among adults in the United States. *Milbank Memorial Fund Quarterly, 6,* 493-508.

Nemoto, T. (1989). Norms toward mobilizing social support among Japenese-American elderly Issei, Nisei, and Shin-Issei. *Journal of the Asian American Psychological Association, 13* (1), 56-71.

Neugarten, B. L., Moore, J. W., & Lowe, J. C. (1965). Age norms, age constraints, and adult socialization. *American Journal of Sociology, LXX*, 710-717.

Newsom, J. T., & Schulz, R. (1996). Social support as a mediator in the relation between functional status and quality of life in older adults. *Psychology and Aging, 11,* 34-44.

Oxman, T. E., & Hull, J. G. (1997). Social support, depression, and activities of daily living in older heart surgery patients. *Journal of Gerontology: Psychological Sciences, 52B*, P1-P14.

Pavalko, E. K., & Artis, J. E. (1997). Women's caregiving and paid work: Causal relationships in late midlife. *Journal of Gerontology: Social Sciences, 52B*, S170-S179.

Pearlin, L. I., & Schooler, C. (1978). Some extensions of "The structure of coping": Reply to comments by Marshall and Gore. *Journal of Health and Social Behavior, 20*, 202-205.

Peters, G. R., Hoyt, D. R., Babchuk, N., Kaiser, M., & Iijima, Y. (1987). Primary-group support systems of the aged. *Research on Aging, 9,* 392-416.

Pfeiffer, E. (1975). A short portable mental status questionnaire for the assessment of organic brain deficit in elderly patients. *The American Geriatric Society, 23,* 433-441.

Pierce, G. R., Lakey, B., Sarason, I. G., Sarason, B. R., & Joseph, H. (1997). Personality and social support processes: A conceptual overview. In G. R. Pierce, B. Lakey, I. G. Sarason, & B. R. Sarason (Eds.), *Sourcebook of Social Support and Personality*. New York: Plenum.

Pineo, P. C. (1961). Disenchantment in the later years of marriage. *Marriage and Family Living, 23*, 3-11.

Pines, A. M., Ben-Ari, A., Utasi, A., & Larson, D. (2002). A cross-cultural investigation of social support and burnout. *European Psychologist, 7* (4), 256-264.

Reifman, A. (1995). Social relationships, recovery from illness, and survival: A literature review. *Annals of Behavioral Medicine, 17,* 124-131.

Revenson, T. A. (1990). All other things are not equal: An ecological perspective on the relation between personality and disease. In H. A. Friedman (Ed.), *Personality and disease* (pp. 65-94). New York: Wiley.

Revenson, T. A. (1994). Social support and marital coping with chronic illness. *Annals of Behavioral Medicine, 16*, 122-130.

Roberts, J. E., & Kassel, J. D. (1997). Labile self-esteem, life-stress, and depressive symptoms: Prospective data testing a model of vulnerability. *Cognitive Therapy and Research, 21*, 569-589.

Roberts, R. E., Kaplan G. A., Shema, S. J., & Strawbridge, W. J. (1997). Prevalence and correlates of depression in an aging cohort: The Alameda County Study. *Journal of Gerontology: Social Sciences, 52B*, S252-258.

Robison, J., Moen, P., & Dempster-McClain, D. (1995). Women's caregiving: Changing profiles and pathways. *Journal of Gerontology: Social Sciences, 50B*, S362-S373.

Rodin, J. & McAvay, G. (1992). Determinants of change in perceived health in a longitudinal study of older adults. *Journal of Gerontology, 47,* P373-P384.

Rook, K. S. (1984). The negative side of social interaction: Impact on psychological well-being. *Journal of Social and Personality Psychology, 46,* 1097-1108.

Rook, K. S., & Schuster, T. L. (1996). *Handbook of social support and the family.* New York: Plenum Press.

Roper, E. A., Molnar, D. J., & Wrisberg, C. A. (2003). No "Old Fool": 88 years old and still running. *Journal of Aging and Physical Activity, 11*, 370-387.

Rosow, I., & Breslau, N. (1966). A Guttman health scale. *Journal of Gerontology, 21,* 556-559.

Rowe & Kahn (1998). *Successful Aging: The MacArthur foundation study.* New York: Random House.

Rowe, J. W., & Kahn, R. L. (1987). Human aging: Usual and successful. *Science, 237,* 143-149.

Rozen, W., Mohs, R., & Davies, R. (1984). A new rating scale for Alzheimer's disease. *American Journal of Psychiatry, 141*, 1356-1364.

Saranson, B. R., Saranson, I. G., Hacker, T. A., & Basham, R. B. (1985). Concomitants of social support: Social skills, physical attractiveness and gender. *Journal of Personality and Social Psychology, 49*, 469-480.

Saranson, I. G., Levine, H. M., Basham, R. B., & Saranson, B. R., (1983). Assessing social support. The social support questionnaire: *Journal of Personality and Social Psychology, 44*, 127-139.

Sarason, B. R., Sarason, I. G., & Gurung, R. A. R. (2001). Close personal relationships and health outcomes: A key to the role of social support. In B. R. Sarason, & S. W. Duck (Eds.), *Personal Relationships: Implications for Clinical and Community Psychology.* Wiley.

Schulz R., & Rau, M. T. (1985). Social support through the life course. In S. Cohen and S. L. Syme (Eds.), *Social support and health* (pp. 129-149). New York: Academic Press.

Schulz, R., Tompkins, C. A., Wood, D., & Decker, S. (1987). The social psychology of caregiving: Physical and psychological costs of providing support to the disabled. *Journal of Applied Social Psychology, 17*, 401-428.

Schuster, T. L., Kessler, R. C., & Aseltine, R. H. (1990). Supportive interactions, negative interactions, and depressed mood. *American Journal of Community Psychology, 18*, 423-438.

Schwarzer, R., & Leppin, A. (1992). Social support and mental health: A conceptual and empirical overview. In L. Montada, S. H. Filipp & M. J. Lerner (Eds.), *Life crises and experiences of loss in adulthood* (pp. 435-458). Hillsdale, NJ: Earlbaum.

Scott, G., Ciarrochi, J., & Deane, F. P. (2004). Disadvantages of being an individualist in an individualistic culture: Idiocentrism, emotional competence, stress, and mental health. *Australian Psychologist, 39*, 143-153.

Seeman, T. E., & Berkman, L. F. (1988). Structural characteristics of social networks and their relationship with social support in the elderly: Who provides support. *Social Science and Medicine, 26,* 737-749.

Seeman, T. E., Berkman, L. F., Blazer, D., & Rowe, J. W. (1994). Social ties and support and neuroendocrine function: The MacArthur studies of successful aging. *Annals of Behavioral Medicine, 16,* 95-106.

Seeman, T. E., Charpentier, P., Berkman, L. F., Tinetti, M. E., Guralnik, J. M., Albert, M., Blazer, D., & Rowe, J. W. (1994). Predicting changes in physical performance in a high-functioning elderly cohort: MacArthur Studies of Successful Aging. *Journal of Gerontology, 49,* M97-M108.

Segrin, C. (2003). Age moderates the relationship between social support and psychosocial problems. *Human Communication Research, 29*, 317-342.

Shumaker, S. A., & Hill, D. R. (1991). Gender differences in social support and health. *Health Psychology, 10,* 102-111.

Shye, D., Mullooly, J. P., Freeborn, D. K., & Pope, C. R. (1995). Gender differences in the relationship between social network support and mortality: A longitudinal study of an elderly cohort. *Social Science and Medicine, 41,* 935-947.

Siebert, D. C., Mutran, E. J., & Reitzes, D. C. (1999). Friendship and social support: The importance of role identity to aging adults. *Social Work, 44*, 522-533.

Simons, R. L. (1983/1984). Specificity and substitution in the social networks of the elderly. *International Journal of Aging and Human Development, 18,* 121-139.

Snyder, M. & Cantor, N. (1998). Understanding personality and social behavior: A functionalist strategy. In D. T. Gilbert, S. T. Fiske, & G. Lindzey (Eds.), *Handbook of social psychology* (Vol. 1, pp. 635-679). New York: McGraw-Hill.

Steele, C. M. (1988). The psychology of self-affirmation: Sustaining the integrity of the self. In L. Berkowitz (Ed.), *Advances in experimental social psychology, Vol. 21: Social psychological studies of the self: Perspectives and programs.* (pp. 261-302). San Diego: Academic Press

Taylor, S. E., Klein, L. C., Lewis, B., Gruenewald, T., Gurung, R. A. R., & Updegraff, J. (2000). The female stress response: Tend and befriend not fight or flight. *Psychological Review, 107,* 411-429.

Tesser, A. (2002). Constructing a niche for the self: A bio-social PDP approach to understanding lives. *Self and Identity*, *1*, 185-190.

Tjosvold, D., Law, K. S., & Sun, H. F. (2003). Collectivistic and individualistic values: Their effects on group dynamics and productivity in China. *Group Decision and Negotiation, 12*, 243-263.

Tompkins, C. A., Schulz, R., & Rau, M. T. (1988). Post-stroke depression in primary support persons: Predicting those at risk. *Journal of Consulting and Clinical Psychology, 56*, 502-508.

Tower, R. B., & Kasl, S. V. (1996). Depressive symptoms across older spouses: Longitudinal influences. *Psychology of Aging, 11*, 683-697.

Triandis, H. C. (1995). *Individualism & Collectivism*. San Francisco: Westview Press.

Triandis, H. C., & Gelfand, M. J. (1998). Converging measurement of horizontal and vertical individualism and collectivism. *Journal of Personality and Social Psychology, 74*, 118-128.

Triandis, H. C., Bontempo, R., Villareal, M.J., Asai, M., & Lucca, N. (1988). Individualism and collectivism: Cross-cultural perspectives on self-ingroup relationships. Journal of Personality and Social Psychology, 54, 323-338.

Triandis, H. C., Leung, K., Villareal, M. J., & Clack, F. L. (1985). Allocentric versus idiocentric tendencies: Convergent and discriminant validation. *Journal of Research in Personality, 19*, 395-415.

U. S. Bureau of the Census (2004). Population Projections. http://www.census.gov/population/www/projections/popproj.html [Online].

Unger, J. B., McAvay, G., Bruce, M. L., Berkman, L., & Seeman, T. (1999). Variation in the impact of social network characteristics on physical functioning in elderly persons: MacArthur studies of successful aging. *Journal of Gerontology, 54B,* S1-S7.

Van Tilburg, T. (1998). Losing and gaining in old age: Changes in personal network size and social support in a four-year longitudinal study. *The Journals of Gerontology, 53B*, S3131-S323.

Vogt, T. M. (1992). Aging, stress, and illness: Psychobiological linkages. In M. G. Ory, R. P. Abeles, and P.D. Lipman (Eds.), *Aging, health, and behavior* (pp. 207-236). Newbury Park, CA: Sage.

Von Dras, D. D., & Siegler, I. C. (1997). Stability in extraversion and aspects of social support at mid-life. *Journal of Personality and Social Psychology, 71*, 233-241.

Von Dras, D. D., Williams, R. B. Jr., Kaplan, B. H., & Siegler, I. C. (1996). Correlates of perceived social support and equality of interpersonal relationships at mid-life. *International Journal of Aging and Human Development, 43,* 199-217.

VonDras, D. D. & Madey, S. F. (2004). The attainment of important health goals throughout adulthood: An integration of the Theory of Planned Behavior and aspects of social support. *International Journal of Aging and Human Development, 56,* 207-236.

VonDras, D. D., Malcore, S. A., Pouliot, G. P., & Iwahashi, S. (2004). Equality of Social Relationships in Different Interpersonal Domains: Effects of Age and Culture. Presentation at the 16th Annual Convention of the American Psychological Society in Chicago, IL.

VonDras, D. D., Siegler, I. C., Barefoot, J. C., Williams, R. B., & Mark, D. B. (2000). Coronary chatherization patient and wife's perceptions of social support: Effects due to characteristics of recipient, provider, and their interaction. *International Journal of Aging and Human Development, 50*, 97-125.

Weiss, R. S. (1974). The provisions of social relationships. In Z. Rubin (Ed.), *Doing unto others* (pp. 17-26). Englewood Cliffs, NJ: Prentice-Hall.

In: Aging and the Elderly: Psychology, Sociology and Health ISBN 1-60021-190-9
Editor: L. O. Randall, pp. 139-151

Chapter 6

ANOREXIA OF AGING

Claudia Savina, Lorenzo M. Donini* and Carlo Cannella
Istituto di Scienza dell'Alimentazione – Università di Roma "La Sapienza," Italy
Casa di Cura Villa delle Querce – Nemi, Rome, Italy

ABSTRACT

Independence and self–esteem are strongly related to physical and mental function which in turn are largely determined by nutritional status and physical activity. Food is an integral part of our well-being and quality of life. It extends beyond simply satisfying hunger and providing nourishment. Specific foods have a symbolic meaning and particular food habits are influenced by religious, cultural, social and emotional experience.

Elderly people showing interest towards food, nourishment and keeping a good appetite, in most cases still are vital human beings full of interests and quite independent. Behavioural characteristics before mentioned describe the picture of the elderly aging with "a good health", known in medical literature as *Healthy Aging*.

Aging is normally associated with body weight gain in individuals who fail to decrease food intake in proportion to the age-related decline in energy expenditure. However, decreases in body weight are common in elderly individuals (over 70 years of age) who do not eat enough to meet energy demands.

Age related reduction in energy intake is largely a physiologic effect of healthy aging and reveals itself with a loss of eating need and pleasure. This reduction intake may predispose to the harmful anorexic effect of psychological, social and physical problems that become increasingly frequent with aging. The physiological anorexia of aging increases the propensity for developing pathological anorexia and weight loss when an older person falls ill with either a medical or a psychological illness [1]. A 10% loss of body weight over 10 years is consistently associated with increased mortality and functional disability [2].

---

* Università di Roma "La Sapienza"; Istituto di Scienza dell'Alimentazione; Ple Aldo Moro, 5 – 00185 Roma (Italia); e-mail: lorenzomaria.donini@uniroma1.it; tel.: +39.06.4969.0216; fax: +39.06.4991.0699

Weight loss is one of the pathognomonic signs of malnutrition (whether energetic or protein-energy) which may negatively influence the clinical outcome of rehabilitation programmes, confirming that a convenient nutritional status helps the achievement of such a condition and it is absolutely essential when recovering from acute illnesses [3].

A further demonstration of the importance of nutritional status has been pointed out by several studies showing that, after sixties of age, weight loss is associated to a decline in muscle mass and consequently in muscle strength. The picture just mentioned is well-known as *sarcopenia*, which plays a main role in the beginning of: frailty, functional and metabolic impairments, physical disabilities that expose the elderly to an increased risk of falls and protein-energy malnutrition. The obese elderly also affected by protein malnutrition configure the so called *fat frail* who obtains worse outcomes in rehabilitation programmes [4].

Epidemiology of Anorexia of Aging in the Elderly

From an epidemiological point of view, nutritional surveys showed a low to moderate prevalence of frank nutrient deficiencies in free living elderly groups. The SENECA-EURONUT study, enrolling cognitively intact and free living elderly from twelve European nations, found that dietary intakes were often below the recommended levels established for younger adults but this was not reflected in the indicators of nutritional status [5]. The National Health and Nutrition Examination Survey has clearly shown a linear decline in food intake from 20 to 80 years in both men and women even if this change could be caused by a greater incidence of pathological causes in elderly people [6]. In another research the authors found that food intake was lower in older persons than in younger: their data showed that the major decrease was due to a decrease in fat (55%) rather than in carbohydrate (40%) [7]. According to different record of cases and nutritional parameters, data are worst in institutionalised older persons whose rates of protein energy malnutrition range from 30 to 60% [8-10].

Definition of Anorexia of Aging

Age-related anorexia may be defined as an unintentional decline in food intake, and, as a result, of body weight, that begins near the end of life; it represents a sign of a failure to preserve steady state levels of body weight and energy stores. The regulation of food ingestion is an extremely complex process with multiple fail-safe mechanisms able to preserve that the feeding drive remains intact. Food intake can be considered to be under the regulation of a central feeding drive influenced by a peripheral satiation system and receiving further feedback signals from fat cells, absorbed nutrients and circulating hormones. Animal and human studies suggest that alterations at multiple levels of this system occur with aging, resulting in the physiologic anorexia of aging.

Absence of obvious pathology associated distinguishes, according to some authors, the *physiological anorexia of aging* (due to appetite, taste and olfactory acuity, dental status, physical activity, ...) from *pathological anorexia*, a phenomenon characterised by increased resting energy expenditure, elevated cytokines and muscle and fat wasting related to disease (acute and chronic diseases, disability, ...). It is however difficult to verify the real absence of underlying disease and this may influence the prevalence, in different settings, of anorexia of aging [2].

A third form of anorexia in elderly is related to *environment* (age, sex, income, cooking facilities, retirement/leisure time, education, distance to food store, availability of transportation, social activity, self-esteem, symbolism of food, mental awareness, ...) and *iatrogenic conditions* (use of drugs, ...).

1. Physiological Anorexia of Aging

Energy Balance in the Elderly

In the elderly we have a disregulation of energy balance and food intake control. After an overnight fast, older tend to be less hungry than younger persons and after a standard meal older persons report a greater degree of satiation than younger.

Older individuals are also less capable of returning to their previous weight after a perturbation of their food intake than younger are and even after refeeding, older persons return to a lower weight than previously. Young people significantly increase their energy intake following underfeeding while elderly do not and their energy needs remain somewhat depressed relative to their previous weight maintenance requirements.

Healthy older persons ingest less energy than younger men do over a single meal. However, when given a preload (e.g. yoghurt) elderly fail to adequately regulate their food intake, overeating 10-30%, whereas younger had a more precise regulation of their food intake.

These findings are consistent with the suggestion that a lack of the normal ability to regulate energy intake contributes to impaired energy regulation in old age. However, rather than a loss of the ability to regulate energy intake, this being an independent factor, weight loss may be caused in the elderly by the combination of a reduction in the ability to regulate food intake and other adverse events [11-13].

Altered Regulation of Food Intake Control

In the elderly, more rapidly acting or more potent inhibitory satiety signals may contribute to the altered regulation of satiation system. The passage of nutrients into the small intestine and their absorption contribute to stimulate the release of hormones. These include cholecystokinin (CCK), glucagon-like peptide-1, glucose-dependent insulinotropic peptide, insulin and amylin, all of them with proven or putative satiating effects. CCK is probably the most important satiating hormone and is thought to be responsible of 20% of the signals responsible for meal termination. It causes simultaneous contraction of the gallbladder and relaxation of the sphincter of Oddi, thus releasing bile into the duodenum, and stimulates pancreatic enzyme secretion. CCK acts together, in a synergic way, with other hormones or neurotransmitters as serotonin, corticotrophin releasing factors, histamine, glucagon and somatostatin. CCK also activates vagal afferent fibres that terminate in the brainstem. The effects of CCK are mediated by an increase in the contractile activity of the pylorus, which slows gastric emptying and increases the sensitivity to gastric relaxation. Animal studies have shown greater levels and an increased satiating effect of CCK in older compared with younger animals. Many authors found that elderly patients with idiopathic senile anorexia had increased plasma concentrations of CCK compared with age-matched controls.

The regulation of the satiation system is under the control of the adaptive relaxation of the stomach fundus: dilatation allows it to act as a reservoir for food before passing along the antrum. In fact gastrointestinal sensory signals induced by relaxation of food contribute to initial sensations of fullness during a meal. With aging, food tends to pass more rapidly from the fundus into the antrum and then to remain longer there, leading to earlier and greater degree of antral relaxation. The degree of antral relaxation is directly proportional to the development of satiation after ingestion of a meal. Most studies suggest that the rate of gastric emptying slows in older compared with younger persons. For this reason, the elderly frequently complain of increased fullness and early satiation during a meal.

The decrease of the adaptive relaxation of the fundus stomach in the elderly is associated with the reduction of the number of neurons in the myenteric plexus and with the reduction of nitric oxide (NO), a short-lived gas produced by the endothelial and neuronal cells and inducible nitric oxide synthase. NO is a transducer of the effects of a number of hormones in the control of feeding like leptin and NPY. NO delays gastric emptying by altering pyloric tone and it seems to play an important role for both receptive and adaptive relaxation of the fundus of the stomach to food. Even if the condition may not be the same in humans, in studies with older animals there is a decrease in messenger RNA for NO-synthase with aging [14-18].

Decline in food intake in the elderly may be due to the altered regulation of peripheral feedback signals as those coming from fat cells. Leptin is produced by fat cells and is responsible for appetite modulation: the effect of elevated leptin levels, especially in men, may cause anorexia. One mechanism whereby leptin inhibits food intake and stimulates energy expenditure involves altered transcription of hypothalamic neuropeptides. Leptin decreases the expression of orexigenic peptides (NPY, agouti-related peptide, melanin-concentrating hormone) and increases mRNA levels of anorexic peptides (propiomelanocortin, cocaine and amphetamine-related transcript). Studies in humans have demonstrated that, after adjustment for body fat, a significant inverse relationship between serum leptin and age exists. However leptin concentrations are not dramatically altered with aging and seem to be more related to body fat than aging per se leaving open the possibility that disrupted leptin signals, as opposed to increased leptin levels, occurs in age-related energy imbalance such as anorexia.

Peripheral feedback signals may come from the rate of peripheral nutrient utilisation and the plasma nutrient concentrations that influence circulating messages relating to overall fuel status. Elderly have difficulty in maintaining their internal state and this can be due to changes in regulatory systems as it happens for example for salt and water homeostasis.

Aging is associated with a decline in homeostatic capabilities so that the elderly is less sensitive to both internal and environmental changes. Circulating glucose is thought to be one of the signals of hunger in younger adults and detection of hypoglycemia may be impaired in older individuals. With aging, even if glucose impairment is not quantitatively important, glucose may still be an important mediator of changes in the regulation of food intake.

Also circulating hormones may influence food intake. Insulin as been suggested to act as a satiety agent by affecting the expression of neuropeptides such as NPY and insulin concentrations increase with aging as a result of increased insulin resistance. At the moment, there are no data supporting the role of insulin in the development of the anorexia of aging.

Nevertheless animal studies have reported that hyperglycemia and or hyperinsulinemia may be causes of the greater satiating effects of glucose in older subjects.

Sex hormones are well recognised to regulate appetite: testosterone increases food intake Thus the reduction of testosterone levels in older males may play a role in the reduction of food intake (increasing leptin levels) and in the loss of muscle mass (sarcopenia) [1, 2, 15, 19, 20].

The opioid feeding drive, mediated in particular by dinorphin (but also by beta-endorphins and enkefalines), plays an important role in driving fat intake in animals and humans, in determining the palatability of food and in initiating and terminating eating. A decrease in concentrations of endogenous opioid peptides and in their effectiveness, related to the decrease in opioid receptors, occurs with aging: elderly patients with idiopathic senile anorexia seem to have lower levels of cerebrospinal fluid and plasma β-endorphin.

Central feeding drive may be influenced also by neuropetide Y (NPY) that is the most potent orexigenic agent. The effects of NPY are predominantly on food rich in carbohydrate. NPY is less effective in increasing food intake in older than in younger animals and its concentrations decline with aging especially in Alzheimer's dementia patients.

In elderly patients with idiopathic senile anorexia some authors found an increased ratio of tryptophan, a serotonin precursor, to large neutral amino acids in the cerebrospinal fluid. Elevated brain serotonin level causes satiety.

The issue concerning the production of interleukin with anorexic action in geriatric age is disputable (IL6, TNFα). Researches, up to now, did not give any univocal result; some of them showed an increased production of IL6 also without any chronic or acute illness in course, while others did not reach similar conclusions. [16, 17, 21-24].

Alterations in the Hedonic Qualities of Food

The enjoyment of food depends not only on its taste but also on its smell as it approaches the mouth and on the release of volatile organic substances within the mouth. In addition food temperature and texture, as well as masticatory sounds, all produce the ultimate sensory experience.

Throat dryness in elderly is frequent and related to either a progressive atrophy of the salivary glands, or to the lack of nutrients (Zn), besides, drugs use (such as diuretics, anticholinergic drugs, drugs for treatment of Parkinson's disease, tricyclic antidepressants...). Poor dentition or ill fitting dentures are often mentioned as a factor affecting the nutrition of elderly people and even masticatory efficiency of removable denture is much less than that of complete natural dentition.

Subtotal or total edentulism is not only an oral disease but also a disease affecting the quality of life and the healthy status since it deeply limits the hedonistic component of feeding that is only apparently a commonplace feature. In particular, edentulism alters food selection, forcing the elderly to change the basket of the basic foods of his own nutrition. In fact, the elderly, even wearing dentures, above all if bad fitting, because of the reduced masticatory efficiency, tend to avoid specific foods such as those of hard, fibrous texture, as meat, fruits (es.: apples, pears, ...) and vegetables (es.: raw carrots, raw fennels, ...). For this reason, both the edentate elderly, who does not wear dentures and whose hula are physiologically sclerous, and the elderly who wear partial or total dentures, even though well fitting, decide to select soft texturing foods in order to reduce or eliminate oral pain. The texture therefore is the main organoleptic characteristic used as coping behaviour. By means of this behaviour the elderly: 1. does not reduce total energy intake since selected foods are generally rich in simple sugar, saturated fats and cholesterol and are even able to cause overweight or obesity in those ones with oral disease; 2. reduces the intake of animal protein, vitamins e minerals.

Also, a reduced masticatory efficiency is thought to lead to a preference for foods of softer consistency, high in sugar content. However few relationships with macronutrients intake have been observed.

According to most studies, a functionally inadequate dental status affects micronutrient intake: for edentulous subjects in the SENECA study intakes of carbohydrates and vitamin B6 especially, but also to a lesser extent for vitamins C and B1, dietary fibre, calcium and iron, were reduced.

Also the masticatory efficiency may be negatively affected by drugs like muscle relaxants or benzodiazepines, in case of illnesses seriously compromising motility (Parkinson's disease, cerebrovascular disease, major depression,…), the musculature efficiency, generally speaking (myasthenia, hypothyroid myopathia, …) or that regarding the mouth in particular (oculo-pharingeal muscular distrophy, cerebrovascular accident, …) [25-26].

Aging is characterized by a reduction in sensorial perceptions: visus sharpness decreases, olfactory and gustative thresholds increases, hearing and tactile discriminative capacity decreases. These changes negatively affect the hedonistic feature of all the step of feeding. Elderly food choice is done in order to: make shopping easier (stocking of great quantity of foods versus variety, precooked food), facilitate meal preparation (cooking a lot of foods which is stocked in the fridge and consumed after being warmed up exposing the elderly to reduced intake of vitamins), facilitate ingestion (soft, easy to chew foods which do not exacerbate oral pain during chewing and swallowing).

Taste and smell are key determinants of the palatability of food. With advancing age and mainly related to chemosensory losses, taste and smell changes occur: this can lead to poor appetite, inappropriate food choices and lower nutrient intake.

In the elderly we have a reduction of taste papillae and an increase in taste thresholds, sweet taste being less affected than other modalities (sour, salt, bitter) and salt showing the highest increase. Similarly older persons are less capable to identify different compounds. Taste dysfunction also results from certain diseases, medications, surgical intervention, malnutrition and environmental exposure, bad oral hygiene or when a dental prosthesis is used.

In contrast with the variability in taste changes, the ability to smell declines progressively with age in relation to diseases or medications while older persons rate flavour as the most important determinant of their food choice. With aging, threshold losses have been reported for multiple odorants and many disorders affecting smell perception like anosmia, hyposmia and dysosmia increase in severity with advancing age. Some authors found that older persons preferred food having a greater flavour concentration. Addition of simulated food flavours to meats, vegetables and other foods to amplify smells to compensate for chemosensory losses has been shown to be helpful in an elderly population resulting in an improved immunity and functional status, palatability and food acceptance.

Sight is basic for eating behaviour. By sight it is possible to evaluate: shape, dimension, appearance, and colour of foods. Colour plays a very important role in food choice since it allows to assess food appearance, it arouses expectations of taste, odour, texture, healthiness; it also provides signs about maintenance of food. In food choice or rejection sight is the first control point parallel working with experiences and memories. In fact, people are reticent when tasting differently coloured food (this fact suggest that food choice or rejection is made up by a complex evaluation based on both sensory perceptions and memories) [27-28].

2. Pathological Anorexia of Aging

Medical Conditions

Despite being apparently healthy most of the elders suffer from one or more chronic conditions, which may produce anorexia, malabsorption and increased metabolism, alone or combined. Anorexia often is an underrated symptom in the clinical management of patients suffering from acute and chronic diseases. Besides what already stated about depression and oral disorders, decline in food intake in the elderly may be due to medical conditions such as disability (even if little information exists on the association of disabilities and macronutrient intakes, limitations in daily life activities are considered a key cause of weight loss), gastrointestinal disorders and malabsorption deficiencies (swallowing disorders are both associated with aspiration and decreased food intake; dyspepsia is extremely common in older persons and is associated with anorexia; persons with intestinal bacterial overgrowth have been shown to lose weight associated with both anorexia and malabsorption; helicobacter pylori infection prevalence increases with age and may play a role in anorexia), acute and chronic infections (chronic obstructive pulmonary disease, for example, produces anorexia secondary to oxygen desaturation and increased metabolism due to increased activity of the respiratory muscles), hypermetabolism and hypercatabolism (causing increased energy and protein requirements and producing their anorectic and wasting effects by releasing cytokines).

In particular these cytokines have a powerful anorectic effect that is mediated by: leptin (release and action on leptin receptor), direct stimulus of Corticothropin Releasing Factor, the increase $PGE_{1\alpha}$ levels, or inhibition o anorectic peptides release (dynorphin, NPY, galanina, MCH).

Leptin is a peptide hormone belonging to the helical cytokines family (IL-6, IL-11, leukmia inhibitory factor, ciliary neurotrophic factor). Further the leptin receptor is homologous to the gp 130 signal-transducing molecule that it is also associated with the IL-6 receptor (transducers 1 e 3 signal activation) which activity decreases with aging. It seems that signal transducers transcription factors may have a basic role in AA pathogenesis. The same postreceptor pathway is activated by endotoxin, lipopolysaccharides e anorectic cytokines.

Among elderly patients Alzheimer's dementia is frequent and it is one of the dwindles of geriatric failure to thrive. It is however still unclear whether weight loss precedes or follows dementia and whether it is caused by low levels of energy intake or by a hypermetabolic state. In people affected by dementia some changes concerning the control of feeding intake (disregulation of the central opioid feeding drive, CCK increase, reduced levels of plasma and brain NPY and brain neuroepinephrine, changes in sensorial perception) add to problems concerning deterioration of mental status, (loss of memory of the latest meal, apraxia of eating, agnosia with difficulties in interpreting sense data related to vision, taste, smell or touch, distraction from eating during mealtime), changes in behavioural function (circadian shift in intake preponderance of calories consumed at breakfast) and the loss of the Activities of Daily Leaving (inability to buy food, to cook meals, to feed themselves and feeding time lengthening) thus creating a serious risk as far as nutrition is concerned.

Patients with Parkinson's disease often exhibit eating problems: most of them show a decrease sense of smell, a cognitive decline, a loss of motivation to eat related to depression, difficulties in starting to eat owing to increased need to external stimulation or in performing the acts of eating. Drugs given for the treatment of Parkinson's disease may cause anorexia and further contribute to decreasing food intake.

Many medical conditions, as those affecting the nervous system (Alzheimer's disease, epilepsy, multiple sclerosis, Parkinson's disease, ...), or those affecting the nutritional sphere (chronic renal failure, cancer, zinc – vitamin B12 – niacin deficiencies, ...), endocrine diseases (diabetes mellitus, hypothyroidism, ...), local inflammations (allergic rhinitis, bronchial asthma, sinusitis, ...) and viral infections (acute viral hepatitis, influenza-like infections, ...) may also affect the sense of taste and smell [29-36].

3. Anorexia of Aging Secondary to Iatrogenic or Environment Conditions

Loss of Motivation to Eat

One of the causes of anorexia of aging is the loss of motivation to eat that may be due to depression and social networks loss or deterioration.

Social factors, like poverty, inability to shop, to feed one's self, to prepare and cook meals, can contribute to decreased food intake in the elderly.

Less energy is acquired during meals taken alone than during meals eaten in company, difference in energy intake being about 30%. An extensive friendship network may be positively related to appetite and nutrient intake while widowhood may cause a decrease in meal enjoyment, poorer appetite and weight loss. Providing nutrition food via specific social programs may not overcome the eating problems associated with social isolation. Such data are generally used to suggest that social eating promotes overeating and obesity, but another interpretation is that eating alone, in the elderly especially, leads to undernourishment and weight loss.

Energy intake is greater when a variety of foods is provided than when only a single food is available. Dietary variety has been shown to decline as age increases, with sensory impairment, poverty, loneliness and widowhood. Variety of foods is positively correlated with nutritional quality and has been associated with health outcomes.

Hospitalisation or the institutionalisation in a nursing home, independently from physical acute illness, forecasts a reduction of feeding intake; all this bounds up to worsening of mood, to the perception of a likely future loss of the family environment besides the loss of all of those non-biological values nevertheless attributed to food intake. The foods we eat as well as when, where and how we eat them are decisions based on individual choices and lifetime habits. In a nursing home or in a hospital these choices are limited. Therefore, many elders refuse to eat because they do not like the food they are served or because the food is of different ethnicity. In a recent survey, only 23% of the residents in a nursing home were very satisfied with the food and 58% stated choice and control over food to be very important. Nursing home residents or hospital patients may also reject food to punish a staff member who has not been kind to them, as a way to manipulate the staff itself, to get more attention or to refuse a dietary prescription.

Depression has been shown to be one of the most important treatable causes of weight loss in both community and institutional settings. Depression is related to loneliness, low self-esteem, intolerance against the environment, retirement from job, loss of a relative or a pet, hospitalisation or retirement in a nursing home.

The mechanism behind anorexia in depression has not been fully elucidated. There are some evidence that depression increases corticotrophin releasing factor (CRF) levels, suggesting a role for CRF causing anorexia and weight loss in the elderly.

The prevalence of depression is high in the elderly. Geriatric Depression Scale (GDS) scores above the cut-off of 5 were found in about 12% of the men and 28% of the women enrolled in the SENECA study. There was a significant negative correlation between GDS score and cholesterol blood levels. Successful treatment of depression in nursing home residents results in reversal of weight loss. Weight loss and anorexia were found to be important symptoms related to increased mortality in depressed elderly.

Refusal to eat can be part of an indirect self-destructive behaviour (ISDB) a form of covert, indirect and perhaps unconscious suicidal behaviour. ISDB is defined as an act of omission or commission that causes self-harm that leads indirectly and over time to the patient's death. Persons can omit behaviours that would sustain life and health like prescribed treatments or food. ISDB has been shown to be associated with a direct suicidal potential, dissatisfaction with the treatment program and life in general, confused reasoning and judgement, poor prognosis for discharge, absence of religious commitment and significant losses in the patient's life. Some older people decrease their food intake few months before dying: for those patients who feel an excessive burden of life, refusing food is an acceptable method for terminating their lives.

Nervous or "tardy" anorexia can recur in older persons who were previously weight restrictors. Eating disorders have been considered illness of adolescence and young adulthood but few cases of later onset (over 50 years of age) presentation have been reported. Patients with belated anorexia have a persistently depressive mood but a lesser degree of disturbed body image and of preoccupation with weight, eating and shape [33-35, 37-46].

Prescription Medicines

Comprising 12% of the population, elderly persons consume 35% of prescription drugs in the United States. Epidemiological studies indicate that the mean number of medications used by community-dwelling elderly over the age of 65 ranges from 2.9 to 3.7 medications [47]. The side effects of these drugs are a major cause of weight loss in older persons both free-living or institutionalised. Drugs can affect nutritional intake by decreasing appetite (digoxin, amiodarone, spironolactone, cimetidine, amitriptyiline, most antibiotics, metronidazole, ...), causing malabsorption, nausea or vomiting (sorbitol, theophyllin elixir, laxatives, ...), increasing metabolism (excess thyroxine replacement, theophylline, ...), depleting body's mineral stores (aluminium or magnesium hydroxide antacids , ...). In addition drug induced depression, cognitive impairment and constipation may cause food refusal [14, 31, 32, 34, 35].

Over 250 drugs have been clinically reported to alter taste and/or smellike drugs to lower cholesterol or lipids in blood (fibrates, statines, ...), antihistamines, drugs to fight infectious diseases (antibiotics, fluoroquinolones, ...), to treat cancer, for arthritis and pain (corticosteroids, …), for asthma and breathing problems (β-adrenergic agonists, …), for hypertension (ACE inhibitors, Ca-channel-blockers, …) and heart disease (nitroglycerin patches, …) besides muscle relaxants and drugs for treatment of Parkinson's disease or epilepsy, drugs to improve mood.

Compared to young individuals, the average detection thresholds for elderly individuals, with one or more medical conditions and taking an average of 3.4 medications, were 11.6 times higher for sodium salts, 4.3 times higher for acids, 7.0 times higher for bitter compounds, 2.7 times higher for sweeteners [27, 36].

MANAGEMENT OF ANOREXIA OF AGING

It is very important to keep into consideration and face anorexia of aging in due time. Consequences, as stated, can be extremely serious and deeply affect both patient's mobility, mortality and quality of life. Therefore, it will be of the utmost importance to insert a special evaluation of the nutritional risk in the Comprehensive Geriatric Assessment, that must be performed in all elderly patients at admission, and constantly evaluate the nutritional status and their feeding intake of the older patients using specific method (Eating Behaviour Scale [47], Blandford Scale [48], Mini Nutritional Assessment [49], …), to identify and treat the underlying disease (acute and chronic infections, depression, …) when possible, to institute environmental and behavioural modifications (changing in atmosphere during mealtime, providing favourite foods, increasing food flavours, seeking companionship during meals, increasing physical activity, …), to both increase staffing levels and to organise staff better to produce higher quality feeding assistance during mealtimes [50], to use, in selected cases, appetite stimulants (megestrol acetate, cyproheptadine, growth hormone, …), to plan early nutrition rehabilitation programs (liquid supplements, enteral feeding) and nutritional education programs for caregivers (using methods such as the Nutritional Calendar [51]; these programs should enable the caregiver to establish a minimal evaluation of the nutritional state, to know the nutritional value of basic food , to cope with eating behaviour disorders, …) [20, 35, 52-54].

CONCLUSION

Food intake can contribute to improve older people well-being and quality of life. Therefore despite some dietary interventions are unlikely to reduce disability or extend life expectancy, they may be still worthwhile if they enhance an elderly individual's well-being or quality of life.

We need further studies to better understand factors contributing to poor nutrition in the elderly, such as changes in various neurotransmitters, to develop preventive (reduction of risk factors, improvement of nutritional assessment, …) and treatment strategies (nucleotides, increased energy and nutrient density food, improving taste and smell, …).

Dietary related interventions in older adults should aim to prevent decline and to extent possible restore or to maintain function and quality of life. Interventions need to be acceptable, so that to integrate other health promoting strategies and be continually monitored and assessed to evaluate their effectiveness.

In elderly people, also relation to their cultural and emotional value, traditional food, even if it is known for not being always nutritionally sound, should be preferred. However innovations in agriculture and food technologies will increasingly allow us to assure a richer content of nutrients and beneficial phytochemical and a reduced content of inhibitory and anti-nutritional factors. These changes also present their risks as nothing in human evolutionary experience have prepared those who are exposed to these novel foods to the particular chemical composition they are made up with.

REFERENCES

[1] Morley JE: Anorexia, body composition and ageing. *Curr Opin Clin Nutr Metab Care* 2001, 4, 9-13Horwitz BA, Blanton CA, McDonald RB: Physiologic determinants of the anorexia og aging. *Annu Rev Nutr* 2002, 22, 417-43.

[3] Gazewood JD, Mehr DR: Diagnosis and management of weight loss in the elderly. *J Fam Pract* 1998, 47, 19-25.

[4] Stevens J: Impact of age on association between weight and mortality. *Nutr Rev* 2000, 58, 129-137.

[5] Euronut-SENECA De Groot CGPM, Van Staveren WA, Hautvast JGAJ eds: A concerted action on nutrition and health in Europe. *Eur J Clin Nutr* 1991, 45 suppl, 3, S1-196.

[6] Anonimous. Daily dietary fat and total food energy intakes. 3rd NHANES, phase III 1988-1991. *MMWR Morb Mortal Wkly Rep* 1994, 43, 116-25Wurtmann JJ , Lieberman H, Tsay R: Calorie and nutrient intakes of elderly young subjects measured under identical conditions. *J Gerontol* 1988, 43, B174-180.

[8] Sullivan DH: The role of nutrition in increased morbidity and mortality. *Clin Geriatr Med* 1995, 11, 661-674.

[9] Elmstahl S, Steen B: Hospital nutrition in a geriatric long-term care medicine. *Age Ageing* 1987, 16, 73.

[10] Ahari M, Kimigiar M: Food intake and body mass index in the privately institutionalised elderly. *Int J Vit res* 1997, 67, 41.

[11] Elia M, Ritz P, Stubbs RJ: Total energy expenditure in the elderly. *Eur J Clin Nutr* 2000, 54, S3, 92-103.

[12] Henry CJK: Mechanisms of changes in basal metabolism during ageing. *Eur J Clin Nutr* 2000, 54, S3, 77-91.

[13] Elia M: Organ and tissue contribution to metabolic rate. In: Energy metabolism. Tissue determinants and cellular corollaries. JM Kinney & HN Tucker Eds, New York, *Raven Press,* 1992, pp 62-8.

[14] Morley JE: Anorexia of aging. *Am J Clin Nutr* 1997, 66, 760-73.

[15] MacIntosh CG, Horowitz M, Verhajen MAMT, Smout AJPM, Wishart J, Morris H, Goble E, Morley JE, Chapman IM: Effect of small intestinal nutrient infusions on appetite, gastrointestinal hormone release and gastric myoelectrical activity in young and older men. *Am J Gastr* 2001, 96, 4, 997-1006.

[16] Martinez M, Arnalich F, Hernanz A: Alterations of anorectic cytokine levels from plasma and cerebrospinal fluid in idiopathic senile anorexia. *Mech Ageing Dev* 1993, 72, 145-53.

[17] Martinez M, Hernanz A, Gomez-Cerezo J: Alterations in plasma and cerebrospinal fluid levels of neuropeptides in idiopathic senile anorexia. *Regul Pept* 1993, 49, 109-117.

[18] MacIntosh CG, Morley JE, Wishart J, Morris H, Jansen JB, Horowitz M, Chapman IM: Effect of exogenous cholecystokinin (CCK)-8 on food intake and plasma CCK, leptin, and insulin concentrations in older and young adults: evidence for increased CCK activity as a cause of the anorexia of aging. *J Clin Endocrinol Metab* 2001 Dec;86(12):5830-7.

[19] Roberts SB: Energy regulation and aging. *Nutr Rev* 2000, 58, 91-7.

[20] Morley JE: Decreased food intake with aging. *J Gerontol A Biol Sci Med Sci* 2001 Oct;56 Spec No 2(2):81-8.

[21] MacINtosh CG, Sheehan J, Davani N, Morley JE, Horowitz M, Chapman IM: Effects of aging on the opioid modulation of feeding in humans. *JAGS* 2001, 49, 1518-1524.

[22] Arnalich F, Hernanz<A, Vazquez JJ, Amores A: Cell mediated immune responses and cytokine production in idiopathic senile anorexia. *Mech Aging Dev* 1994, 77, 67-74.

[23] Beharka AA, Meydani M, Leka LS, Meydani A, Meydani SN: Interleukin-6 production does not increase with age. *J Gerontol* 2001, 56A, B81-8.

[24] Yeh SS, Wu SY, Levine DM, Parker TS, Olson JS, Stevens MR, Schuster MW: The correlation of cytokine levels with body weight after megestrol acetate treatment in geriatric patients. *J Gerontol A Biol Sci Med Sci* 2001 Jan;56(1):M48-54.

[25] De Groot CPGM, van Staveren WA, de Graaf C: Determinants of macronutrients intake in elderly people. *Eur J Clin Nutr* 2000, 54, S3, 70-6.

[26] Haller J, Weggemans RM, Lammi-Keefe CJ, Ferry M: Changes in the vitamin status of elderly Europeans. *Eur J Clin Nutr* 1996, 50, S2, 32-46.

[27] Schiffman SS, Graham BG: Taste and smell perception affect appetite and immunity in the elderly. *Eur J Clin Nutr* 2000, S3, 54-63.

[28] Mulligan C, Moreau K, Brandolini M, Livingstone B, Beaufrère B, Boire Y: Alterations of sensory perceptions in healthy elderly subjects during fasting and refeeding. *Gerontology* 2002, 48, 39-43.

[29] Reynish W, Andrieu S, Nourhashemi F, Vellas B: Nutritional factors and Alzheimer's disease. *J Gerontol A Biol Sci Med Sci* 2001 Nov;56(11):M675-80.

[30] Young KW, Greenwood CE: Shift in diurnal feeding patterns in nursing home residents with Alzheimer's disease. *J Gerontol A Biol Sci Med Sci* 2001 Nov;56(11):M700-6.

[31] Chrischilles EA, Foley DJ, Wallace RB, Lemke JH, Semla TP, Hanlon JT: Use of medications by persons 65 and over. *J Gerontol* 1992, 47, M137-144.

[32] Carr-Lopez SM, Phillips SM: The role of medications in geriatric failure to thrive. *Drugs Aging* 1996, 9, 221-5.

[33] Bernstein M, Tucker K, Ryan M: Higher dietary diversity is associated with better nutritional status in frail elders. *FASEB J* 1999, A695.

[34] Kane RA, Caplan AL, Urv-Wong EK: Everyday matters in the lives of nursing home residents. *JAGS* 1997, 45, 1086-93.

[35] Marcus EL, Berry EM: Refusal to eat in the elderly. *Nutr Rev* 1998, 56, 163-171.

[36] Schiffman SS: Perception of taste and smell in elderly persons. *Crit Rev Food Science Nutr* 1993, 33, 17-26.
[37] De Castro JM, De Castro ES: Spontaneous meal patterns of humans. *Am J Clin Nutr* 1989, 50, 237-47.
[38] Mclntosh WA, Shifflett PA, Picou JS: Social support, stressful events, strain ,dietary intake and the elderly. *Med Care* 1989, 27, 140-53.
[39] Rosenbloom CA, Whittington FJ: The effects of bereavement on eating behaviours and nutrient intakes in elderly widowed persons. *J Gerontol* 1993, 48, S223-9.
[40] Thompson MP, Morris LK: Unexplained weight loss in the ambulatory elderly. *JAGS* 1991, 39, 497-500.
[41] Morley JE, Kraenzle D: Causes of weight loss in a community nursing home. *JAGS* 1994, 42, 583-5.
[42] Yesavage JA, Brink TL, Rose TL: Development and validation of a geriatric depression rating scale. *J Psych Res* 1983, 17, 27.
[43] Haller J, Weggemans RM, Ferry M, Guigoz Y: Mental health: MMSE and GDS of elderly Europeans in the SENECA study of 1993. *Eur J Clin Nutr* 1996, 50, S2, 112-6.
[44] Morley JE, Kraenzle D: Weight loss. *JAGS* 1995, 43, 82-3.
[45] Pulska T, Pahkala K, Laippala P; Kivela SL: Depressive symptoms predicting six-year mortality in depressed elderly finns. *Int J Geriatr Psych* 2000, 15, 940-6.
[46] Mclntoch JL, Hubbard RW: Indirect self-destructive behaviour among the elderly. *J Gerontol Soc Work* 1988, 13, 37-48.
[47] Tully MW, Lambros Matrakas K, Muir J, Musallam K: The Eating Nehaviour Scale. *J Geront Nurs* 1997, july, 9-15.
[48] Blandford G, Watkins LB, Mulvihill MN, Taylor B: Assessing abnormal feeding behaviour in late stage dementia. Research and Practice in Alzheimer Disease: Weight loss & Eating behaviour in Alzheimer's patients. B. Vellas, Rivière S, Fitten J Eds, Serdi, Paris, 1998, pag. 47-64.
[49] Guigoz Y, Vellas B, Garry PJ: Mini Nutritional Assessment. *Facts and Research in Gerontology,* 1994, 4 (suppl 2), 113-43.
[50] Simmons SF, Osterweil D, Schnelle JF: Improving food intake in nursing home residents with feeding assistance: a staffing analysis. *J Gerontol A Biol Sci Med Sci* 2001 Dec;56(12):M790-4.
[51] Riviere S, Lauque S, Vellas B: Health promotion programme: nutrition and Alzheimer's disease. Research and Practice in Alzheimer's Disease, Serdi ed, Paris, pag. 93.
[52] Rivière S, Gillette-Guyonnet S, Voisin T, Reynish E, Andrieu S, Lauque S, Salva A, Frisoni G, Nourhashemi F, Micas M, Vellas B: A nutritional education program could prevent weight loss and slow cognitive decline in Alzheimer's disease. *J Nutr Health Aging* 2001, 5, 295-9.
[53] Thomas DR, Ashmen W, Morley JE, Evans WJ: Nutritional management in long-term care: development of a clinical guideline. Council for Nutritional Strategies in Long-Term Care. *J Gerontol A Biol Sci Med Sci* 2000 Dec;55(12):M725-34.
[54] Wilson MM, Purushothaman R, Morley JE: Effect of liquid dietary supplements on energy intake in the elderly. *Am J Clin Nutr* 2002 May;75(5):944-7.

In: Aging and the Elderly: Psychology, Sociology and Health ISBN 1-60021-190-9
Editor: L. O. Randall, pp. 153-175

Chapter 7

AGING, ATHEROSCLEROSIS AND THE LIVER SIEVE

David G. Le Couteur[1], Victoria C. Cogger[1], Sarah N. Hilmer[1], Michael Muller[1], Matthew Harris[1], David Sullivan[2], Allan J. McLean[3] and Robin Fraser[4]

[1]Centre for Education and Research on Ageing and ANZAC Research Institute, University of Sydney and Concord RG Hospital, Sydney NSW, Australia
[2]Royal Prince Alfred Hospital, Sydney NSW, Australia
[3]National Ageing Research Institute, University of Melbourne, Parkville VIC, Australia
[4]Christchurch School of Medicine and Health Sciences, University of Otago, Christchurch, New Zealand

ABSTRACT

Old age is the major risk factor for vascular disease, and as the population ages, is also becoming the most prevalent risk factor. There are few mechanistic explanations for the association of old age with vascular disease. Old age is associated with changes in the endothelium within the hepatic sinusoid, consisting of loss of fenestrations, thickening of the endothelium, deposition of basal lamina and increased expression of various antigens such as von Willebrands factor. These endothelial changes have been observed in humans, non-human primates and rats and may have a unique pathogenesis because of the role of the liver in detoxification and its exposure to gut-derived toxins and dietary substances. The age-related loss of hepatic sinusoidal endothelial fenestrations is particularly significant because fenestrations have an important role in the transfer of lipoproteins, especially chylomicron remnants, from sinusoidal blood to the hepatocytes (the 'liver sieve'). The loss of fenestrations with old age may explain the association of old age with impaired chylomicron remnant clearance and postprandial hyperlipidaemia. Given the ability to modulate fenestrations with various pharmacological and endogenous substrates, the hepatic sinusoidal endothelium may be a therapeutic target for the prevention and treatment of age-related dyslipidaemia and vascular disease.

1. Old Age: The Dominant Risk Factor for Vascular Disease

The contemporary increase in the number of older people in the World is a true demographic revolution, with an impact on human society that is rivaling and will exceed that of the Industrial Revolution. [1] The proportion of the population over the age of 60 years doubled during the last hundred years and it is projected that this will increase two- to three-fold during the next century as the 'baby boomer' generation reaches old age. The numbers of very elderly people aged more than eighty years will increase even more dramatically. [2]

Although this demographic shift has been dubbed 'the aging crisis' [3] it should be emphasised that aging is usually a positive experience and older people generally rate their health as good, or better and live independently in the community. [4] However, old age is unquestionably associated with increased vulnerability and susceptibility to disease and disability. There are several diseases that are relatively specific to old age such as dementia and osteoporosis. Old age is also the most important risk factor for many other diseases of the Western world including atherosclerosis, cancer, arthritis, visual impairment and depression. As lifestyle modification, medical interventions, and environmental factors minimize the risk factors for many diseases, the aging process now largely determines the chances of death and age-related diseases after the third decade of life. [5]

The incidence of atherosclerosis and disease secondary to atherosclerosis increases dramatically with aging. [6-8] For example, the incidence of stroke in 15 studies increases from 0.1-0.3 cases per 1000 per annum in people under the age of 45 years to 15-40 cases per 1000 per annum in people over the age of 85 years. [9] According to the Framingham data, the annual incidence of heart failure increases from 1-2 per 1000 at ages 45-54 years to about 30 per 1000 at ages 64-85 years. [10] Likewise, coronary heart disease increases from 1-5 per 1000 at ages 35-44 years to 22-30 per 1000 at 75-84 years. [7]

Although not acknowledged, old age is the main risk factor for atherosclerosis and cardiovascular disease in the Western world. [7, 11-14] Lakatta [7] concludes: "although epidemiological studies have discovered that lipid levels, diabetes, sedentary lifestyle, and genetic factors are risk factors for coronary disease, hypertension, congestive heart failure and stroke, the quintessential cardiovascular diseases within our society, advancing age unequivocally confers the major risk". Accordingly, the Framingham study attributes a vascular risk to aging that is more than two to three times greater than that of smoking, hypertension, diabetes mellitus and hypercholesterolaemia (Figure 1). [12] As people age, the importance of hypertension, fasting cholesterol levels and smoking as major risk factors for ischaemic heart disease decline as the influence of chronological age becomes dominant. [12] For instance, the risk of thromboembolic stroke in the presence of hypertension declined from a seven-fold excess in men aged 45 to 54 years to a 1.4-fold excess in men older than 75 years. [15] Low total serum cholesterol is paradoxically associated with reduced survival in the oldest old, with each 1 mmol/L increase in total cholesterol corresponding to a 15% decrease in mortality. [16,17] Furthermore, there is a reduced impact of the strategies used to prevent vascular disease such as smoking cessation in old age. [18]

Despite the close association between aging and vascular disease, there is no mechanism linking aging and atherosclerosis that is generally accepted and this presents "... a conundrum of significant proportions to clinicians and basic scientists alike". [6] The broader issues of

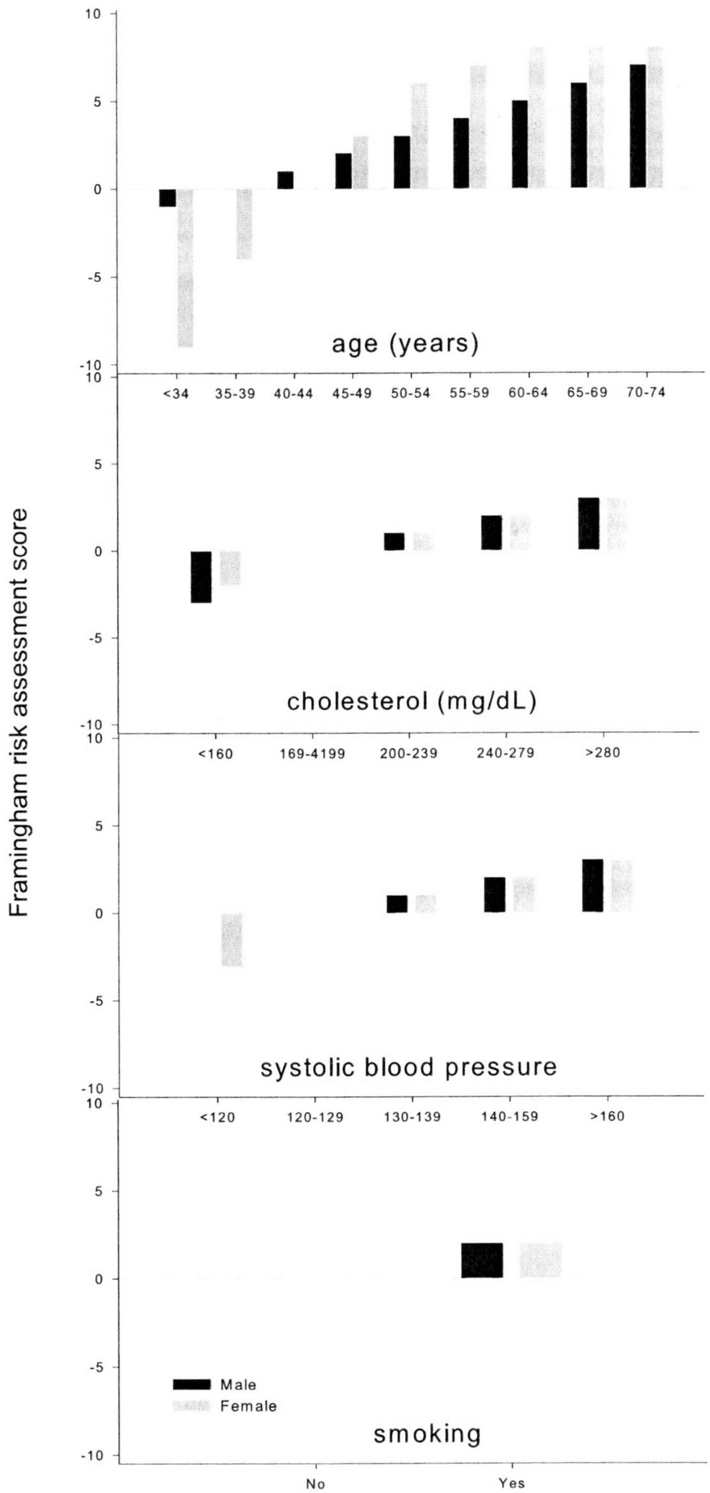

Figure 1. Assessment of cardiovascular risk by use of multiple risk factor assessment. The Global Risk Assessment scores by age, cholesterol, systolic blood pressure and smoking. The dominant effect of age is apparent. [12]

whether vascular disease is part of the primary aging process, secondary to some specific yet undefined age-related susceptibility or merely the accumulation of plaque burden and various risk factors with the passage of time, remain debated. [8] Indeed, the relationship between aging and *any* disease is complex, as yet poorly defined and rarely investigated.

2. Aging and Blood Vessels

There are several mechanisms that have been postulated for the association of old age with vascular disease:

Vascular and, more specifically, endothelial change is part of the aging process and secondary to biological processes recognised as intrinsic to aging. This implies that aging and vascular disease have the same mechanisms and defining aging and disease is simply a semantic issue.

Old age is associated with increased opportunity for, and duration of, exposure to known risk factors for vascular disease. There is a gradual accumulation of atherosclerotic plaques with aging. [13] This implies that healthy aging is not associated with vascular changes and that the occurrence of atherosclerosis and vascular changes in old age reflects a disease process using the current definitions of disease.

The underlying aging process increases the impact of risk factors for disease and severity of disease. [7] This assumes that there is an "aging process × exposure to risk factor interaction" and that primary aging changes in the cardiovascular system increase the risk and severity of cardiovascular disease. [7]

Aging is the major risk factor for cardiovascular disease, which is the major cause of morbidity and mortality in the Western World, therefore it is surprising that the understanding of the mechanisms linking aging and vascular disease is still debated at this rudimentary level. [19]

2.1. Primary Aging

From the cellular and biochemical perspective, there are several mechanisms that are considered to underlie the primary aging process: oxidative stress, mitochondrial dysfunction, telomere shortening, altered apoptosis and various genetic mechanisms. These aging mechanisms have not been studied widely in relationship to vascular and endothelial aging but overall it appears that aging changes seen in other tissues are present in endothelial cells. Whether these changes contribute to altered function or atherosclerosis is unknown.

Oxidative Stress

There is substantial evidence that aging is associated with, if not the consequence of, free radical damage by various endogenous oxidants. [5, 20] Oxidants include superoxide and hydroxyl radicals and other activated forms of oxygen such as hydrogen peroxide and singlet oxygen as well as reactive nitrogen species such as peroxynitrite. The primary sites of production of reactive oxygen species are probably mitochondria, as a by-product of oxidative metabolism. [21] Endothelial cells are exposed to oxidant stress because of their luminal exposure to oxidized lipids, reactive nitrogen species and oxygen. [22] Aging is associated with increased vascular production of the superoxide and peroxynitrate radicals [23] and altered vascular levels of endogenous antioxidants. [24]

Mitochondria

Mitochondria are both producers and targets of oxidative stress. This forms the basis for the mitochondrial theory of aging. [25, 26] Accumulation of somatic mutations of mitochondrial DNA, induced by exposure to reactive oxygen species generated within mitochondria, leads to errors in the mitochondrial DNA-encoded polypeptides and subsequent defective electron transfer activity and oxidative phosphorylation. Such respiratory chain defects lead to increased reactive oxygen species production, thus establishing a vicious cycle with aging. [27, 28] Impairment of mitochondrial function has been identified in senescent endothelial cells in vitro, [29] and mitochondrial DNA mutations have been reported from endothelial cells in older humans. [30]

Telomeres and Cellular Senescence

After a finite number of divisions (the Hayflick limit), primary cell cultures enter a state of replicative senescence, refractory to further mitogenic stimuli. [31] This might determine the maximum life span of an organism. [32] One explanation for cells reaching this limit arises from the shortening of telomeres with each mitotic division. The maximal number of times that human fibroblast can divide in culture decreases with the age of the donor and is reduced in premature aging conditions such as Werner's syndrome. [33] Telomere shortening has been identified in endothelial cells undergoing in vitro senescence and from older humans and, thus, has been implicated in vascular aging and atherosclerosis. [34, 35]

Apoptosis

Aging is associated with dysregulation of apoptosis [36] and overall it has been suggested that aging is mostly associated with upregulation of apoptosis. [37] It is not clear whether age-related dysregulation of apoptosis is the result of genetic programming or stochastic aging processes such as oxidative stress. [37] Apoptosis is increased in endothelial cells undergoing in vitro senescence. [38]

Genetic Mechanisms

The role of genetically programmed aging is controversial. [39, 40] Evidence for a primary role for genetic programming includes the observations that lifespan of a given species is relatively fixed and human aging has a hereditary component. Single mutations in humans can produce premature aging syndromes and altered expression of single genes may increase maximum lifespan in lower organisms. [41] Aging is associated with altered expression of some genes, but usually these have not been unexpected changes. [32, 42] A role for DNA methylation has been proposed for vascular aging. [43]

2.2. Aging Changes in Systemic Vessels

Vascular changes have been observed in old age in rats and rabbits and since these species do not develop atherosclerosis spontaneously, the changes are considered to reflect the primary aging process rather than concurrent disease. These include thickening of the intima associated with increased intimal expression of transforming growth factor-beta (TGF-β), intercellular adhesion molecule (ICAM-1), angiotensin converting enzyme (ACE) and type 2 matrix-metalloproteinase MMP-2. [14] There is increased collagen and fibronectin in the extracellular matrix. [14, 19]

Similar changes have been reported with aging in humans. Intimal thickening has been found in older people even in the absence of significant atherosclerosis and this can be in the order of two-to three-fold increases in thickness. [7, 44] This is associated with the well-established changes of luminal dilatation, increased vascular stiffness and reduced compliance. [7]

3. Aging and the Hepatic Sinusoidal Endothelium

In the past, the liver has been considered to be relatively unaffected by the primary aging process and spared the effects of age-related diseases. [45, 46] Functional changes, particularly related to impaired drug metabolism, have been attributed to age-related reduction in blood flow and liver mass. [46, 47] At the light microscopic level, aging is associated with lipofuscin accumulation and an increase in multinucleate hepatocytes. [45] Motivated by the observation that such changes cannot fully explain the age-related impairment of hepatic drug metabolism, [46] we examined the structures lying between the blood and the hepatocyte that could impose a barrier to substrate transfer, ie the hepatic sinusoidal endothelium and extravascular space of Disse. The sinusoidal endothelium occupies a strategic position regulating and balancing the catabolism of dietary lipids with the synthesis of hepatic lipids, which will have profound effects on systemic lipoprotein levels and atherogenesis.

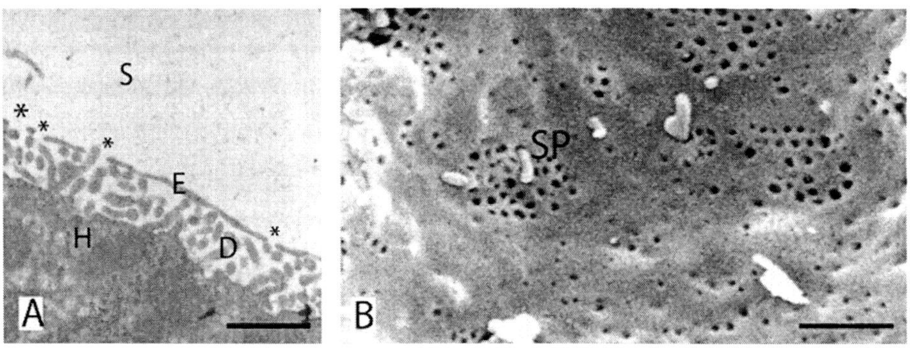

Figure 2. Transmission electron micrograph (A) and scanning electron micrograph (B) of the hepatic sinusoidal endothelium in a young rat. The endothelium (E) is attenuated and perforated with fenestrations (asterisk). The space of Disse (D) contains microvilli and separates the sinusoid (S) from the hepatocyte (H). The scanning electron micrograph shows a sinusoid perforated with fenestrations grouped into liver sieve plates (SP). Scale bars = 1 μm. [52]

Hepatic sinusoidal endothelial cells are highly specialized endothelial cells lining the wall of the hepatic sinusoid, which separate the sinusoidal blood derived primarily from the portal vein, from hepatocytes (Figure 2). [48, 49] Hepatic sinusoidal endothelial cells are perforated with fenestrations. Fenestrations are pores approximately 100-200 nm in diameter and grouped together in clusters known as liver sieve plates. Unlike other capillaries, fenestrations in hepatic sinusoidal endothelial cells are true discontinuities in the endothelium, lacking either a diaphragm or underlying basal lamina. [48, 50] The cytoplasmic extensions of hepatic sinusoidal endothelial cells are extremely attenuated, with widths in the order of 100-300 nm. Atomic force microscopy has shown that hepatic sinusoidal endothelial cells are the softest cells yet studied. [51]

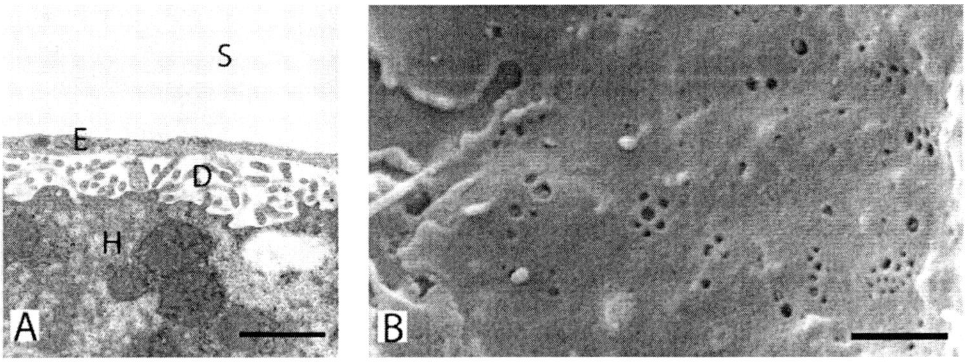

Figure 3. Transmission electron micrograph (A) and scanning electron micrograph (B) of the hepatic sinusoidal endothelium in an old rat. The endothelium (E) is thickened and is defenestrated, impeding transfer of substances from the sinusoid (S) into the space of Disse (D) and subsequently, the hepatocytes (H). The scanning electron micrograph clearly illustrates the defenestration of the sinusoidal endothelium associated with old age in the liver. Scale bars = 1 μm.

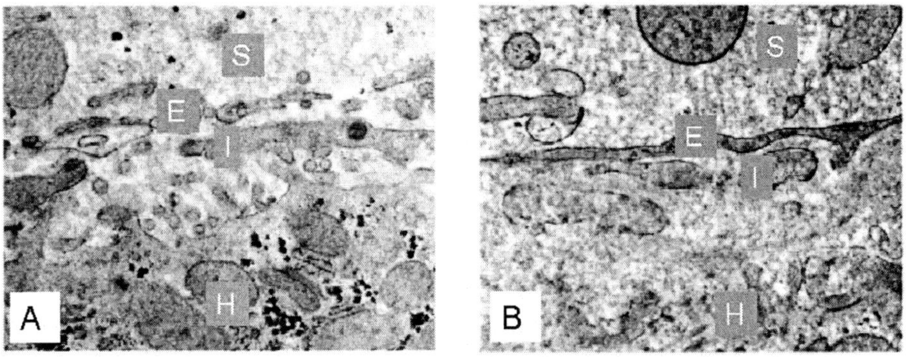

Figure 4. Transmission electron microscopy of the hepatic sinusoidal endothelium from a young human (A) and an old human (B). The endothelium from the older human is defenestrated. H hepatocyte, E endothelial cell, I stellate cell, S sinusoid. [53]

Recently we reported that aging is associated with marked changes in the hepatic sinusoidal endothelium and space of Disse in the rat (Figure 3), [52] surgical and post mortem specimens from human livers (Figure 4), [53] and the non-human primate, *Papio hamadryas* (Figure 5). [54] These changes were termed "pseudocapillarization" because the aging sinusoidal endothelium has lost its porous liver sieve structure and becomes more like capillaries seen in other vascular beds. [52]

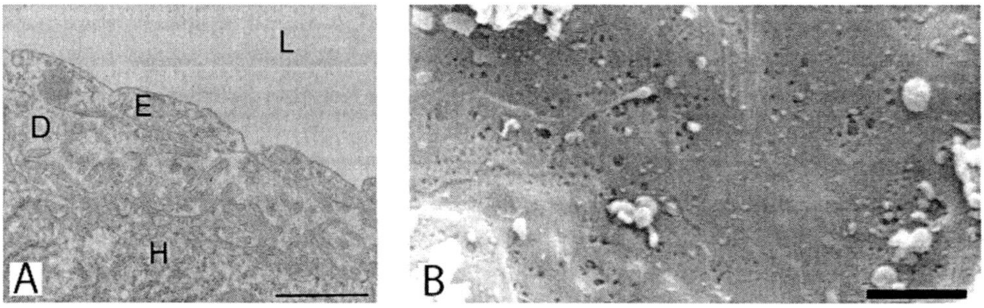

Figure 5. Transmission electron micrograph (A) and scanning electron micrograph (B) from an old baboon. The endothelium (E) is thickened and defenestrated and the space of Disse (D) is dense secondary to extracellular matrix deposition. L, lumen of the sinusoid, H hepatocyte. Scale bar = 1 μm. The scanning electron micrograph shows defenestration of the endothelium with age in the baboon. Scale bar = 2 μm.

The first observation we made was that there is substantive thickening of the sinusoidal endothelium. Specifically, there was a 40% increase in thickness in the sinusoidal endothelium from 130 ± 8 nm to 186 ± 9 nm in baboons, [54] and from 230 ± 50 nm to 320 ± 80 nm in rats. [52] In humans, endothelial thickness increased by 75% from 165 ± 17 nm to 289 ± 9 nm. [53]

In addition, we noted a reduction in the number of fenestrations in the sinusoidal endothelium ('defenestration'). In the aged baboon, the porosity of the endothelium determined on scanning electron microscopy was reduced from 4.2 ± 0.5% to 2.4 ± 0.4% [54] and was very similar to the reduction of porosity in old age in the rat from 4.1 ± 2.3% to 2.5 ± 1.2%. [52] In human tissue, we were unable to perform scanning electron microscopic analysis, however, the fenestration count determined on transmission electron microscopy was reduced by approximately 80%. [53]

This age-related change in the ultrastructure of the sinusoidal endothelium was associated with an increased expression of vWF in baboons, humans and rats (Figure 6). [52-54] Endothelial cells in tissue beds outside the liver express vWF, a glycoprotein mediating attachment of platelets after endothelial injury, but it is not expressed in sinusoidal cells of normal young liver. The upregulation of vWF in old age confirms that significant biological changes are occurring in the endothelium and is consistent with the electron microscopic analysis.

There were some differences between baboons, rats and humans in terms of extracellular matrix changes. In baboons we noted that there was age-related upregulation of laminin, but not of collagen, and, likewise, transmission electron microscopy did not reveal any major changes in collagen deposition in the space of Disse. Only two of the old baboons demonstrated any basal lamina formation. In contrast, there was substantive deposition of collagen and basal lamina formation in the livers from older humans and this was associated with increased perisinusoidal staining of Masson trichrome and collagen. Rats had changes intermediate between those we saw in humans and baboons. These species differences in extracellular matrix changes may indicate differences in co-existent diseases or 'rates of aging' between species.

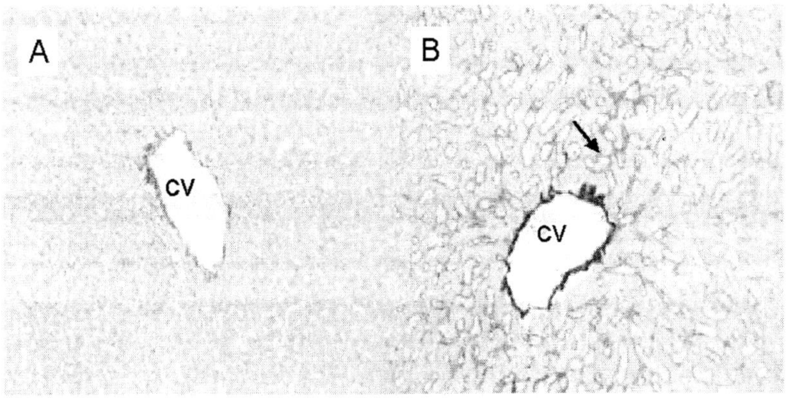

Figure 6. Immunohistochemistry of von Willebrands factor in the human liver. The staining in the young liver (A) is mostly around the central vein (cv) whereas there is extensive perisinusoidal staining (arrow) in the old liver (B).

Major age-related changes in the liver appear to be confined to the perisinusoidal regions, in particular the endothelium. Old age was found to be associated with some deposition of lipofuscin and multinucleate cells in the hepatic parenchyma, however no other major morphological changes were observed on light microscopy or electron microscopy.

The aging changes in the sinusoidal endothelium are consistent with aging changes documented in other systemic blood vessels. There are clear parallels with the age-related intimal thickening and extracellular matrix changes that have been documented in blood vessels from several species including humans. The effects of aging on fenestrations in other fenestrated vessels (eg glomerular, lymphatic) are unknown.

4. Mechanisms for Age-Related Pseudocapillarization

The fenestrations in hepatic sinusoidal endothelial cells are dynamic structures whose diameter and number vary in response to numerous other stimuli. [48] These include a broad range of factors such as endotoxins, alcohol, nicotine, adrenaline, acetylcholine, endothelin, tumor necrosis factor-alpha (TNF-α), pressure and temperature - over 40 agents were listed in the review by Braet and Wisse. [48] Furthermore, the pathogenesis of structural changes in the hepatic sinusoidal endothelium and especially fibrosis in the space of Disse in hepatic fibrosis and cirrhosis are complex and have been the focus of intensive research. Therefore, the range of possible mechanisms for the development of age-related pseudocapillarization is diverse. In addition, the unique anatomy and function of the liver provides alternative mechanisms for aging vascular changes compared with other vascular beds.

There are several possible mechanisms for age-related changes in the hepatic sinusoidal endothelium:

- primary aging
- systemic vascular disease
- occult liver disease
- portal toxins

- dietary factors
- age-related vascular inflammation

In order to explore the possibility that pseudocapillarization is the consequence of primary aging biological processes, we have studied the effects of oxidative stress on the hepatic endothelium. Rat livers were perfused ex vivo, in situ with hydrogen peroxide via the portal vein. The livers were then fixed and the ultrastructure of the liver tissue examined with transmission and scanning electron microscopy. The effects of hydrogen peroxide were largely confined to the perisinusoidal areas (Figure 7). The sinusoidal endothelial cells became swollen and more porous, with large gaps replacing sieve plates. The space of Disse showed an increase in volume and the density of hepatocyte projections decreased. Activation of Kupffer cells was noted. Little or no ultrastructural change was observed within the hepatocytes. [55] Although these changes in the liver sieve do not replicate aging, it is possible that after acute oxidative injury with loss of sieve plates, there may be a delayed scarring process with defenestration and deposition of collagen and basal lamina proteins.

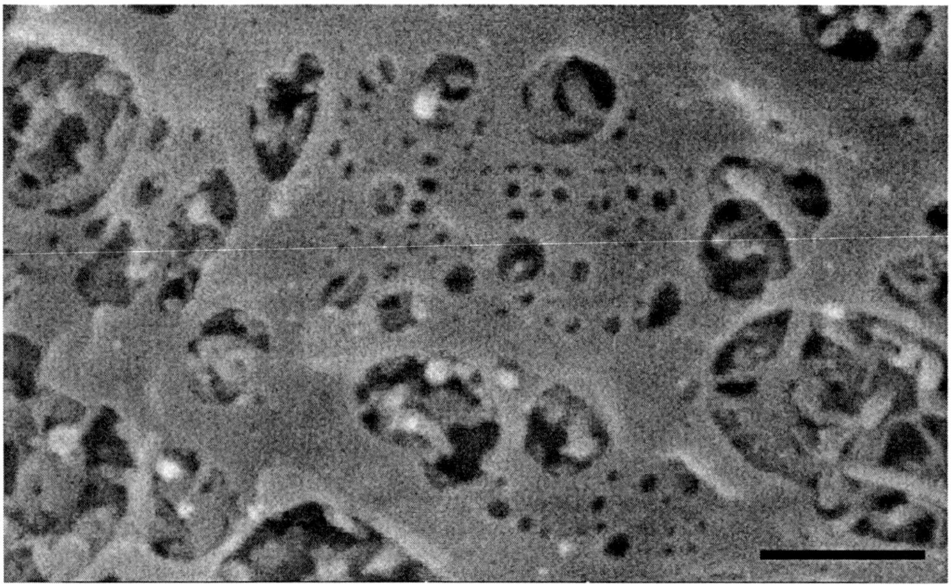

Figure 7. Scanning electron micrograph of the sinusoidal endothelium following acute exposure to H_2O_2. The sieve plates have been opened up to form large gaps. Scale bar = 1 μm.

Aging is associated with bioenergetic disruption in the liver. Using magnetic resonance spectroscopy, ATP levels were found to be reduced from 2.81 ± 0.33 to 2.25 ± 0.26 μmol/g in young versus old rat livers, respectively ($P < 0.001$). [52] Therefore we studied the effects of mitochondrial inhibition and intracellular hypoxia on fenestration. Treatment of hepatic sinusoidal endothelial cells with the mitochondrial inhibitor, antimycin-A led to marked defenestration associated with F-actin disruption and the formation of unusual structures in the centre of the liver sieve plates, 'defenestration associated structures' (Figure 8). [56]

It is also possible that hepatic pseudocapillarization is a manifestation of widespread systemic vascular disease, such as atherosclerosis. However, atheroma is rare in venous systems. Furthermore, rats and baboons are relatively free of atherosclerosis in other blood vessels and the presence of age-related endothelial changes in these species is more likely to represent aging. [14]

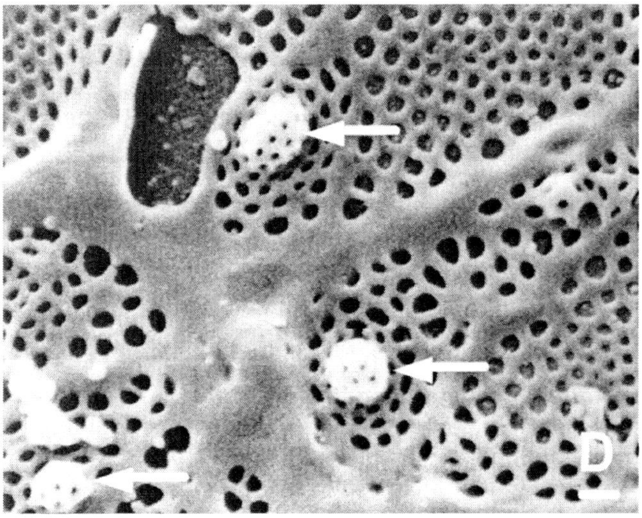

Figure 8. Scanning electron microscopy of an isolated hepatic endothelial cell following administration of antimycin A. Several defenestration associated structures are apparent above the liver sieve plates (arrow). [56]

Various liver diseases are associated with changes in the liver sinusoidal endothelium and space of Disse. In cirrhosis these changes are termed 'capillarization' [57] and consist of defenestration, collagen deposition and basal lamina formation. Although these ultrastructural changes are somewhat similar to those of age-related pseudocapillarization, aging is not associated with the extensive disruption of hepatic architecture that defines cirrhosis. The sinusoidal changes in many liver diseases are often associated with activation of stellate cells, usually assessed by increased expression of αSMA (smooth muscle antigen). [58, 59] We have not noted in increase in the expression of αSMA with aging, which suggests that stellate activation is not present, but does not preclude the possibility that stellate cell activation has occurred at a younger age. However, we did note a novel, presumptively age-related cell in the baboon. [54] These cells had a ring-like appearance on light microscopy and were in the perisinusoidal regions. Electron microscopy and immunohistochemistry indicated that these cells are most likely to be abnormal stellate cells that are engorged with a single fat globule. The significance of these perisinusoidal ring cells for aging is not clear but presumably they indicate that some process of hepatic stellate cell modification is occurring in old baboons. [54]

The hepatic endothelial cells are exposed to various toxins from the gut delivered by the portal vein. In this respect, the hepatic endothelial cells are unique amongst endothelial cells in their potential exposure to dietary constituents (including xenobiotics, oxidized fats) and endotoxins from gut microflora. Endotoxin has been shown to induce defenestration in rat sinusoidal endothelium. [60]

Finally, age-related vascular inflammation may be implicated. It has been observed that with increasing age there is an increase in chronic systemic inflammation that is independent of overt disease states. [61] This view is based on the consistent finding from several studies that an age-dependent elevation in plasma cytokine levels occurs. In particular, plasma levels of tumour necrosis factor-alpha (TNF-α) [62] and interleukin 6 (IL-6) [63] are elevated with increasing age. Plasma levels of IL-6, while low to undetectable in the majority of healthy young people, begin to increase at approximately 50 to 60 years of age with the response becoming pronounced after 70 years. [62] Differences in cytokine production by mitogen-stimulated peripheral blood mononuclear cells from young and elderly subjects have been reported. Significant increases in TNF-α, IL-1β and IL-6 production were detected from elderly donors compared to younger persons. [64, 65] Similarly, a positive age-dependent association between increased production of reactive oxygen species by peripheral blood neutrophil and mononuclear cells has been reported. [66] Monocytes play an important role in the aetiopathogenesis of atherosclerosis and the presence of inflammatory infiltrates in atherosclerotic lesions was recognised early in the study of the disease eventually leading to the recognition of atherosclerosis as an inflammatory process. [67] Pro-inflammatory cytokines, such as TNF-α and IL-1, induce oxidative stress by up-regulating NAD(P)H oxidase, eNOS and iNOS, resulting in increased production of reactive oxygen and nitrogen species. Transcriptional activators, particularly activator protein 1 (AP-1) and nuclear factor kappa B (NF-κB), play important roles in the up-regulation of these enzymes. [68] Cytokines and reactive oxygen species, through transcription factor regulation, induce expression of adhesion molecules that further promote the inflammatory response. [69]

The role of systemic or local inflammatory mediators in the defenestration of the hepatic sinusoidal endothelium, with or without the effects of aging, has received little attention. Nevertheless, several studies suggest a role for inflammation in the defenestration process. Treatment of rodents with the pro-inflammatory cytokine, TNF-α, results in a decreased number of fenestrae [70] and an increase in the expression of endothelial ICAM-1. [71] Further insight into the role of inflammatory mediators and defenestration has been obtained by studying the role of endotoxin in hepatic injury. Treatment of rats with endotoxin results in marked defenestration [72] but not if hepatic Kupffer cells (a resident macrophage population) are inactivated prior its administration. [73] Endotoxin is known to be a potent inducer of Kupffer cell pro-inflammatory mediators, including TNF-α, IL-1 and IL-6.

A study of inflammatory liver diseases provides further associations between the role of cytokines and the defenestration process. Hepatic fibrosis is a condition characterised, in part, by defenestration of the sinusoidal endothelium and is associated with markedly enhanced plasma levels of TNF-α, a key component in the progression of the disease. [74] Similarly, fenestrae numbers were reported to be decreased in subjects with fatty liver disease. Of interest was the observation that the process of defenestration was reversible following successful treatment of the condition. [75] Both changes in diet and exercise are beneficial in the treatment of this disease, factors that reduce the inflammatory response.

The influence of diet on the maintenance and numbers of hepatic fenestrae is not known. However, aging is associated with a prolongation in the postprandial hyperlipidemic state with age-related defenestration of the hepatic sinusoids believed to be a contributing factor. [76] Hyperlipidemia is a recognised independent risk factor for atherosclerosis and is associated with increased levels of circulating cytokines, particularly CRP and IL-6. [77] Hyperlipidemia may induce defenestration by cytokine mediators and/or by promoting oxidative stress or intracellular redox changes secondary to the presence of oxidized fatty acids.

5. The Liver Sieve and Lipoprotein Metabolism

On the basis of the unusual and unique structure of the hepatic sinusoidal endothelium, we postulated that the fenestrated endothelium acts like a dynamic filter and termed this 'the liver sieve'. [78] Fenestrations permit the passage of plasma and substrates within plasma, plasma proteins including albumin, and smaller lipoproteins into the extravascular space of Disse. Blood cells massage fluid through the fenestrations by virtue of the fact that their diameter is greater than that of a typical sinusoid (4.09 μm in zone 1 to 5.67 μm in zone 3). [79, 80] The thinness of hepatic endothelial cells and the lack of basal lamina and collagen in the space of Disse ensure that any permeability barriers to the diffusion of substrates between blood and hepatocytes are minimized. The nature of the portal blood (containing gut-derived nutrients, xenobiotics, and microbial contaminants) and the role of the liver (regulation of systemic metabolism, detoxification) dictate that hepatic sinusoidal endothelial cells must allow unimpeded access of substrates in sinusoidal blood to hepatocytes. Of course, traffic through the fenestrations is likely to be bi-directional for larger substrates synthesized in the liver and released into the systemic circulation, such as albumin and VLDLs.

The liver is the main site for lipoprotein metabolism. The biochemical and receptor-based mechanisms regulating lipoprotein disposition in the liver have been extensively studied and are established. [81] However, prior to receptor binding and hepatocellular metabolism, circulating lipoproteins must traverse the hepatic sinusoidal endothelium, presumably via the fenestrations. This provides an opportunity for regulation of lipoprotein metabolism on the basis of size. [49]

The first stage in the metabolism of dietary fats is the production of chylomicrons. Chylomicrons are triglyceride-rich, spherical lipoproteins formed in the intestine from dietary lipids. They are large particles with diameters of 100-1000 nm that are unable to pass through the fenestrations of the hepatic sinusoidal endothelium. [49, 78] Furthermore, chylomicrons are diverted from the liver by the thoracic duct, possibly because large particles are frequently implicated in the activation of Kupffer cells. Chylomicrons are then metabolized to chylomicron remnants by lipoprotein lipase present on the endothelium of systemic capillaries. In hepatectomized rats, there is accumulation of chylomicron remnants in the blood [82] indicating the importance of the liver in the metabolism of chylomicron remnants. Chylomicron remnants are smaller particles (30-80 nm) that have acquired apoE. These particles pass through fenestrations of the sinusoidal endothelium [49, 83] and are sequestered within the space of Disse where they undergo further metabolism by hepatic lipase. Chylomicron remnants bind to hepatocyte membrane receptors that recognize apoE (low density lipoprotein receptor, low density lipoprotein receptor-related protein) allowing uptake into and subsequent metabolism by hepatocytes.

The role of the fenestrations in the steric selection of chylomicrons and chylomicron remnants has been established in vivo. [49, 83] Wisse first postulated that fenestrations filter chylomicrons and other lipoproteins according to size. [84] Membranes isolated from hepatocytes cannot differentiate between chylomicrons and chylomicron remnants whereas in vivo, livers selectively take up chylomicron remnants. [85] Electron microscopy has demonstrated that large chylomicrons are found in the sinusoidal blood compared with smaller chylomicron remnants observed in the space of Disse. [78] An example is shown in Figure 9. There is differential trapping by the liver of radiolabelled chylomicrons of different sizes such that smaller particles are trapped to a greater extent than those larger than 100 nm. [78]

The effect of defenestration on lipid metabolism has also been investigated. Nicotine, endotoxins, and dimethylnitrosamine induce defenestration and are associated with increased susceptibility to dietary cholesterol. [49] Likewise, rabbits and chickens, which have reduced fenestrations compared to man and rodents, are vulnerable to dietary cholesterol, resulting in hyperlipidaemia and atherosclerosis. [49] In humans, there is a correlation between alcohol consumption, defenestration and hyperlipidaemia and we have postulated that the loss of the liver sieve contributes to alcohol-induced hypertriglyceridaemia. [86] As well as effects on lipid metabolism, morphological changes in the liver sieve that occur in aging and liver disease have been linked to impaired transfer of many substrates including albumin, drugs and oxygen. [87]

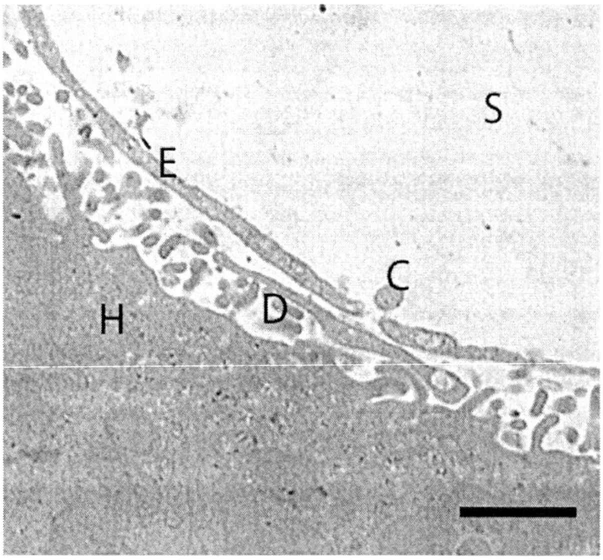

Figure 9. A transmission electron micrograph of the sinusoidal endothelium from a young rat. The lipoprotein (C) is, on morphological criteria, a chylomicron and lies beside a fenestration in the endothelium (E). Scale bar = 1 μm.

Similar results indicating exclusion of the basis of size have been reported for large and small liposomes [88] and colloidal gold particles of different diameters. [89] An expression that has been used to describe the manner by which the liver sieve allows passage of smaller particles and prohibits passage of large particles, especially with respect to lipoproteins, is 'steric hindrance'. [85] In general it has been observed that passage of particles through pores in membranes ceases when the radius of the particle exceeds 30% of the radius of the pore [90] and presumably this applies to fenestrations within the hepatic endothelium, suggesting that only the smallest remnants can pass.

Defenestration causes impaired clearance of chylomicron remnants after meals because the circulating chylomicron remnants produced from dietary fat are unable to enter the space of Disse. [49] Because remnants are still relatively rich in triglycerides, this is manifested as postprandial hypertriglyceridaemia. It is possible to quantitate the effects of defenestration on the transfer of substrates such as lipoproteins by application of the engineering principles related to membrane filtration. There are several, pressure-driven, membrane processes including microfiltration (particles 0.1-0.5 μm), ultrafiltration (10-100 nm), nanofiltration (1-10 nm) and reverse osmosis (<1 nm). Therefore, ultrafiltration is the best term to describe the passage across hepatic endothelial fenestrations, with diameters around 100 nm. The hydraulic pressure driving filtration is the sinusoidal pressure, which is very low and in the order of a few centimeters of water, [91] and in the axial direction consistent with tangential flow ultrafiltration. In ultrafiltration, the volume flux (J) is described by the Hagen-Poiseuille formula:

$$J = \frac{fR^2 \Delta P}{8\eta l}$$

where f is the porosity of the membrane, R diameter of the pores, ΔP the pressure gradient across the membrane, η viscosity, and l the thickness of the membrane. [90] In old age, it is unlikely that there is a substantial change in the sinusoidal pressure. [91] However, we have documented changes in the geometry of the endothelium including a reduction in porosity from 4.1 to 2.5%, a decrease in fenestration diameter from 73 to 60 nm and an increase in thickness from 0.23 to 0.32 μm. [52] By application of the Hagen Poiseuille law, it can be estimated that pseudocapillarization of the hepatic sinusoidal endothelium will be associated with a reduction in flux across the endothelial in the order of 70%.

6. Aging and Lipid Metabolism

Aging generally is associated with hyperlipidaemia [6] however some studies have shown that cholesterol levels are reduced in the very elderly near death, perhaps as a result of severe comorbidities associated with weight loss and cachexia. [16, 17]

A few studies have shown that postprandial hyperlipidaemia is more common in old age and may occur in the absence of fasting hyperlipidaemia. [92-94] The degree of postprandial hypertriglyceridaemia after a fat-rich meal correlates with age in humans. Fasting triglycerides levels are greater in older people and the increase after a meal is two times greater in older subjects compared to younger subjects. Old age is associated with increased postprandial retinyl-ester concentrations, which is a marker of chylomicron remnants, and a two-fold prolongation of the residence time for retinyl-esters in triglycerides-rich lipoproteins. [92-94]

Aging is also associated with reduced hepatic expression of low-density lipoprotein receptor and LDL receptor-related protein and this has been proposed as one explanation for the reduced clearance of chylomicron remnants in old age. [95] However, the effects of any age-related changes in the expression of low-density lipoprotein receptor and LDL receptor-related protein (and other lipid binding substrates in the space of Disse such as apolipoprotein E (apoE) and heparan sulphate proteoglycan) will be constrained if chylomicron remnants are unable to enter the space of Disse because of loss of fenestrations. Because the effects of old age on expression and distribution of apoE in the liver had not been reported, we studied the effect of old age on the immunohistochemistry of hepatic apoE. Overall, old age was not associated with marked changes in the expression of apoE between adult and old humans. However, there was a change in the distribution of apoE staining. The livers of older humans displayed increased hepatocyte cytoplasmic staining and reduced peri-sinusoidal staining. Similar trends were noted in the livers from older baboons (Figure 10). [96] Such findings are suggestive of altered apoE recycling in old age and have several possible mechanisms, including potentially reduced access by lipids into the space of Disse.

The hypothesis that postprandial hyperlipidaemia, rather than other forms of hyperlipidaemia, is the root cause of atherosclerosis was proposed by Moreton, [97] Fraser, [98] and Zilversmit. [99] This concept seems to be well accepted. [83] The clinical evidence for the association includes the observation that coronary artery disease is associated with elevated postprandial hypertriglyceridaemia independent of fasting LDL and HDL concentrations. [83, 100] The clearance of chylomicron remnants is reduced substantially in normolipidaemic subjects with coronary artery disease. [100] At the level of mechanism, chylomicron remnants and retinyl esters are taken up by the arterial vessel wall by transcytosis and have been observed in atherosclerotic plaques. [99, 101] However, research into the role of chylomicron remnants in atherosclerosis, and the role of the liver in the metabolism of chylomicron remnants has been limited by technical difficulties involved in the measurement of chylomicron remnants and the generation of labeled remnants.

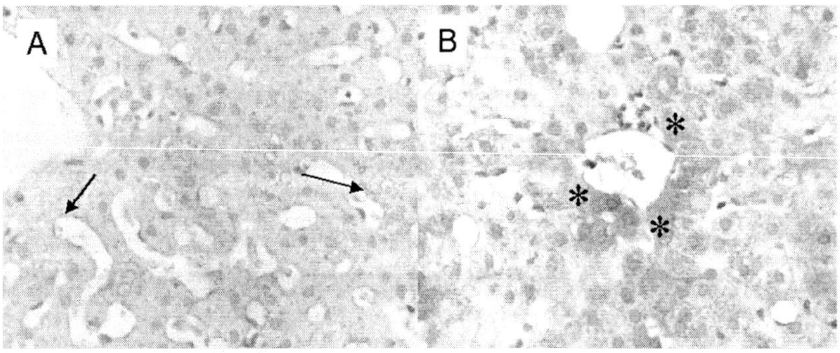

Figure 10. The immunohistochemistry of apolipoprotein E in the baboon liver. In the young liver (A), staining is primarily perisinusoidal (arrow). Compared with the young baboon, in the old baboon (B), staining is less in the perisinusoidal regions and greater in the cytoplasm (asterisk). This suggests an age-related change in the cellular trafficking of apolipoprotein E. [96]

7. Aging, Atherosclerosis and the Liver Sieve

We have proposed that the age-related changes in the hepatic sinusoidal endothelium, particularly the reduction in fenestrations [52-54] leads to age-related impairment of lipoprotein transfer across the endothelium. The systemic consequence is impaired lipoprotein metabolism, manifest as postprandial hyperlipidaemia, and with time, atherosclerosis (Figure 11). [76] The hypothesis is simple with each step in the pathogenic chain essentially proven. The hepatic sinusoidal endothelium contains pores ('fenestrations') that permit the passage of particles of certain size ('chylomicron remnants'). With old age the diameter and frequency of fenestrations diminishes, with an increase in matrix in the space of Disse, so leading to reduced porosity of the liver sieve and a consequent reduction in the clearance of chylomicron remnants. Impaired clearance of chylomicron remnants is linked to atherosclerosis. [76]

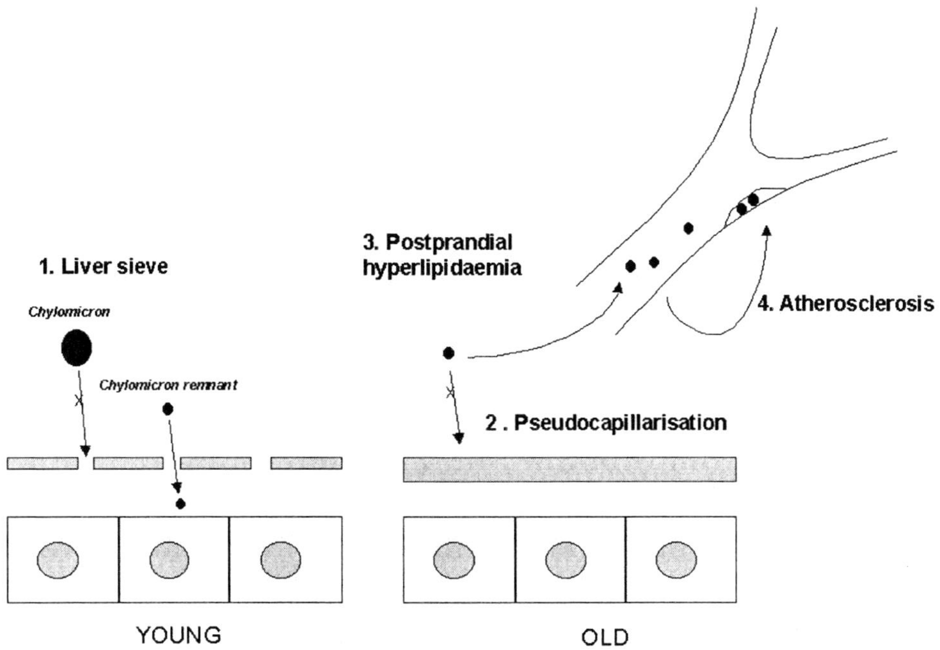

Figure 11. The relationship between the age-related decrease in porosity of the hepatic sinusoidal endothelium, impaired chylomicron remnant clearance and the development of atherosclerosis. [76]

8. Conclusions

As the Western World ages, there is an imperative to increase our understanding of the mechanisms linking old age to atherosclerosis. Furthermore, old age has become the major risk factor for atherosclerosis, particularly as other risk factors for atherosclerosis such as smoking, hypertension and hyperlipidaemia are effectively managed.

Recently, age-related changes in the hepatic sinusoidal endothelium, termed pseudocapillarization, have been reported. Although these changes parallel many of the aging changes seen in other blood vessels, the unique ultrastructure of the hepatic sinusoidal endothelial cells and anatomy of the portal circulation indicate unique pathogenic mechanisms and systemic implications.

In particular, fenestrations within the hepatic sinusoidal endothelium are involved in the disposition of lipoproteins, regulating transfer of lipoproteins between the systemic circulation and hepatocytes on the basis of size. Loss of fenestrations as occurs in old age, would be expected to be associated with impaired hepatic metabolism of lipoproteins that have a large diameter, such as chylomicron remnants and LDLs. Indeed old age is associated with hyperlipidaemia, impaired clearance of chylomicron remnants and post-prandial hyperlipidaemia.

Strategies to maintain integrity of the hepatic sinusoidal endothelium or to induce refenestration of the aged hepatic endothelium are plausible targets for the prevention and treatment of age-related atherosclerosis. The development of dietary or pharmacological interventions based on this mechanism is feasible given the dynamic nature of fenestrations, the increasing understanding of the cellular mechanisms of fenestration and defenestration and the diverse range of interventions that have been found to influence their number and diameter.

ACKNOWLEDGMENTS

We acknowledge the support of the National Health and Medical Research Council of Australia, the Department of Veterans Affairs, and the Aging and Alzheimers Research Foundation.

REFERENCES

[1] United Nations. Implications of an Ageing Society. *www.un.org/esa/socdev/ageing/ageimpl.htm*; 2000.

[2] United Nations. A demographic revolution. *www.un.org/esa/socdev/ageing/agewpop1.htm*; 2000.

[3] Watts J. Report urges swift action on global ageing "crisis". *Lancet* 2001;358:731.

[4] Strawbridge WJ, Wallhagen MI, Cohen RD. Successful aging and well-being: self-rated compared with Rowe and Kahn. *Gerontologist* 2002;42:727-33.

[5] Harman D. Aging: overview. *Ann NY Acad Sci* 2001;928:1-21.

[6] Hazzard W. Dyslipoproteinemia in the elderly. *Clin Geriatr Med* 1992;8:89-102.

[7] Lakatta EG, Levy D. Arterial and cardiac aging: major shareholders in cardiovascular disease enterprises: Part I: aging arteries: a "set up" for vascular disease. *Circulation* 2003;107:139-46.

[8] Lakatta EG. Cardiovascular aging research: The next horizons. *J Am Geriatr Soc* 1999;47:613-25.

[9] Feigin VL, Lawes CM, Bennett DA, Anderson CS. Stroke epidemiology: a review of population-based studies of incidence, prevalence, and case-fatality in the late 20th century. *Lancet Neurol* 2003;2:43-53.

[10] Wilson PW. An epidemiological perspective of systemic hypertension, ischemic heart disease, and heart failure. *Am J Cardiol* 1997;80 (9B):3J-8J.

[11] Hazzard WR, Bierman EL. Delayed clearance of chylomicron remnants following vitamin- A-containing oral fat loads in broad-beta disease (type III hyperlipoproteinemia). *Metabolism* 1976;25:777-801.

[12] Grundy SM, Pasternak R, Greenland P, Smith S, Fuster V. Assessment of cardiovascular risk by use of multiple-risk factor assessment equations. A statement for healthcare professionals from the American Heart Association and the American College of Cardiology. *J Am Coll Cardiol* 1999;34:1348-59.

[13] Grundy SM. Age as a risk factor: you are as old as your arteries. *Am J Cardiol* 1999;83:1455-7, A7.

[14] Lakatta EG. Arterial and cardiac aging: major shareholders in cardiovascular disease enterprises: Part III: cellular and molecular clues to heart and arterial aging. *Circulation* 2003;107:490-7.

[15] Abbott RD, Curb JD, Rodriguez BL, Masaki KH, Popper JS, Ross GW, et al. Age-related changes in risk factor effects on the incidence of thromboembolic and hemorrhagic stroke. *J Clin Epidemiol* 2003;56:479-86.

[16] Weverling-Rijnsburger AW, Blauw GJ, Lagaay AM, Knook DL, Meinders AE, Westendorp RG. Total cholesterol and risk of mortality in the oldest old. *Lancet* 1997;350:1119-23.

[17] Weverling-Rijnsburger AW, Jonkers IJ, van Exel E, Gussekloo J, Westendorp RG. High-density vs low-density lipoprotein cholesterol as the risk factor for coronary artery disease and stroke in old age. *Arch Intern Med* 2003;163:1549-54.

[18] Doll R, Peto R, Wheatley K, Gray R, Sutherland I. Mortality in relation to smoking: 40 years' observations on male British doctors. *Bmj* 1994;309:901-11.

[19] Lakatta EG. Cardiovascular aging research: the next horizons. *J Am Geriatr Soc* 1999;47:613-25.

[20] Finkel T, Holbrook NJ. Oxidants, oxidative stress and the biology of ageing. *Nature* 2000;408:239-47.

[21] Harman D. The biological clock: the mitochondria? J Am Geriatr Soc 1972;20:145-47.

[22] Yu BP, Chung HY. Oxidative stress and vascular aging. *Diabetes Res Clin Pract* 2001;54:S73-80.

[23] van der Loo B, Labugger R, Skepper JN, Bachschmid M, Kilo J, Powell JM, et al. Enhanced peroxynitrite formation is associated with vascular aging. *J Exp Med* 2000;192:1731-44.

[24] van der Loo B, Labugger R, Aebischer CP, Skepper JN, Bachschmid M, Spitzer V, et al. Cardiovascular aging is associated with vitamin E increase. *Circulation* 2002;105:1635-8.

[25] Miquel J, Economos AC, Fleming J, Johnson JE, Jr. Mitochondrial role in cell aging. *Exp Gerontol* 1980;15:575-91.

[26] Linnane AW, Marzuki S, Ozawa T, Tanaka M. Mitochondrial DNA mutations as an important contributor to ageing and degenerative diseases. *Lancet* 1989;i:642-45.

[27] Papa S. Mitochondrial oxidative phosphorylation changes in the life span. Molecular aspects and physiopathological implications. *Biochim Biophys Acta* 1996;1276:87-105.

[28] Ozawa T. Genetic and functional changes in mitochondria associated with aging. *Physiol Rev* 1997;77:425-64.

[29] Zhang J, Block ER, Patel JM. Down-regulation of mitochondrial cytochrome c oxidase in senescent porcine pulmonary artery endothelial cells. *Mech Ageing Dev* 2002;123:1363-74.

[30] Kumazaki T, Sakano T, Yoshida T, Hamada K, Sumida H, Teranishi Y, et al. Enhanced expression of mitochondrial genes in senescent endothelial cells and fibroblasts. *Mech Ageing Dev* 1998;101:91-9.

[31] Hayflick L. Mortality and immortality at the cellular level. A review. *Biochemistry* (Mosc) 1997; 62:1180-90.

[32] Fossel M. Cell senescence in human aging and disease. *Ann NY Acad Sci* 2002;959:14-23.

[33] Martin GM, Oshima J. Lessons from human progeroid syndromes. *Nature* 2000;408:263-66.
[34] Minamino T, Komuro I. Role of telomere in endothelial dysfunction in atherosclerosis. *Curr Opin Lipidol* 2002;13:537-43.
[35] Aviv H, Khan MY, Skurnick J, Okuda K, Kimura M, Gardner J, et al. Age dependent aneuploidy and telomere length of the human vascular endothelium. *Atherosclerosis* 2001;159:281-7.
[36] Warner HR. Aging and regulation of apoptosis. *Curr Top Cell Regul* 1997;35:107-21.
[37] Higami Y, Shimokawa I. Apoptosis in the aging process. *Cell Tissue Res* 2000;301:125-32.
[38] Hoffmann J, Haendeler J, Aicher A, Rossig L, Vasa M, Zeiher AM, et al. Aging enhances the sensitivity of endothelial cells toward apoptotic stimuli: important role of nitric oxide. *Circ Res* 2001;89:709-15.
[39] Hayflick L. The future of ageing. *Nature* 2000;408:267-96.
[40] Guarente L, Kenyon C. Genetic pathways that regulate ageing in model organisms. *Nature* 2000;408:255-62.
[41] Armbrecht HJ. The biology of aging. *J Lab Clin Med* 2001;138:220-25.
[42] Weindruch R, Kayo T, Lee CK, Prolla TA. Gene expression profiling of aging using DNA microarrays. *Mech Ageing Dev* 2002;23:177-93.
[43] Dong C, Yoon W, Goldschmidt-Clermont PJ. DNA methylation and atherosclerosis. *J Nutr* 2002;132:2406S-09S.
[44] Lakatta EG. Cardiovascular regulatory mechanisms in advanced age. *Physiol Rev* 1993;73:413-67.
[45] Popper H. Aging and the liver. *Prog Liver Dis* 1986;VIII:659-83.
[46] Le Couteur DG, McLean AJ. The aging liver: drug clearance and an oxygen diffusion barrier hypothesis. *Clin Pharmacokinet* 1998;34:359-73.
[47] Woodhouse KW, Wynne HA. Age-related changes in liver size and hepatic blood flow. The influence on drug metabolism in the elderly. *Clin Pharmacokinet* 1988;15:287-94.
[48] Braet F, Wisse E. Structural and functional aspects of liver sinusoidal endothelial cell fenestrae: a review. *Compar Hepatol* 2002;1:1-17.
[49] Fraser R, Dobbs BR, Rogers GW. Lipoproteins and the liver sieve: the role of fenestrated sinusoidal endothelium in lipoprotein metabolism, atherosclerosis, and cirrhosis. *Hepatology* 1995;21:863-74.
[50] Braet F, De Zanger R, Crabbe E, Wisse E. New observations on cytoskeleton and fenestrae in isolated rat liver sinusoidal endothelial cells. *J Gastroenterol Hepatol* 1995;10:S3-7.
[51] Braet F, de Zanger R, Seynaeve C, Baekeland M, Wisse E. A comparative atomic force microscopy study on living skin fibroblasts and liver endothelial cells. *J Electron Microsc* (Tokyo) 2001;50:283-90.
[52] Le Couteur DG, Cogger VC, Markus AM, Harvey PJ, Yin ZL, Ansselin AD, et al. Pseudocapillarization and associated energy limitation in the aged rat liver. *Hepatology* 2001;33:537-43.
[53] McLean AJ, Cogger VC, Chong GC, Warren A, Markus AM, Dahlstrom JE, et al. Age-related pseudocapillarisation of the human liver. *J Pathol* 2003;200:112-17.

[54] Cogger VC, Warren A, Fraser R, Ngu M, McLean AJ, Le Couteur DG. Hepatic sinusoidal pseudocapillarization with ageing in the non-human primate. *Exp Gerontol* 2003;38:1101-07.

[55] Cogger VC, Mross PE, Hosie MJ, Ansselin AD, McLean AJ, Le Couteur DG. The effect of acute oxidative stress on the ultrastructure of the perfused rat liver. *Pharmacol Toxicol* 2001;89:306-11.

[56] Braet F, Muller M, Vekemans K, Wisse E, Le Couteur DG. Antimycin A-induced defenestration in rat hepatic sinusoidal endothelial cells. *Hepatology* 2003;38:394-402.

[57] Popper H, Elias H, Petty DE. Vascular pattern of the cirrhotic liver. *Am J Clin Pathol* 1952;22:717-29.

[58] Burt AD. Cellular and molecular aspects of hepatic fibrosis. *Journal of Pathology* 1993;170:105-14.

[59] Friedman SL. The cellular basis of hepatic fibrosis. *New England Journal of Medicine* 1993;328:1828-35.

[60] Dobbs BR, Rogers GW, Xing H-Y, Fraser R. Endotoxin-induced defenestration of the hepatic sinusoidal endothelium: a factor in the pathogenesis of cirrhosis? *Liver* 1994;14:230-33.

[61] Brod SA. Unregulated inflammation shortens human functional longevity. *Inflamm Res* 2000;49:561-70.

[62] Paolisso G, Rizzo M, Mazziotti G, Tagliamonte M, Gambardella A, Rotondi M, et al. Advancing Age And Insulin Resistance: Role Of Plasma Tumor Necrosis Factor-A. *Am. J. Physiol.* 1998;275:E294-E99.

[63] Hager K, Machein U, Krieger S, Platt D, Seefried G, Bauer J. Interleukin-6 and selected plasma proteins in healthy persons of different ages. *Neurobiol Aging* 1994;15:771-72.

[64] Born J, Uthgenannt D, Dodt C, Nunninghoff D, Ringvolt E, Wagner T, et al. Cytokine production and lymphocyte subpopulations in aged humans. An assessment during nocturnal sleep. *Mech Ageing Dev* 1995;84:113-26.

[65] Fagiolo U, Cossarizza A, Scala E, Fanales-Belasio E, Ortolani C, Cozzi E, et al. Increased cytokine production in mononuclear cells of healthy elderly people. *Eur J Immunol* 1993;23:2375-8.

[66] Kukovetz EM, Bratschitsch G, Hofer HP, Egger G, Schaur RJ. Influence of age on the release of reactive oxygen species by phagocytes as measured by a whole blood chemiluminescence assay. *Free Radic Biol Med* 1997;22:433-8.

[67] Munro J, Cotran R. The pathogenesis of atherosclerosis: atherogenesis and inflammation. *Lab Invest* 1988;58:249-61.

[68] Lavrovsky Y, Chatterjee B, Clark RA, Roy AK. Role of redox-regulated transcription factors in inflammation, aging and age-related diseases. *Exp Gerontol* 2000;35:521-32.

[69] Sellak H, Franzini E, Hakim J, C. P. Reactive oxygen species rapidly increase endothelial ICAM-1 ability to bind neutrophils without detectable upregulation. *Blood* 1994;83:2669-77.

[70] Persidsky YU, Frolov A, Barshtein YU. Tumor necrosis factor action on the various types of mouse liver cell in vivo. In: Knook DL, Wisse E, editors. Cells of the hepatic Sinusoids. 4 ed. Leiden: *Kupffer Cell Foundation;* 1993. p. 82-84.

[71] Ohira H, Ueno T, Sakamoto M, Torimura T, Inuzuka S, Sata M, et al. Expression of intercellular adhesion molecule-1 (ICAM-1) on cultured rat liver sinusoidal endothelial

cells by tumor necrosis factor-a and interleukin-1. In: Knook DL, Wisse E, editors. Cells of the hepatic Sinusoids. 4 ed. Leiden: *Kupffer Cell Foundation;* 1993. p. 79-81.

[72] Fraser R, Rogers GWT, Sutton LE, Dobbs BR. Single dose models of defenestration: tools to explore mechanisms, modulation and measurement of hepatic sinusoidal porosity. In: Wisse E, Knook DL, Wake K, editors. Cells of the hepatic Sinusoids. Leiden: *Kupffer Cell Foundation;* 1995. p. 263-66.

[73] Sarphie TG, D'Souza NB, Deaciuc IV. Kupffer cell inactivation prevents lipopolysaccharide-induced structural changes in the rat liver sinusoid: an electron-microscopic study. *Hepatology* 1996;23:788-96.

[74] Khoruts A, Stahnke L, McClain CJ, Logan G, Allen JI. Circulating tumor necrosis factor, interleukin-1 and interleukin-6 concentrations in chronic alcoholic patients. *Hepatology* 1991;13:267-76.

[75] Madarame T, Nagaoka T, Inomata M, Kaneta H, Yoshida T, Suzuki K, et al. Relationship between endothelial structure and capillarisation in fatty liver. In: Knook DL, Wisse E, eds. Cells of the hepatic Sinusoids 4 Leiden: Kupffer Cell Foundation, 191-192, 1993., editors. Cells of the hepatic Sinusoids. 4 ed. Leiden: *Kupffer Cell Foundation;* 1993. p. 191-92.

[76] Le Couteur DG, Fraser R, Cogger VC, McLean AJ. Hepatic pseudocapillarisation and atherosclerosis in ageing. *Lancet* 2002;359:1612-15.

[77] Lundman P, Eriksson MJ, Silveira A, Hansson LO, Pernow J, Ericsson CG, et al. Relation of hypertriglyceridemia to plasma concentrations of biochemical markers of inflammation and endothelial activation (C-reactive protein, interleukin-6, soluble adhesion molecules, von Willebrand factor, and endothelin-1). *Am J Cardiol* 2003;91:1128-31.

[78] Fraser R, Bosanquet AG, Day WA. Filtration of chylomicrons by the liver may influence cholesterol metabolism and atherosclerosis. *Atherosclerosis* 1978;29:113-23.

[79] Wisse W, De Zanger RB, Charels K, Van Der Smissen P, McCuskey RS. The liver sieve: considerations concerning the structure and function of endothelial fenestrae, the sinusoidal wall and the space of Disse. *Hepatology* 1985;5:683-92.

[80] Popescu D, Movileanu L, Ion S, Flonta ML. Hydrodynamic effects on the solute transport across endothelial pores and hepatocyte membranes. *Phys Med Biol* 2000;45:N157-65.

[81] Terpstra V, van Amersfoort ES, van Velzen AG, Kuiper J, van Berkel TJ. Hepatic and extrahepatic scavenger receptors: function in relation to disease. *Arterioscler Thromb Vasc Biol* 2000;20:1860-72.

[82] Redgrave TG. Formation of cholesteryl ester-rich particulate lipid during metabolism of chylomicrons. *J Clin Invest* 1970;49:465-71.

[83] Yu KC, Cooper AD. Postprandial lipoproteins and atherosclerosis. *Frontiers Biosci* 2001;6:332-54.

[84] Wisse E. An electron microscopic study of the fenestrated endothelial lining of rat liver sinusoids. *J Ultrastruct Res*· 1970;31:125-50.

[85] Floren CH. Binding of apolipoprotein E-rich remnant lipoproteins to human liver membranes. *Scand J Gastroenterol* 1984;19:473-79.

[86] Clark SA, Cook HB, Oxner RB, Angus HB, George PM, Fraser R. Defenestration of hepatic sinusoids as a cause of hyperlipoproteinaemia in alcoholics. *Lancet* 1988;ii:1225-27.

[87] Le Couteur DG, Fraser R, Hilmer S, Rivory LP, McLean AJ. The hepatic sinusoid in aging and cirrhosis: effects on hepatic substrate disposition and drug clearance. *Clin Pharmacokinet* 2003:(in press).
[88] Romero EL, Morilla MJ, Regts J, Koning GA, Scherphof GL. On the mechanism of hepatic transendothelial passage of large liposomes. *FEBS Lett* 1999;448:193-96.
[89] Hardonk MJ, Harms G, Koudstaal J. Zonal heterogeneity of rat hepatocytes in the in vivo uptake of 17 nm colloidal gold granules. *Histochemistry* 1985;83:473-7.
[90] Cherkasov AN. Selective ultrafiltration. *J. Membr. Sci.* 1990;50:109-30.
[91] Le Couteur DG, Rivory LP, Roberts MS, Pond SM. Aging and the response of the isolated perfused rat liver to vasoactive drugs. *Biochem Pharmacol* 1992;43:913-15.
[92] Cassader M, Gambino R, Rulu G, Marena S, Bodoni P, Pagano G. Postprandial triglyceride-rich lipoprotein changes in elderly and young subjects. *Aging Clin Exp Res* 1996;8:421-28.
[93] Cohn JS, McNamara JR, Cohn SD, Ordovas JM, Schaefer EJ. Postprandial plasma lipoprotein changes in human subjects of different ages. *J Lipid Res* 1988;29:469-79.
[94] Krasinski SD, Cohn JS, Schaefer EJ, Russell RM. Postprandial plasma retinyl ester response is greater in older subjects compared with younger subjects. Evidence for delayed plasma clearance of intestinal lipoproteins. *J Clin Invest* 1990;85:883-92.
[95] Field PA, Gibbons GF. Decreased hepatic expression of the low-density lipoprotein (LDL) receptor and LDL receptorrelated protein in aging rats is associated with delayed clearance of chylomicrons from the circulation. *Metabolism* 2000;49:492-98.
[96] Hilmer SN, Warren A, Cogger VC, Fraser R, McLean AJ, Sullivan DR, et al. The effect of aging on the immunohistochemistry of apolipoprotein E in the liver. *Exp Gerontol* 2003;in press.
[97] Moreton JR. Atherosclerosis and dietary hyperlipemia. *Science* 1947;106:190-91.
[98] Fraser R. The role of dietary triglycerides in cholesterol metabolism. *Atherosclerosis* 1974;19:327-36.
[99] Zilmersmit DB. Atherogenesis: a postprandial phenomenon. *Circulation* 1979;60:473-85.
[100] Weintraub MS, Grosskopf I, Rassin T, Miller H, Charach G, Rotmensch HH, et al. Clearance of chylomicron remnants in normolipidaemic patients with coronary heart disease: case control study over three years. *BMJ* 1996;312:935-39.
[101] Rapp JH, Lespine A, Hamilton RL, Chaumeton AH, Tweedie-Hardman J, Kotite L, et al. Triglyceride-rich lipoproteins isolated by selected affinity anti-apolipoprotein B immunosorption from human atherosclerotic plaque. *Arterioscler Thromb* 1994;14:1767-74.

In: Aging and the Elderly: Psychology, Sociology and Health ISBN 1-60021-190-9
Editor: L. O. Randall, pp. 177-196

Chapter 8

TOPICS IN AGING: INCOME AND POVERTY AMONG OLDER AMERICANS IN 2004[1]

Debra Whitman and Patrick Purcell

ABSTRACT

Older Americans are an economically diverse group. In 2004, the median income of individuals age 65 and older was $15,199, but incomes varied widely around this average. Twenty-eight percent of Americans 65 or older had incomes of less than $10,000 in 2004, while 10% had incomes of $50,000 or more. As Congress considers reforms to Social Security and the laws governing pensions and retirement savings plans, it may be helpful to consider how changes to one income source would affect each of the others, and thus the total income of older Americans.

Older persons receive income from a variety of sources, including earnings, pensions, personal savings, and public programs such as Social Security and Supplemental Security Income. Using data from the March 2005 *Current Population Survey,* this report describes the number of elderly receiving income from each of these sources and the extent to which income from each source is either concentrated at the high- or low-end of the income distribution or is evenly distributed.

Retirement benefits from Social Security and pensions are the most common source of income among the aged. In 2004, Social Security paid benefits to 88% of Americans age 65 and older. Social Security is also the largest single source of income among the aged. Sixty-nine percent of Social Security beneficiaries age 65 or older receive more than half of their income from Social Security. For 39% of elderly recipients, Social Security contributes more than 90% of their income, and for nearly one-quarter of recipients, it is their *only* source of income. In 2004, 35% of people age 65 and older received income from a private or public pension. Among people age 65 and older who reported income from a government pension, the median annual amount was $15,600. Among recipients of private pensions, the median amount received in 2004 was just $6,720.

---

[1] Excerpted from CRS Report Number RL32697, dated November 7, 2005

Many Americans prepare for retirement by saving and investing some of their income while they are working. Of the 35.2 million Americans age 65 or older who were living in households in 2004, 19.7 million (56%) received income from assets, such as interest, dividends, rent, and royalties. Most received small amounts of income from the assets they owned. Of all individuals age 65 or older who received income from assets in 2004, half received less than $952.

Earnings from work continue to be an important source of income for older Americans, especially those under age 70. Although there was a trend toward earlier retirement from about 1960 to 1985, over the past 20 years more Americans have continued to work at older ages. In 2004, median earnings for individuals age 55-6 1 who worked were $34,000, while median earned income for workers age 62-64 was $27,000. For workers 65 and older, the median earned income was $15,000. Poverty among those age 65 and older has fallen from one-in-three older persons in 1960 to one-in-ten today. While the overall rate of poverty is relatively low, it remains high for women, minorities, the less-educated, and those older than 80.

INTRODUCTION

This report describes the income and poverty status of the 35.2 million Americans age 65 and older living in the community in 2004.[1] Older persons receive income from a variety of sources, including earnings, pensions, personal savings, and public programs such as Social Security and Supplemental Security Income. The substantial variation in the number of people receiving income from each source and the amounts they receive from each source are the main topics of this report. Using data from the March 2005 *Current Population Survey,* we describe both the number of elderly receiving income from each of 10 major sources and the extent to which income from each source is either concentrated at the high- or low-end of the income distribution or is more evenly distributed among the elderly population.

In addition to looking at sources and amounts of income, the report examines the income of the elderly relative to the federal poverty thresholds. In 2004, 9.8% of Americans 65 and older had family incomes below the federal poverty threshold. This was lower than both the poverty rate for the population 18 to 64 years old (11.3%) and the poverty rate among children under age 18 (17.8%).[2]

Although income is an important measure of a person's economic well-being, it is not the only such measure, nor is it always the best one. Individuals with the same cash income may have significantly different levels of financial assets or other forms of wealth. Some own their own homes while others rent. Some receive non-cash benefits from their former employer — such as fully or partially paid health insurance — while others have to pay for health services or insurance out-of-pocket. The federal and state governments also provide many non-cash benefits and services such as Medicaid, Food Stamps, and the Low-Income Home Energy Assistance Program that improve the financial circumstances of lower-income families, but which do not show up in measures of cash income. Finally, some older Americans live with family members or receive considerable non-financial assistance from their families, while others live alone and pay someone to perform household chores or to provide personal care services. Even with these limitations, however, the amount of income that older Americans receive is an important measure of their ability to purchase the goods and services that contribute to their economic well-being.

THE DATA

The findings in this report are based on data collected in the March 2005 *Current Population Survey* (CPS), conducted by the Bureau of the Census. The CPS is a survey of approximately 100,000 households comprising a representative sample of the civilian, non-institutionalized population of the United States. Each March, the survey includes detailed questions on sources and amounts of income received during the previous calendar year. The CPS is widely used by researchers in government, academia, and the private sector, and it is the source of the official statistics published annually by the Census Bureau on median family income, the number of Americans living in poverty, and the number of people without health insurance. Like any survey, the CPS is subject to error. *Sampling error* occurs if the households selected to participate in the survey are not representative of the population. *Non-sampling error* occurs if survey participants provide inaccurate information or if their responses are incorrectly recorded.

How Income was Counted

All income figures in this report are for *individual* elderly persons. Focusing on the income of individuals rather than families or households may overstate the resources available to some elderly and underestimate the resources available to others within the same family. For example, an elderly couple may receive a pension from a husband's former employer. The pension income would only be attributed to the husband and not his wife even though she may share in the benefits of that income. While the income figures may not reflect the total income available within a family, the advantage of this methodology is that it provides an accurate count of the number of older Americans who receive income from specific sources such as pensions or public assistance. To calculate poverty rates, however, income was combined for all family members before comparing it to the official federal poverty thresholds.[3]

TOTAL INCOME

Both the sources of income and the amounts received from each source differ among elderly in different age groups. For example, individuals 80 and older are more likely to receive income from pensions and Social Security and are less likely to work than the elderly who are between the ages of 65 and 69. (See Table 1) Comparing those 80 and older to those age 65 to 69, the older group received, on average, \$9,428 less in earnings, \$6,000 less in public pensions, \$3,888 less in private pensions, and \$100 less in asset income. The older group received \$336 more in Social Security than their younger counterparts. Total income also declined with age. Median total income in 2004 was $18,249 for persons 65 to 69 years old, $14,857 for those age 70 to 79, and $13,999 for individuals age 80 or older.

Table 1. Percentage of Older Americans with Income in 2004, Mean and Median Amounts, by Source

	Age					
	Total, 55+	**55 to 64**	**Total, 65+**	**65 to 69**	**70 to 79**	**80+**
Total number of people (000s)	64,745	29,532	35,213	10,124	15,860	9,230
Percentage with no income	4.4	6.3	2.9	3.3	3.0	2.3
Earnings						
Percentage with earnings	40.2	66.5	18.0	32.6	16.2	5.1
Mean	$41,010	$44,673	$29,672	$32,792	$27,256	$21,101
Median	$29,000	$32,000	$15,000	$19,428	$12,000	$10,000
Social Security						
Percentage with Social Security	56.0	17.7	88.2	83.1	89.6	91.2
Mean	$10,578	$9,952	$10,683	$10,586	$10,636	$10,858
Median	$10,399	$9,516	$10,399	$10,303	$10,399	$10,639
Public pensions						
Percentage with public pensions	9.2	6.3	11.6	11.5	11.9	11.4
Mean	$20,948	$23,538	$19,765	$21,865	$19,548	$17,840
Median	$16,824	$19,200	$15,600	$19,200	$16,200	$13,200
Private pensions or annuities						
Percentage with private pensions	17.2	9.4	23.8	20.7	24.5	26.1
Mean	$11,906	$16,453	$10,402	$12,535	$10,493	$8,395
Median	$7,428	$11,134	$6,720	$9,000	$6,960	$5,112
Income from assets						
Percentage with income from assets	57.1	58.3	56.0	57.2	56.2	54.5
Mean	$5,111	$4,810	$5,374	$5,890	$5,244	$5,009
Median	$777	$600	$952	$1,000	$947	$900
Veterans' benefits						
Percentage with veterans' benefits	2.8	2.3	3.2	2.3	3.1	4.3
Mean	$10,512	$13,363	$8,802	$10,169	$8,651	$8,172
Median	$6,599	$9,995	$5,639	$7,919	$4,799	$5,746
Public assistance[a]						
Percentage with public assistance	3.5	3.5	3.5	3.8	3.2	3.7
Mean	$5,057	$6,024	$4,238	$4,639	$3,933	$4,241
Median	$4,800	$6,540	$3,600	$3,600	$3,156	$3,600
Other income[b]						
Percentage with other income	4.2	6.2	2.6	3.6	2.4	1.9
Mean	$7,815	$7,732	$7,983	$8,583	$7,723	$7,289
Median	$4,000	$4,080	$3,600	$4,000	$4,000	$3,600
Total Income						
Percentage with any income	95.6	93.7	97.1	96.7	97.0	97.7
Mean	$31,490	$40,894	$23,878	$29,641	$23,052	$19,028
Median	$19,255	$28,600	$15,199	$18,249	$14,857	$13,999

Source: The Congressional Research Service (CRS) analysis of the March 2005 Current Population Survey.

[a] Includes mainly Supplemental Security Income, Temporary Assistance for Needy Families, and state general assistance.

[b] Includes unemployment compensation, workers' compensation, and income from unidentified sources.

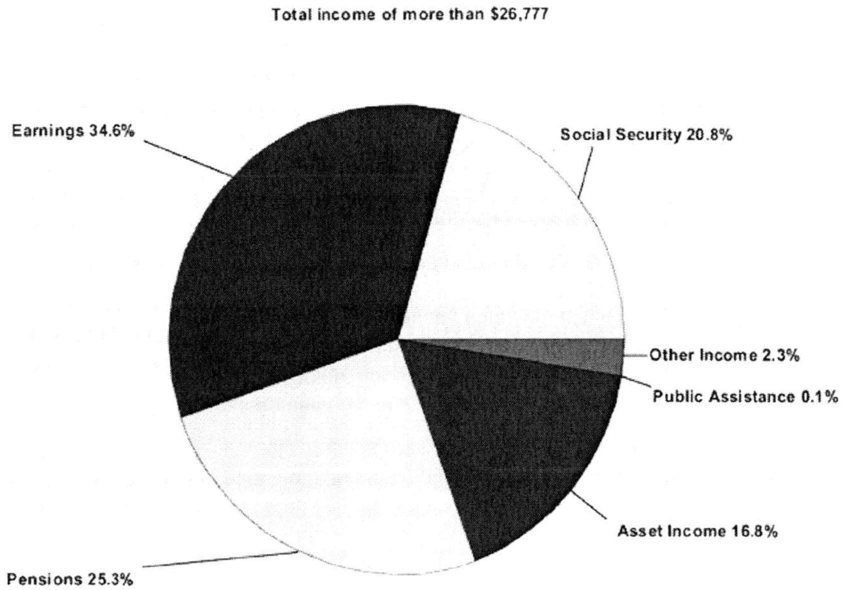

Figure 1. Income Sources of People Age 65+ in 2004, First (Highest) Quartile.

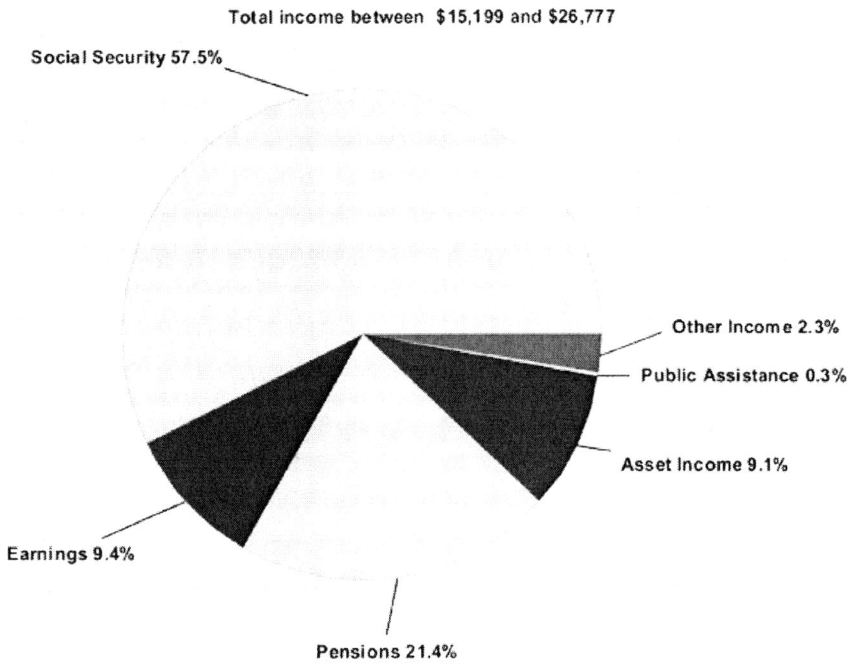

Figure 2. Income Sources for People Age 65+ in 2004, Second Quartile.

Personal savings, Social Security, and employer-sponsored pensions are sometimes referred to as the "three-legged stool" of retirement income. While this term may be useful as a metaphor, for many older Americans, at least one of the legs of the stool is missing. Figure 1 and Figure 4 illustrate this point for individuals in the highest and lowest quartiles of the income distribution. In 2004, 86% of the income received by elderly individuals in the lowest income quartile (those with less than $9,390 in total income) came from Social Security. For this group, less than 5% of their income came from savings and only 2% was received from pensions. Older Americans with higher incomes had more diversified sources of income. In 2004, 21% of income received by individuals in the highest quartile of the income distribution (those with $26,800 or more in income) came from Social Security. These individuals also were more likely to have wage income and to receive income from pensions and assets. They received, on average, three-fourths of their income from these three sources. Figure 2 and Figure 3 show that Social Security comprised 58% and 82% of income, respectively among older Americans in the second and third income quartiles in 2004.

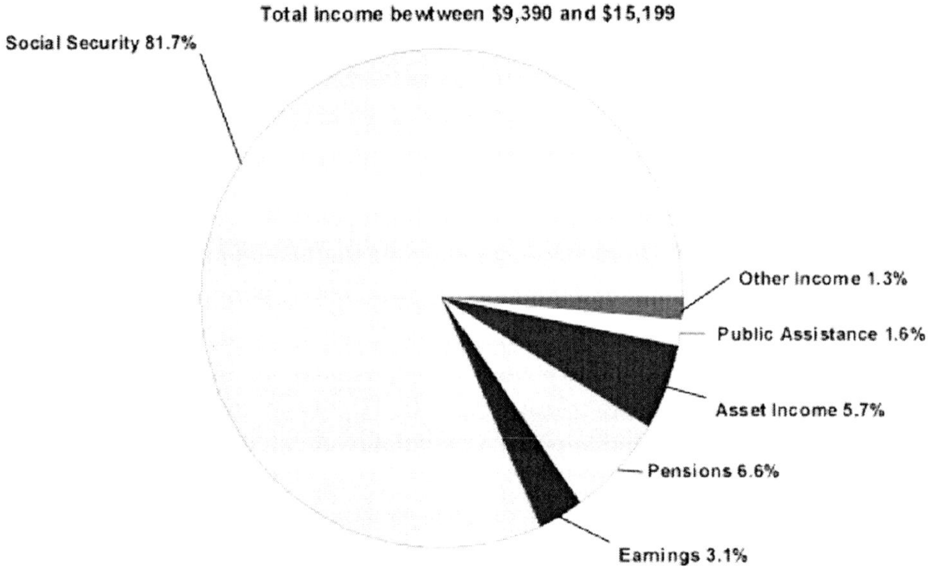

Figure 3. Income Sources of People Age 65+ in 2004,Third Quartile.

The average amount received in 2004 from each income source by people in the lowest and highest income quartiles is shown in Figure 5. Those in the poorest quarter of the elderly population received an average of $5,470 from Social Security, $79 from earnings, $153 from pensions, and $297 from assets. Older Americans in the highest income quartile received on average $11,847 from Social Security, $19,681 from earnings, $14,392 from pensions, and $9,571 from assets. There are significant financial advantages from continuing to work past age 65. On average, members of the highest income brackets received $1 out of $3 of their income from working.

Income of the elderly varied significantly by age, sex, race, education and marital status. Figure 6 shows that in 2004, individuals between the ages of 65 and 69 had a median income of $18,250 while those who were 80 or older had a median income of $14,000. Men 65 and older had a median income of $21,200, compared to $12,079 for women. The median income of older African Americans, $11,450, was 71% of the median income of older white Americans — $16,170. The median income of older Americans increases substantially with their educational level. Those without high-school diplomas had a median income of $10,800 in 2004 while college graduates had incomes nearly three times as high. Married individuals had median incomes $1,800 higher than single individuals.

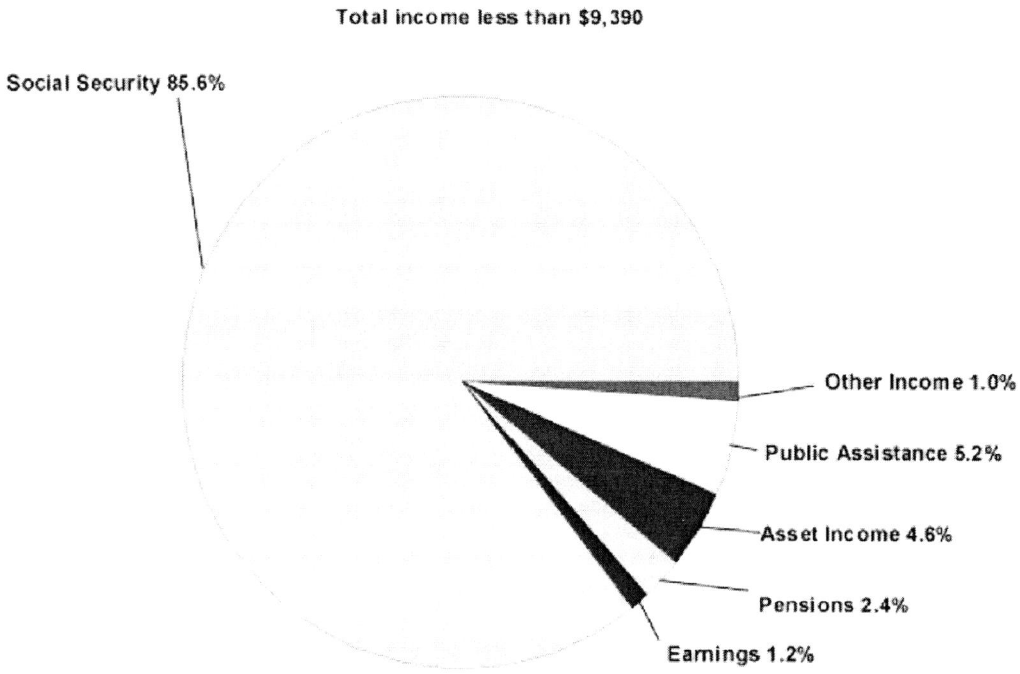

Figure 4. Income Sources of People Age 65+ in 2004, Fourth (Lowest) Quartile.

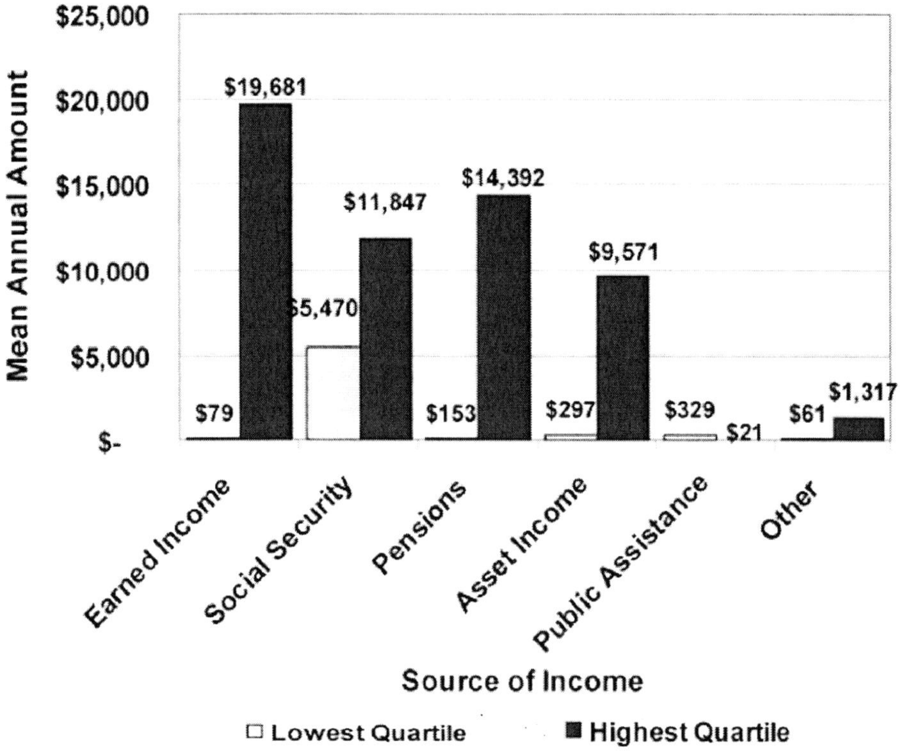

Figure 5. Mean Income by Source and Income Quartile, 2004.

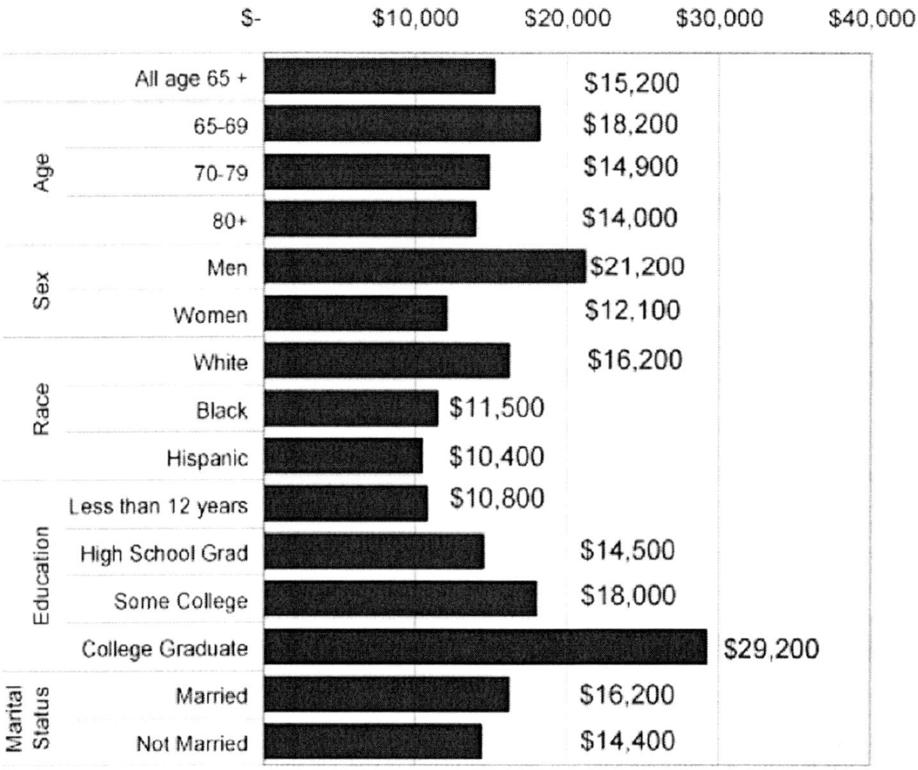

Figure 6. Median Total Income of Group in 2004.

POVERTY

Poverty among the elderly has decreased dramatically over the past four decades. In 1959 the poverty rate of those age 65 and older was 35%. Largely due to increases in Social Security benefits, the elderly poverty rate fell dramatically between the mid-1960s and mid-1970s, declining to about 15% by 1975. The percentage of older Americans in poverty has stayed steady at roughly 10% since the mid 1 990s. Although a smaller percentage of the elderly are in poverty than are people under 65, in 2004 nearly 3.5 million older Americans had family incomes below the federal poverty threshold.[4,5]

While the poverty rate for all persons age 65 and older was 9.8% in 2004, the poverty rates among women, minorities, single individuals, those with low education, and the oldest old were higher. (See Figure 7.) Twelve percent of women age 65 and older were in poverty in 2004 compared to only 7% of men. Because women live longer, the number of poor older women in 2004 (2.4 million) was more than twice the number of poor older men (1.1 million). Poverty rates were especially high among minorities. In 2004, nearly one-quarter of elderly African-Americans and almost one-fifth of elderly Hispanics were in poverty. About 81% of all older Americans identify themselves as white. Thus, while only 7.5% of older white Americans were poor, poor whites comprised 62% of all poor elderly in 2004. Older individuals with low education also had high poverty rates. Nineteen percent of those without a high school education had family incomes below the poverty line in 2004 compared to only

5% of those with a college degree. There is a significant difference in the poverty rates of married persons and single elderly individuals. Married couples, who often have more than one source of income, had a poverty rate of only 4.5% in 2004. In contrast, 16.2% of unmarried individuals age 65 and older had incomes less than the official poverty threshold in 2004. The oldest Americans had the highest poverty rates. Eleven percent of individuals age 80 and older were poor in 2004 compared to 9% of individuals between the ages of 65 and 69. Nearly half of all Americans age 80 and older had family incomes of less than twice the poverty threshold in 2004.

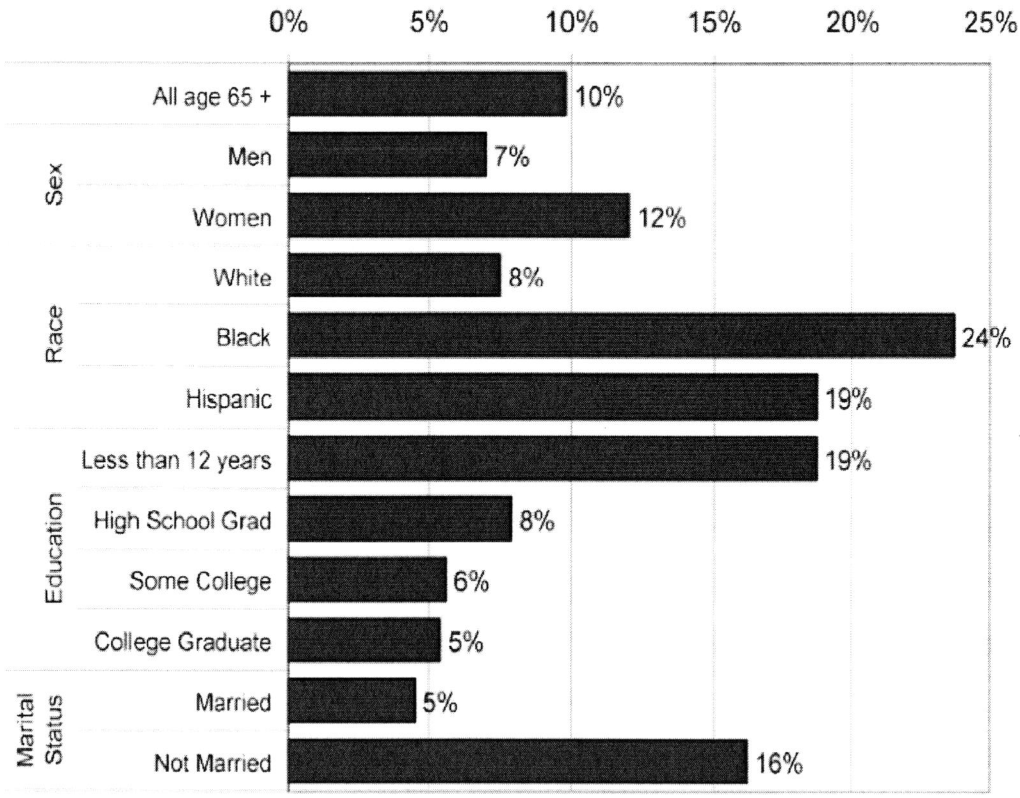

Source: CRS analysis of the March 2005 Current Population Survey.

Figure 7. Percentage of People Age 65 and Over in Poverty in 2004.

The Near-Poor

Many older Americans have family incomes that put them just above the official poverty threshold. In 2004, while 9.8% of people age 65 and older had incomes below the poverty thresholds of $9,060 for an individual and $11,418 for a couple, 24% of older Americans had family incomes below 150% of the thresholds ($13,590 for an individual,$ 17,127 for a couple). Thirty-eight percent of people 65 and older had incomes less than twice the poverty thresholds ($18,120 for an individual, $22,836 for a couple).

INCOME FROM RETIREMENT BENEFITS

Social Security[6]

Retirement benefits from Social Security are the most common source of income among the aged. Social Security is a social insurance program designed to protect workers, their dependent children, and surviving spouses in the event that a worker dies, becomes disabled, or reaches retirement age. In 2004, Social Security paid benefits to 88% of Americans age 65 and older. Social Security is the largest single source of income among the aged. Sixty-nine percent of Social Security beneficiaries age 65 or older receive more than half of their income from Social Security. For 39% of elderly recipients, Social Security contributes more than 90% of their income, and for nearly one-quarter of recipients, it is their *only* source of income. (See Table 2) While Social Security is an important source of income for a majority of the elderly, the benefit amounts paid by Social Security are relatively small compared to many recipients' pre-retirement incomes. According to the Social Security Administration, Social Security retired worker benefits replace approximately 56% of the earnings of a career-long low-wage earner, 42% of the earnings of a career-long average-wage earner, and 27% of the earnings of a career-long high-wage earner. Average monthly Social Security benefits in 2005 are $963 for a retired worker and $1,583 for an elderly couple. As Figure 8 shows, 46% of all beneficiaries received less than $10,000 from Social Security in 2004 and 3% received more than $20,000 in Social Security benefits.

Table 2. Social Security as a Percentage of Income among Recipients Age 65 and Older in 2004

Percent of Income from Social Security	Recipients (thousands)	Percentage of Recipients
Less than 20%	2,470	8.0%
20% to 39%	4,613	14.9
40% to 49%	2,495	8.0
50% to 69%	4,818	15.5
70% to 89%	4,433	14.3
90 to 99%	4,804	15.5
100% of income	7,411	23.9

Source: CRS analysis of the March 2005 *Current Population Survey.*

Note: In 2004, 31.0 million people age 65 or older received income from Social Security and 4.2 million people had no Social Security income.

Pensions

Since the late 1 970s, the proportion of American workers who participate in employer-sponsored retirement plans has remained fairly stable at about half of the workforce. In 2004, 49% of wage and salary workers between the ages of 21 and 64 participated in employer-sponsored retirement plans; however, a pointin-time snapshot of pension participation is a poor indicator of who will receive pension income in retirement. Some workers not covered by a pension plan today may have earned a pension at a previous job, or they may earn a pension benefit in the future. Others who are currently participating in a pension plan may never fully vest in their pension benefit, or they might take their accrued benefit as a lump sum before retirement and spend all or part of the distribution.[7]

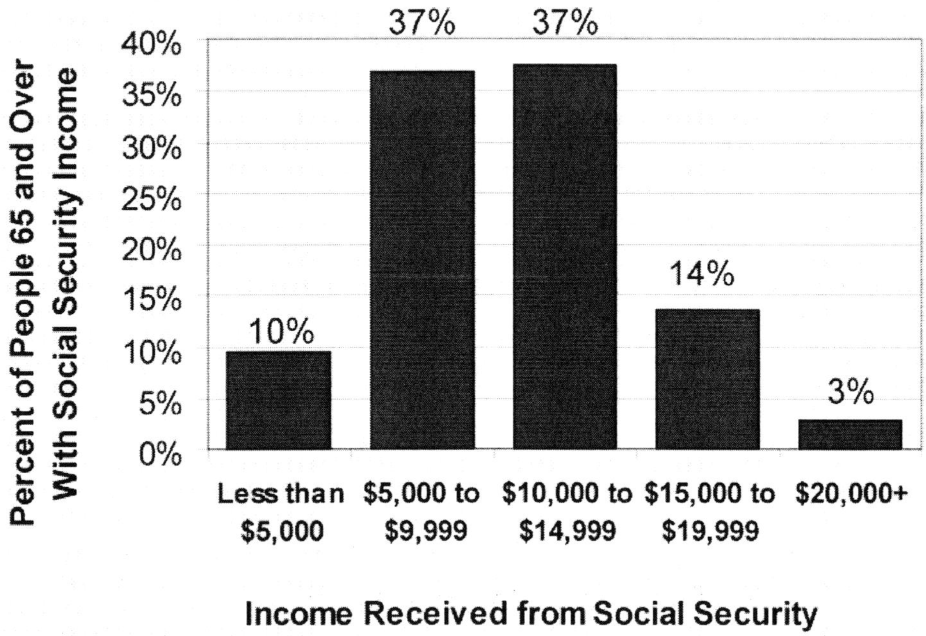

Source: CRS analysis of the March 2005 *Current Population Survey.*

Figure 8. Amount of Social Security Income in 2004.

To receive pension income in retirement, an individual must remain a participant in the plan long enough to earn a pension benefit and must not spend the accrued benefit before retirement. In 1986, Congress shortened the maximum vesting period — the length of time it takes to earn a pension benefit — from ten years to five years, thus making it easier for employees whose employer sponsors a pension to earn a benefit under the plan.[8] On the other hand, many employers offer separating employees the opportunity to take their accrued retirement benefit as a lump-sum distribution. Most defined contribution plans — such as those authorized under §401(k) of the Internal Revenue Code — as well as a growing number of defined benefit plans, now permit departing employees to take a lump-sum distribution. While many employees roll these distributions into another employer-sponsored retirement plan or into an individual retirement account, some spend all or part of the distribution and thereby reduce the income that will be available to them in retirement.[9]

In 2004, 12.2 million people age 65 and older — 34.5% of that age group — received income from a private or public pension.[10] Of this number, 4.1 million had income from a public-sector pension — i.e., from previous employment in the federal, state, or local government — and 8.4 million received income from private-sector pension plans.[11] Together, the federal, state, and local governments account for only about a sixth of all jobs in the U.S. In 2004, for example, only 16.9% of wage and salary workers between the ages of 21 and 64

— roughly one in six — were employed at all levels of government. Nevertheless, nearly *one-third* of pension recipients age 65 and older received income from government-sponsored pension plans. The disparity between the percentage of jobs that are in the government sector and the percentage of retirees with government pensions is accounted for mainly by two factors, both of which make it more likely that a government employee will earn a pension benefit than will a worker in the private sector. First, more government jobs than private-sector jobs offer pension benefits to their employees. In 2004, for example, 85% of all government employees worked at jobs that offered retirement benefits, compared to 56% of private-sector employees whose employers sponsored retirement plans. Second, government employees tend to stay in their jobs longer than private-sector workers, making it more likely that the government employee will fully vest in the pension benefits he or she has earned. The Department of Labor reports that in 2004, the median tenure of government workers with their current employer was nearly double the median tenure of workers in the private sector. Public-sector employees had a median tenure of 6.9 years, while private-sector workers had a median tenure of 3.5-years.[12]

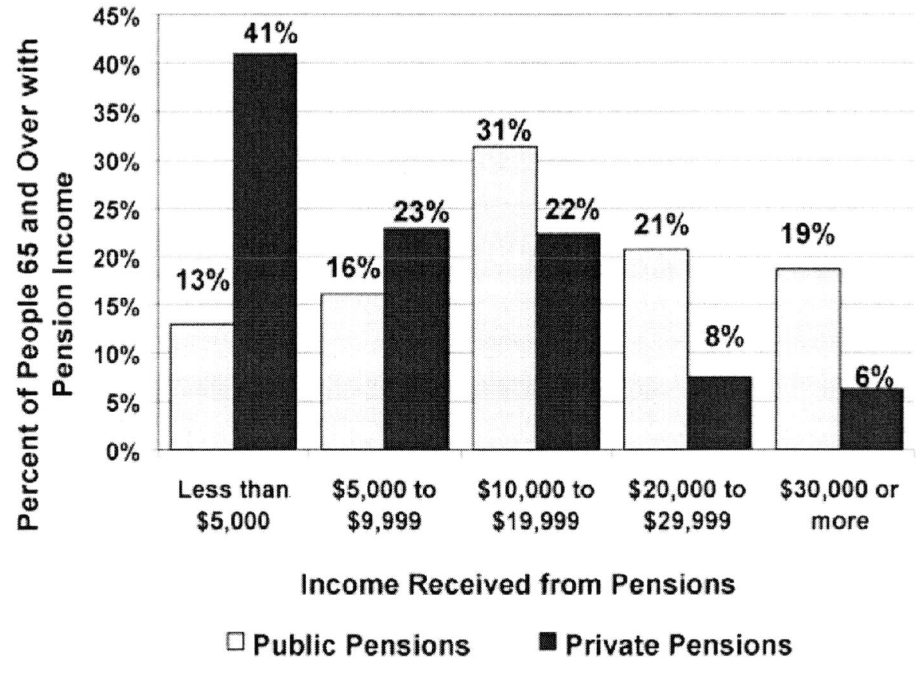

Source: CRS analysis of the March 2005 *Current Population Survey.*

Figure 9. Income from Pensions in 2004.

Public-sector employees not only are more likely to receive a pension in retirement than are workers in the private-sector; they also receive larger pensions than those who worked in the private sector. Among the 4.1 million people age 65 and older who reported income from a government pension in 2004, the median annual amount was $15,600. Thirteen percent of government pension recipients reported that their pension income was less than $5,000 in 2004, while 18.7% reported pension income of more than $30,000. (See Figure 9) Among the 8.4 million people age 65 and older who reported income from a private-sector pension in 2004, the median annual amount was $6,720. Forty-one percent of private pension recipients reported that their pension income was less than $5,000 in 2004 and 6.3% reported pension income of more than $30,000.

Two Types of Pension Plans

Over the past 25 years, there has been a shift in the distribution of retirement plans and of plan participants from *defined benefit* plans to *defined contribution* plans. A defined benefit or "DB" plan usually pays as a lifelong annuity based on the employee's length of service and average salary. Most DB plans are funded entirely by employer contributions and investment earnings. Defined contribution or "DC" plans are much like savings accounts maintained by employers on behalf of each participating employee. The employer contributes a specific dollar amount or percentage of pay, which is invested in stocks, bonds, or other assets. The employee usually contributes to the plan, too. In a DC plan, it is the employee who bears the investment risk. At retirement, the balance in the account is the sum of all contributions plus interest, dividends, and capital gains — or losses. The account balance is usually distributed as a single lump sum. Many large employers recently have converted their traditional DB pensions to hybrid plans that have characteristics of both DB and DC plans, the most popular of which has been the *cash balance plan.* In a cash balance plan, the benefit is defined in terms of an account balance. The employer makes contributions to the plan and pays interest on the accumulated balance. However, these account balances are merely bookkeeping devices. They are not individual accounts owned by the participants. Legally, therefore, a cash balance plan is a defined benefit plan.

INCOME FROM ASSETS

Many Americans prepare for retirement by saving and investing some of their income while they are working.[13] Of the 35.2 million Americans age 65 or older who were living in households in 2004, 19.7 million (56%) received income from assets (interest, dividends, rent, and royalties). Most received small amounts: half of those who had income from assets in 2004 received less than $952. The data displayed in Figure 10 show that low-income individuals were less likely to have received income from assets. Among individuals age 65 or older whose total income in 2004 was less than $20,000, 47% had asset income. In contrast, of those whose total income was more than $20,000, 76% had asset income.

Median income from assets also differed between the lower-income and higher-income elderly. Among people 65 and older with total annual incomes under $5,000, the median amount of asset income was only $200. For roughly one-third of the older population — those with total annual incomes between $10,000 and $19,999 — the median amount of asset income in 2004 was $643. (See Table 3) Those with the highest total incomes were more likely to receive asset income and also received higher amounts. Over 85% of those with total incomes of $50,000 or more received asset income in 2004. Their median income from assets was $7,784.

Table 3. Income from Assets Among People 65 and Older, 2004

Total Income, 2004	Number of People (thousands)	Percent with Asset Income	Mean Asset Income	Median Asset Income
Less than $5,000	1,866	42.6%	$670	$200
$5,000 to $9,999	7,569	36.9	850	300
$10,000 to $19,999	12,143	54.4	1,906	643
$20,000 to $29,000	5,216	69.0	3,430	1,212
$30,000 to $49,999	4,110	76.2	5,862	2,192
$50,000 or more	3,287	85.4	21,324	7,784
All persons with any income[14]	34,190	57.7	$5,374	$952

Source: CRS analysis of the March 2005 *Current Population Survey.*

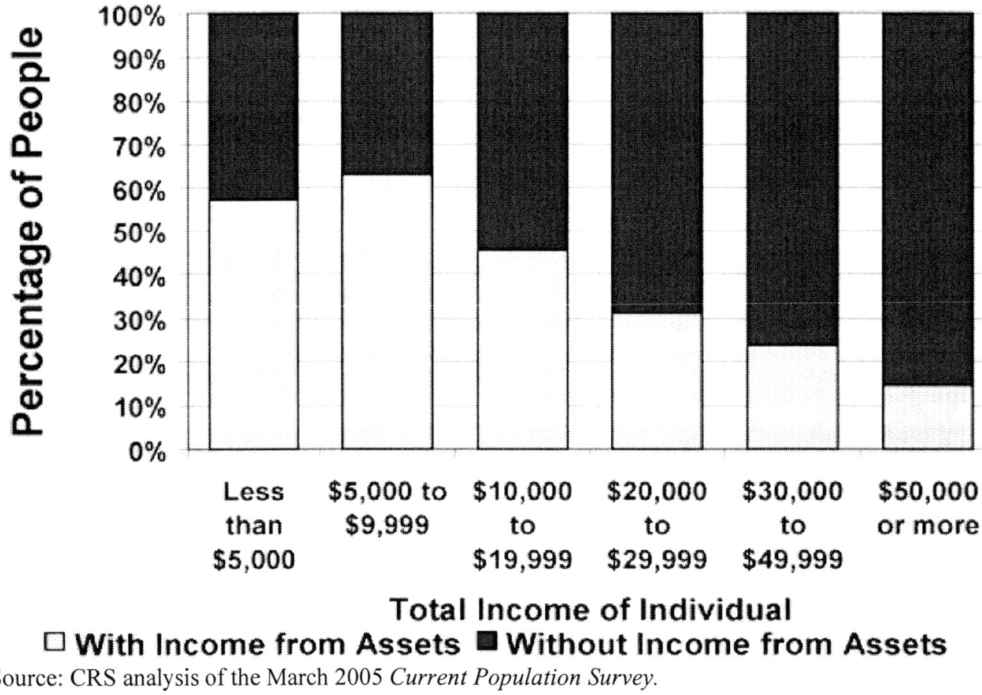

Source: CRS analysis of the March 2005 *Current Population Survey.*

Figure 10. Percentage of People Age 65 and Over with Income from Assets, by Total Income in 2004.

WORK-RELATED INCOME[15]

Earnings

While some Americans continue to work into their 60s and beyond, the labor force participation rate of older individuals drops dramatically as they age. Although there was a trend toward earlier retirement from about 1960 to 1985, the trend for the past 20 years has been that more Americans have continued to work at older ages.[16] In March 2005, 76% of men and 67% of women age 55 were working either full-time or part-time. Of those age 60, 69% of men and 54% of women were employed. Among 65-year olds, 34% of men and 26% of women were employed in March 2005. While the share of older Americans who work declines rapidly after age 65, Figure 11 shows that 21% of men and 19% of women who were 70 years old in March 2005 were still working.

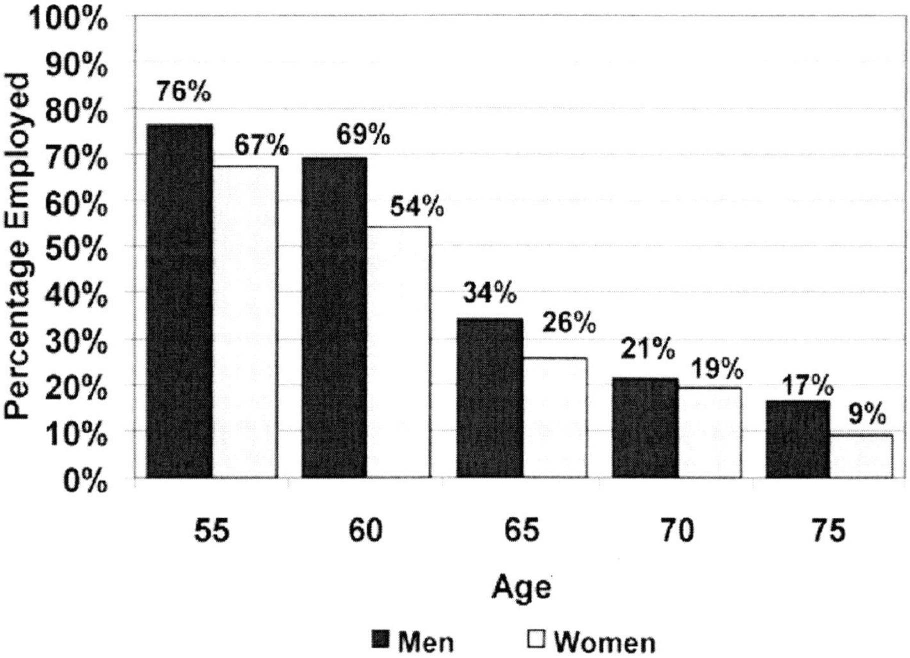

Source: CRS analysis of the March 2005 Current Population Survey.

Figure 11. Employment Rates by Age and Gender, March 2004.

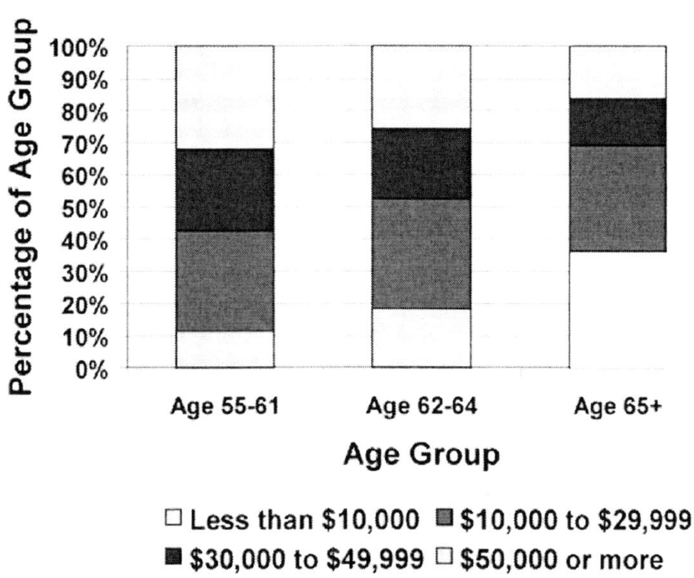

Source: CRS analysis of the March 2005 *Current Population Survey.*

Figure 12. Earned Income by Age, 2004.

Despite the trend to longer working lives, people are progressively less likely to work as they pass age 55 and the average annual earnings of those who continue to work begin to decline at about the same age. This decline can be attributed to two factors: decreases in wages and decreases in the number of hours worked.[17,18] In 2004, the median earnings of workers age 55-61 were $34,000, while median earnings of workers age 62-64 were $27,000. For those over age 65 who continued working, median earnings were only $15,000 in 2004. Figure 12 shows the decline in workers' annual earnings as they age. At the top of the earnings scale, 32% of workers age 55-61 earned $50,000 or more in 2004, while only 16% of those age 65 or older had earned income totaling more than $50,000 in that year. In contrast, while only 6% of Americans age 55-61 who worked in 2004 had total earnings of less than $5,000, 22% of workers age 65 or older had earnings of $5,000 or less.

Unemployment Compensation

Unemployment Compensation (UC) is provided through a joint federal-state system that provides temporary, partial wage replacement to active job seekers who are involuntarily out of work. In 2004, just over one million individuals age 55 and older — about 1.6% of people in this age group — received income from unemployment insurance at some time during the year. Most received UC benefits for six months or less. The median amount of unemployment compensation received by individuals 55 and older was about $2,650.

The percentage of individuals receiving unemployment compensation decreases with age. One reason for this is that older workers are less likely to be unemployed than younger workers. Also, as workers age they are more likely to be eligible for other sources of income, such as pensions and Social Security. In addition, the unemployment benefit an individual receives usually is reduced by the amount of other income he or she receives.[19] This can make the UC benefit particularly small for those age 65 and older. In 2004, the median income from UC benefits for recipients age 65 and older was $2,400, and three-quarters of all individuals age 65 and older who received unemployment compensation received less than $5,265. Although older workers are less likely to be unemployed than younger workers, studies suggest that they take longer to find a new job. Consequently, older workers are more likely than younger workers to exhaust their UC benefits, which typically are limited to 26 weeks.[20]

Workers' Compensation

Workers' compensation provides income replacement and medical benefits to workers who become disabled by work-related injuries and diseases or, in cases of death, their dependents. Workers' compensation benefits are set by state legislatures and the benefit formulas differ from state to state. The benefit generally provides partial wage-replacement for temporary and partial disability, as well as long-term disability.[21] In 2004, 4 17,00 individuals age 55 and older received income through workers' compensation. While few individuals receive workers' compensation benefits after age 65, for those who do, it represents a substantial source of income. For the 106,000 people age 65 and older who received workers' compensation in 2004, the median annual benefit was $5,376.[22]

Income from Veterans' Compensation and Veterans' Pensions

Disabled veterans, their dependents, and survivors are eligible for an array of benefits including income support, medical services, educational benefits and housing assistance. In 2004, roughly 1.1 million Americans age 65 and older received supplementary income from two disability-based programs: the veterans' compensation and veterans' pensions program.

The veteran's compensation program provides payments for veterans with disabilities incurred or aggravated while in the Armed Forces. The compensation program provides payments to disabled veterans in amounts designed to compensate the veteran for loss of earnings capacity. Higher benefits are paid for more severe disabilities than for less severe disabilities. Veterans' pensions are provided through a separate program to wartime veterans and their survivors who have disabilities which are not related to or caused by military duties of the veteran but which render them unable to work.[23] Veterans' pensions are means-tested: payments are decreased by amounts received from other sources such as Social Security, pensions, and income from a spouse. Pensions are not paid to veterans with substantial assets, and veterans' pension benefits are usually small amounts. Taken together, the median veterans' compensation or pension benefit was $5,639 in 2004, or about $470 per month. A quarter of recipients received compensation or pension benefits of $11,800 or more.

Income from Public Assistance

An estimated 1.2 million Americans age 65 or older received public assistance income in 2004. Most received Supplemental Security Income (SSI), a federal program for low-income individuals who are aged, blind, or disabled. Some who were the caretaker relatives of dependent children received income through Temporary Assistance for Needy Families (TANF), which is jointly administered by the federal and state governments and pays benefits to low-income families with children. A small number of elderly received state general assistance payments for those in poverty. The median public assistance payment from all sources to recipients age 65 or older in 2004 was $3,600, or $300 per month.

The largest source of cash assistance for the elderly is Supplemental Security Income (SSI). SSI is a means-tested program administered by the Social Security Administration which provides monthly cash payments to eligible aged, blind, and disabled persons. Aged individuals and couples are eligible for SSI if their incomes fall below the federal maximum monthly SSI benefit. In 2004, the monthly standards were $564 for an individual and $846 for a couple. An individual does not have to be totally without income to be eligible for SSI benefits, but the income standards are significantly lower than the poverty threshold for both individuals and couples.[24] Eligibility for SSI is restricted to qualified persons who have resources of less than $2,000 for an individual or $3,000 for a couple. The resource limit for a couple applies even if only one member of a couple is eligible. Together, these income and asset limits restrict the number of people 65 and older who are eligible for SSI to less than half of the number who have incomes below the federal poverty threshold.

A state may choose to provide an optional supplement to Federal SSI payments. These supplements can help individuals meet needs which are not fully met by the federal payment. Each state determines whether it will make such a payment, to whom, and in what amount. Currently, all but six states make some form of SSI supplemental payments.[25]

CONCLUSION

Americans age 65 and older receive income from a variety of sources. While Social Security benefits, pensions, and income from assets are the most common income sources, earnings also are important, especially for those under age 70.

There are large disparities in the amount and type of income that older Americans receive. Income from assets in the form of interest and dividends, for example, make up a significant percentage of the aggregate income of the elderly population. However, most elderly individuals receive only modest amounts of interest and dividend income and a relatively small number of people receive very large amounts of income from these sources. Social Security, on the other hand, is both the largest source of aggregate income among the elderly and the biggest single source of income for a majority of Americans age 65 and older. Compared to the great disparity in interest and dividend income, there is relatively little difference between the average monthly Social Security benefit and the highest monthly benefit. This is because the Social Security benefit formula limits the maximum amount paid to a retired high-wage earner to about 150% of the amount paid to an average-wage worker.

Public assistance and other public programs play an important role in supporting many older Americans who otherwise would be living in poverty. The importance of each source of income varies across the income distribution. Public programs provide over 90% of all income for the poorest 25% of the population. This contrasts with the wealthiest 25% of the elderly population who receive only one-fifth of their income from public programs.

The reduction in poverty among older Americans is one of the most significant public policy successes of the past half-century. Poverty among those age 65 and older has fallen from one-in-three older persons in 1960 to one-in-ten today. While the overall rate of poverty is relatively low, it remains high for women, minorities, the less-educated, single persons, and those over age 80.

As Congress considers reforms to Social Security and the laws governing pensions and retirement savings plans, it may be helpful to consider how changes to one income source would affect each of the others, and thus the total income of older Americans. Future challenges will include maintaining the fiscal solvency of Social Security and Medicare and developing strategies in the public and private sectors to finance the increased need for long-term care services as the number of older Americans rises in the years ahead

ENDNOTES

[1] This number does not include approximately 1.6 million elderly who live in nursing homes.

[2] U.S. Census Bureau, *Income, Poverty, and Health Insurance Coverage in the United States, 2004;* P60-229, Table 3, p. 10, [http://www.census.gov/prod/2005pubs/p60-229.pdf].

[3] Calculations using the same survey and income categories but based on an *aged unit* — a mix of couples and individuals — can be found in the Social Security Administration's *Income of the Population 55 or Older,* at [http://www.ssa.gov/policy/docs/statcomps/].

[4] This Section combines the total income of each family member and compares it to the official poverty threshold based on the size of the family. The official poverty threshold in 2004 for a single person age 65 or older was $9,060. The poverty threshold for a couple in

which at least one member was 65 or older was $11,418. See *Poverty Thresholds for 2004 by Size of Family and Number of Related Children Under 18 Years,* available at [http://www.census.gov/hhes/poverty/threshld/thresh04.html].

[5] Note that there are two slightly different official government versions of the level of income at which one is considered poor. The first — and the one used in this analysis — is the poverty *threshold* which the Census Bureau uses to count the number of poor in the United States. The second measure, the poverty *guideline,* is used by the Department of Health and Human Services to set eligibility criteria for a number of federal programs.

[6] For a complete description of the Social Security program, see the House Committee on Ways and Means, committee print, WMCP: 108-6, 2004, *2004 Green Book,* Chapter 1, at [http://waysandmeans.house.gov/media/pdf/greenbook2003/Section1.pdf].

[7] To *vest* in a pension or other benefit is to earn a legally enforceable right to receive it.

[8] *Tax Reform Act of 1986,* P.L. 99-514.

[9] See CRS Report RL30496, *Pension Issues: Lump-sum Distributions and Retirement Income Security,* by Patrick Purcell.

[10] As reported here, "pension income" includes payments from a company or union pension, payments from a federal, state, or local government pension, military retirement pay, regular payments from an annuity or paid-up insurance policy, and regular payments from an IRA, Keogh account, or a §401(k)-type account.

[11] These numbers sum to 12.5 million. About 300,000 people had both types of pension.

[12] U.S. Department of Labor, Bureau of Labor Statistics, news release USDL 04-1829, *Employee Tenure in 2004,* Sept. 21, 2004, at [ftp://ftp.bls.gov/pub/news.release/tenure.txt].

[13] In 2001, the median value of financial assets among families headed by a person between the ages of 65 and 74 that owned any financial assets was $51,400. The median for families headed by someone age 75 or older that owned any financial assets was $40,000. The median *net worth* of all families headed by a person between the ages of 65 and 74 was $176,300. The median *net worth* of all families headed by someone age 75 or older was $151,400. Net worth is the value of all assets (including a home) minus all liabilities. See Ana M. Aiscorbe, Arthur B. Kennickell, et. al., "Recent Changes in U.S. Family Finances: Evidence from the 1998 and 2001 Survey of Consumer Finances," available at [http://www.federalreserve.gov/pubs/bulletin/2003/0 1 03lead.pdf].

[14] Of 35.213 million individuals age 65 and older in 2004, 34.190 million (97.1%) reported income from one or more sources and 19.731 million (56.0%) reported income from assets.

[15] Because labor force participation rates begin to fall steadily beginning at about age 55, this section includes information on individuals age 55 and older rather than age 65 and older.

[16] Joseph Quinn, "Retirement Trends and Patterns Among Older American Workers" in Stuart Altman and David Shactman (eds.), *Policies for an Aging Society* (Baltimore: Johns Hopkins University Press, 2002), pp. 293-315.

[17] As a worker ages, the likelihood that he or she will experience a decline in physical or cognitive capacity increases. Increased incidences of illness and disability are partly responsible for the decline in earned income that some workers experience after age 55. For a discussion of the effects of aging on the ability to continue working, see C. Schooler, L. Caplan, and G. Oates, "Aging and Work: An Overview," in *Impact of Work on Older Adults,* K.W. Schaie and C. Schooler, eds. (New York: Springer Publishing, Inc., 1997).

[18] While 72% of people age 55-61 were in the labor force in 2004, the labor force participation rate was 33% among those age 65 to 69 and 12% among people age 70 and

older. Similarly, while 85% of workers age 55-6 1 were employed full time in 2004, only 59% of workers age 65-69 and 42% of workers age 70 and older worked full time. For more information on the labor force participation of older workers, see CRS Report RL30629, *Older Workers: Employment and Retirement Trends,* by Patrick Purcell.

[19] Federal law (P.L. 96-364) requires that when the earnings from an employer are used to calculate the UC benefit, the UC benefit must be reduced if retirement income is received from that employer. States are permitted to reduce benefits on less than a dollar-for-dollar basis by taking into account the contributions made by the worker to finance the plan. Also, the requirement applies only to those payments made on a periodic (not lump-sum) basis. This is to ensure that workers who retires do not also collect UC benefits from the job from which they retired. For more details see CRS Report 95-1180, *Unemployment Benefits Reduced by Pensions and Social Security: A Fact Sheet,* by Celinda Franco.

[20] See CRS Report RL321 11, *Unemployment Compensation /Unemployment Insurance: Trends and Contributing Factors in UC Benefit Exhaustion,* by Julie Whittaker.

[21] For a more thorough discussion of workers' compensation programs, see the House Committee on Ways and Means, committee print, WMCP: 108-6, 2004, *2004 Green Book,* Chap. 15, [http://waysandmeans.house.gov/media/pdf/greenbook2003/WorkersComp.pdf].

[22] Figures include payments from employer-sponsored workers' compensation insurance.

[23] Veteran's pensions are means-tested benefits for low-income veterans, and should not be confused with military retirement benefits — also called "retired pay" — paid to retired officers and enlisted personnel who have completed at least 20 years of service. For this analysis, military retirement benefits are included as part of public pensions.

[24] In 2004, the poverty threshold for a single person age 65 or older was $755 per month. For a couple in which one or both people were over 65, the monthly poverty threshold was $952.

[25] Arkansas, Georgia, Kansas, Mississippi, Tennessee, and West Virginia pay no supplement.

INDEX

A

C

D

E

F

G

H

I

J

K

L

M

N

O

P

T

U

V